P9-DIE-691

I Love Your Style

I Love Your Style

How to Define and Refine

Your Personal Style

by

Amanda Brooks

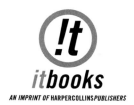

itbooks

AN IMPRINT OF HARPERCOLLINS*PUBLISHERS*

*it*books

I LOVE YOUR STYLE. Copyright © 2009 by Amanda Brooks. All rights reserved. Printed in the United States of America. No part of this book may be used or reproduced in any manner whatsoever without written permission except in the case of brief quotations embodied in critical articles and reviews. For information address HarperCollins Publishers, 10 East 53rd Street, New York, NY 10022.

HarperCollins books may be purchased for educational, business, or sales promotional use. For information please write: Special Markets Department, HarperCollins Publishers, 10 East 53rd Street, New York, NY 10022.

FIRST EDITION

Designed by William Loccisano/Pandiscio Co.

Library of Congress Cataloging-in-Publication Data is available upon request.

ISBN 978-0-06-183312-0

09   10   11   12   13   DT/WCT   10   9   8   7   6   5   4   3   2

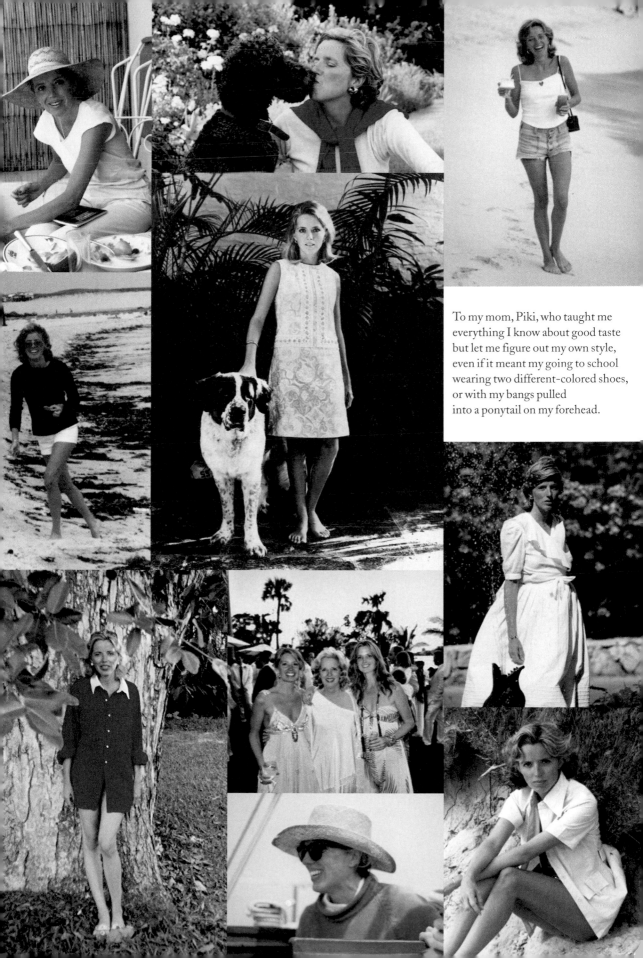

To my mom, Piki, who taught me
everything I know about good taste
but let me figure out my own style,
even if it meant my going to school
wearing two different-colored shoes,
or with my bangs pulled
into a ponytail on my forehead.

CONTENTS

III. Shopping

BASICS

CHEAP CHIC

DESIGNER

VINTAGE

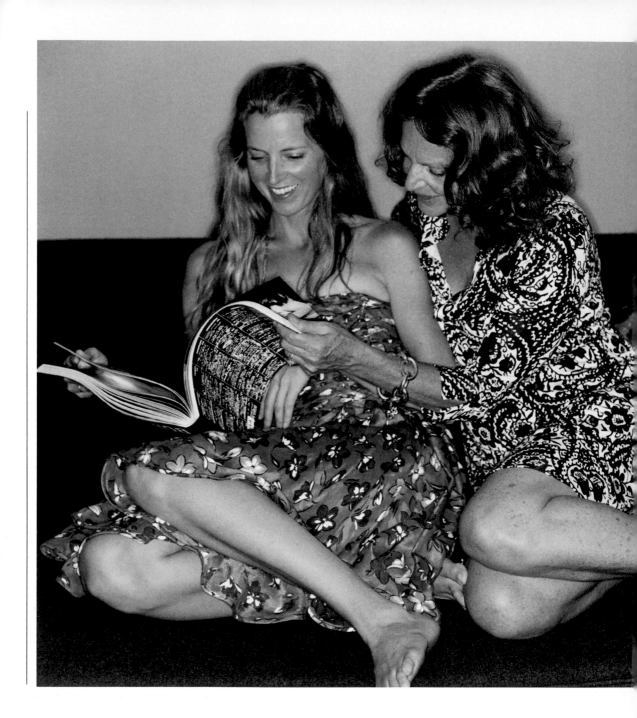

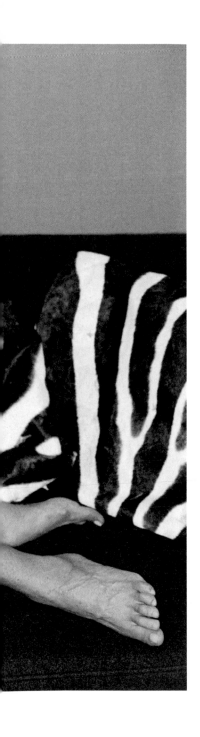

Foreword

by DIANE VON FURSTENBERG

"PERSONAL STYLE IS ACCEPTING WHO YOU ARE."

What is style? It is an effortless confidence in being yourself; it is a way of putting yourself together according to your mood and what you want to project. Personal style appears to come naturally for some, but for others it can take a while to find it!

I grew up in Belgium as an odd duck—with curly dark hair when everyone else had blond straight hair. I hated the way I looked, but slowly I realized that the thing I hated most could actually be an asset, because it was *me*! Finding my own style was about accepting and liking myself . . . it was not always an easy process, but it was the only one.

Amanda Brooks was born, bred, and raised in *style*! She's experimented with it as a child, as a teenager, and soon she became a real pro. She has a true eye and a natural instinct for understanding fashion. She loves design, relates with designers, and has been a muse to many. I love *her* style because it is easy and effortless: her walk, her allure is confident and light; it is never forced. Fashion is a mysterious thing to express, but if anyone is qualified to write a book on style, Amanda is. She has the unique talent of sensing trends, feeling the moment, and knowing what to mix with what. This book is fun, informative, and very clever. I am sure it will inspire many and reassure others.

After all, style is something each of us already has—all we need to do is find it.

Diane von Furstenberg and me looking at photos in Bob Colacello's book Out.

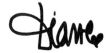

My Style History

When I was a little girl growing up in Palm Beach, my friends and I used to stroll down Worth Avenue to Paris Sorbet, our favorite ice cream shop. Along the way we often stopped to say hello to the ladies who worked in the stores, or wandered into my dad's real estate office to get candy from his secretary. I can still picture us—a towheaded band with nicknames like Honey and Celerie, dressed in Lilly Pulitzer bathing suits, with sandy feet or handmade Jack Rogers sandals, waving at the friendly women who spent most of their days catering to the town's stylish matrons. It was a much more casual time in Palm Beach—we knew virtually everyone in town—but there was still one store too intimidating, too fancy for us to approach: Chanel. Even as children we could sense the force field of pristine chic emanating from those interlocked C's. Instead of greeting the people who worked there, we simply glanced longingly at the mannequins in the window and respectfully went on our way.

If you had told me then that in a decade or so I would be photographing a Chanel fashion show in the garden of the Rodin Museum in Paris—a job that would introduce me to some of the most talented and inspiringly stylish people in the world—I probably would have laughed and gone on daydreaming and licking my ice cream cone. But amazingly, that's exactly what happened, and it was—like so much of what style has brought into my life—extremely exhilarating, challenging, overwhelming, and richly rewarding.

Me, at home, in Bronxville, New York, 1982.

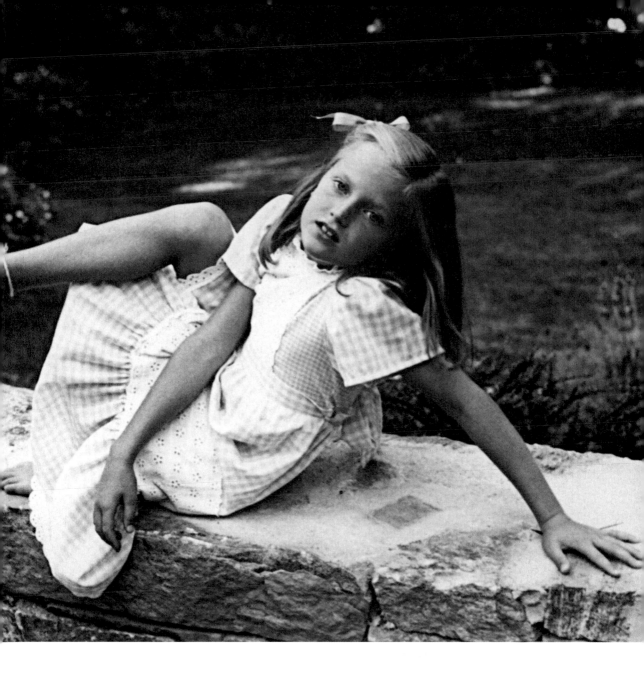

THERE WAS STILL ONE STORE TOO INTIMIDATING,
TOO FANCY FOR US TO APPROACH: CHANEL. EVEN AS CHILDREN
WE COULD SENSE THE FORCE FIELD OF
PRISTINE CHIC EMANATING FROM THOSE INTERLOCKED C'S.

INTRODUCTION
My Style History

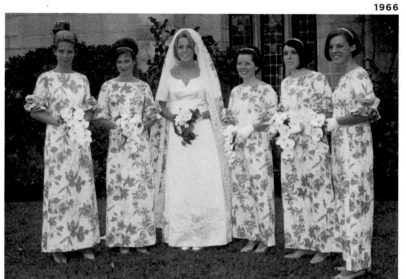

WHEN MY MOM AND DAD GOT MARRIED, LILLY PULITZER . . . DESIGNED A NEW GREEN AND WHITE FLORAL PRINT FOR ALL THE BRIDESMAIDS' DRESSES.

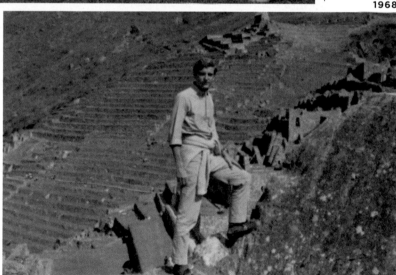

1968

*This page:
(Top)
My mom,
Elizabeth
Stewart, on her
wedding day
with
bridesmaids in
custom Lilly
Pulitzer floral-
printed gowns,
1966.*

*(Bottom)
My dad,
Stephen Cutter,
climbing
Machu Picchu
in his Gucci
loafers, 1968.*

*Opposite:
My mom and
dad at the Palm
Beach Polo
Club, 1966.*

I was born in Palm Beach in the 70s. My mother, an interior designer, wore oversized sunglasses, exaggerated bell-bottoms, and an ostrich-skin Gucci purse. My father, the president of his family's real estate firm, had a perfectly ordered rainbow of neatly pressed pants in his closet with grosgrain ribbon belts to match. (See above for a picture of my dad climbing Machu Picchu in his Gucci loafers!) When my mom and dad got married, Lilly Pulitzer (who had introduced them) designed a new green and white floral print for all the bridesmaids' dresses, which they wore with beehives, white lipstick, and matching green pumps—very 60s chic. It seems obvious now that one way or another style was going to be a part of my story.

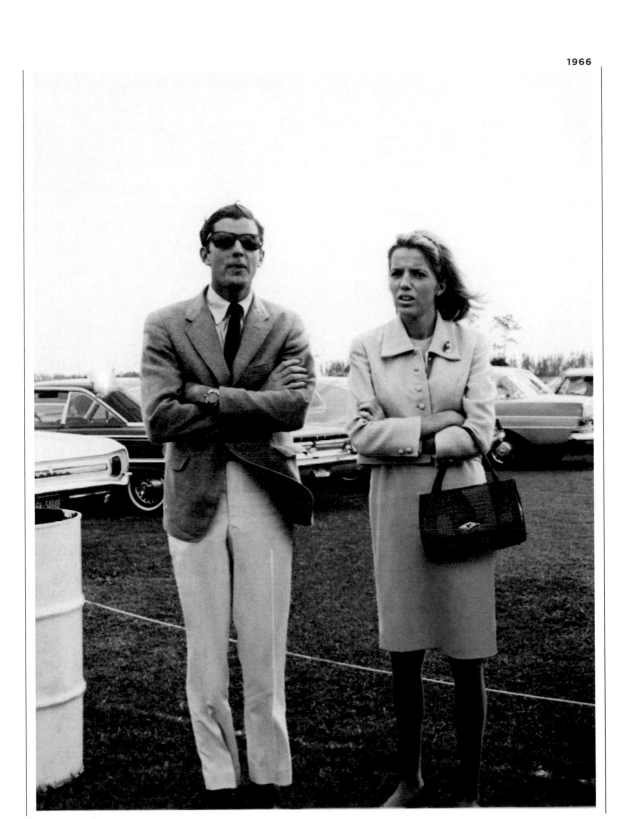

Amanda Brooks

INTRODUCTION
My Style History

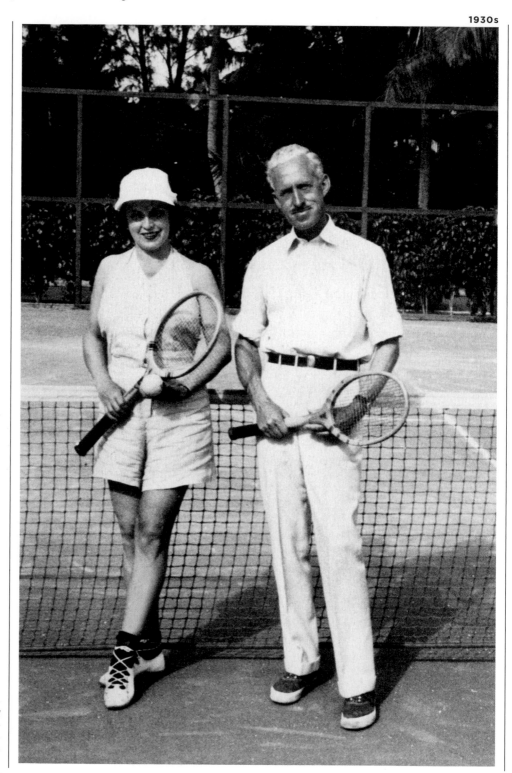

My grandparents Beatrice and Harry playing tennis at the Seaspray Beach Club in Palm Beach, c. late 1930s.

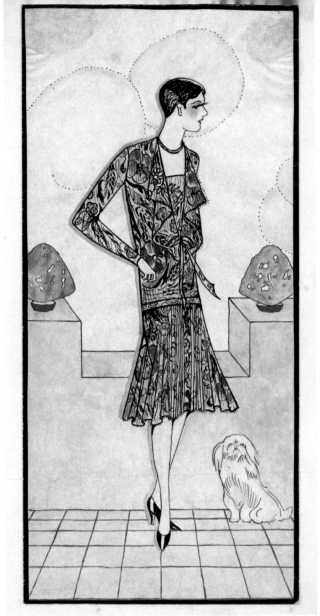

1930s

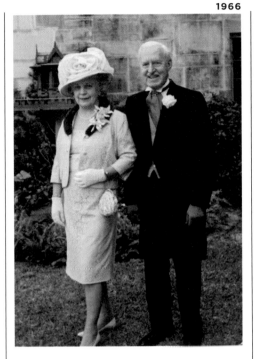

IT'S OBVIOUS THAT MY GRANDMOTHER... HAD SOME GENETIC INFLUENCE ON ME.

*Above:
A fashion
illustration by my
grandmother,
c.1930s.*

*Above right:
My grandparents
at my mom and
dad's wedding in
Palm Beach,
1966.*

Even though she died when I was six, it's obvious that my grandmother Beatrice Bowry had some genetic influence on me. She was the director of the Clothes Institute at Filene's in Boston, as well as a skilled illustrator and an exceedingly stylish dresser. She taught women how to learn to dress themselves, she conducted a modeling school, she presented fashion shows, she gave illustrated lectures, and she even had a vast following on her daily radio address. She also served on the advisory committee for the Costume Institute at the Rhode Island School of Design. My dad tells me that in the 1930s, she was the highest-paid woman in Boston.

Here are a few samples of her philosophy:

"Women can all be made to look charming with proper study of dress."

"Anybody can learn fashion by reading fashion magazines, but that doesn't interpret fashion for the individual."

"There are only certain things everyone can wear. It's more important that a thing be becoming than that it be in the very latest trend of fashion."

"A limited purse is not a valid excuse to dress poorly."

Amanda Brooks

INTRODUCTION
My Style History

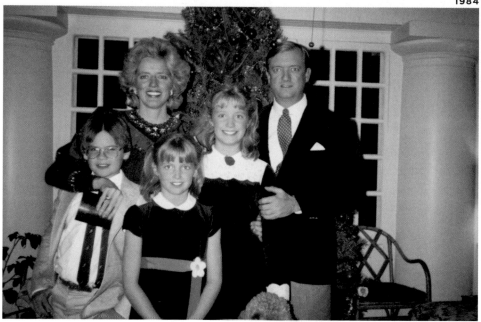

When I was five my parents divorced and my mother married my wonderful stepfather, Will, an old-school Long Island WASP. We moved to Bronxville, a suburban town in Westchester County, New York. It was the opposite of overtly stylish Palm Beach. In Westchester, a spree at Talbot's was really splashing out. Everyone was conservative. Oddly, this only encouraged my mother's interest in high fashion, and she would wear 80s leather Alaia skirts to PTA meetings or ruched Vicky Tiel couture dresses to local cocktail parties. Even more oddly, I felt proud of her rather than embarrassed. I liked that she didn't assimilate into the mass of reserved "good taste." At the local public elementary school, however, I followed the preppy, understated style of my new friends with heart-printed turtlenecks, Laura Ashley floral dresses, and Tretorn sneakers.

In the summers of the early 80s I would visit my father and my stepmother, Hilary, in Palm Beach. Hilary was a total hippie, and also very creative. She got a kick out of scouring thrift stores to find designer treasures cast off by Palm Beach socialites and cutting them up and resewing them to suit her own more romantic style. She introduced me to the joys and infinite possibilities presented by secondhand stores and flea markets, and my passion for thrift shopping was born. I could try a new look with one week's allowance—just a few dollars. After that I didn't like to look like anybody else. If my friends were doing the preppy thing, I was a skater girl; when they went NYC cool and wore black, I was in satin and rhinestones; and when they got into New Wave, I was back to preppy.

Going off to college challenged my sense of myself as someone who loved fashion. Girls at Brown actually wore Marc Jacobs for Perry Ellis "grunge" to class! One of my friends was Tracee Ross, Diana's daughter, who famously raided her mother's closet for glamorous vintage Halston to wear to college parties. How was I supposed to cope with my modest budget and my mostly suburban pedigree? I watched what my friends wore, I kept thrifting, I begged my mother for the very occasional "special treat" purchase, and I discovered Contempo Casuals—the first of the really good, cheap chic trendy stores. It was a humbling moment between my closet and me, but it was a momentous influence, and it gave me my lust for designer clothing.

This page: Our new family (including my stepfather William and stepbrother Angus) in Bronxville for Christmas, 1984. I wish you could see more of my mom's colored-pearl-encrusted sweater.

Opposite: (Left) Me, with my stepfather Will, at my debutante party in Rye, New York, 1992. My mom designed the dress.

(Right) Me, in Patmos, Greece, in my "art gallery girl" phase, 1999.

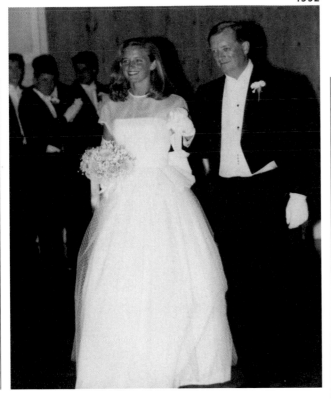

While at Brown studying art history and photography, I landed a summer job as an assistant to famed fashion photographer Patrick Demarchelier. Thank God I'd been reading lots of fashion magazines, because I recognized him in a restaurant and just walked up to introduce myself. He invited me to visit his studio and the next day his manager hired me as an intern. I traveled all over the world assisting on magazine shoots, designer ads, and album covers—Madonna and Janet Jackson included. I was overwhelmed. I was eighteen years old. This was the life of my dreams—but it just seemed too much too soon, and I couldn't find my place in all of it.

I took some time off from the fashion scene and went to work as the assistant to the director at Gagosian Gallery. Yet, even as I spent time with many wonderful artists—Cy Twombly, Nan Goldin, Sally Mann, Seydou Keita, Francesco Clemente—

MY PASSION FOR THRIFT SHOPPING WAS BORN. I COULD TRY A NEW LOOK WITH ONE WEEK'S ALLOWANCE— JUST A FEW DOLLARS.

the inspiration I took (and still take) from them couldn't make up for how much I missed my relationship with fashion—one of nerves and excitement. So I dove back in.

A friend at *Vogue* recommended me as someone who could help Frederic Fekkai develop a handbag collection. I didn't really know what I was doing but definitely knew what I liked. I learned a ton, and we actually made some really cute bags. As a result, Diego Della Valle recruited me to be the creative director at Hogan, the Italian accessories company. For two years I did my thing there: made inspiration presentations, edited the collection, and traveled to the factories in Italy to see my ideas as they were realized. In these two jobs I learned about developing creative ideas and then applying them to the style of the company I worked for. It helped me see my own style more objectively, and it also taught me how to evolve my own style without taking away its essence.

And then in the late 90s I discovered Tuleh. Josh Patner and Bryan Bradley's clothes were exactly what I was in the mood for: color and bold prints and vintage and femininity and drama. If I had created a label that married

INTRODUCTION
My Style History

all the aspects of my fashion personality at that time, it would have been Tuleh. But luckily Josh and Bryan had already done it, and it felt like a miracle. The perfection of the match was confirmed when they told me they felt the same way about me.

Josh and I met for the first time sitting in the front row of one of his shows. He later recalled that after he looked me over and chatted with me for a few minutes he ran backstage and said to Bryan, "I just met Tuleh!!" And so for three wonderfully happy years I worked there as creative director and muse. Each morning I indulged my deepest fantasies in getting dressed—the Revlon "Charlie" girl, a 70s YSL runway model, a modern-day Veronica Lake—then made my way over to Tuleh to discuss what I was wearing, look at fabric swatches, develop new prints, talk about the proportion I was craving, hand over the best of my mom's hand-me-downs, try on half-sewn samples, talk about the shape of a perfume bottle, and bring in old books and photos for inspiration. That only touches the surface of my duties, but all in all I was there to provide a woman's appetite, to seduce them with my desires.

After leaving Tuleh to create a career for myself in my own vision—as a fashion writer and consultant—my style broke free from the constraints of focusing my attention on one brand, and I embraced all the possibilities I found compelling. I bought or borrowed clothes from every designer I knew or admired. I spent more money on clothes than I had ever spent in the past. Just as my career was evolving into one with more freedom, so was my fashion style. Who knows if I will ever settle down into one definitive style. It's hard to imagine giving up on the highs and lows of trying new things. I guess only time will tell.

So, in simple terms, I have been studying fashion and style—and how they apply to both me and the world—for most of my life. For me, learning how to use clothes to express myself has been greatly empowering and occasionally humbling. Some people find

their style groove and stick with it throughout the decades. I have great respect for these people, but for me, the pursuit of style is constantly evolving. It's like being a perpetual teenager—studiously employing trial and error to figure out who I am, and how I want to feel on any given day. Some days the result is spot-on—a perfect combination of my roots in a classic aesthetic mixed with something ironic or unexpected, maybe a bohemian moment and a little hint of trend thrown in. Yet other days my complicated mix of far-flung references seems to amount to a muddled overdose of ideas, or just doesn't come together the way I saw it in my mind. As I get older, my experiences with dressing by trial and error have brought me to a place of greater self-assurance and given me a better shot at getting it right—not that I am immune to the occasional fashion disaster.

My greatest belief about clothes is that style does not come to you unless you pay attention to it. You can have the chicest mother in the world, but none of that will rub off on you unless you are interested and invested in learning. And conversely, you can spend your life surrounded by people who truly have no fashion sense at all, but end up the next Kate Moss, Catherine Deneuve, or Marisa Berenson through thoughtful attention and a fearlessness to try new things. No matter who you are, where you come from, or how fat (or thin) your bank account is, you can and should establish your own personal style.

We women today have a lot on our plates. We *want* to look good, but do we really want to reinvent the wheel in a state of panic every time we have to find something to wear to a big meeting, a date, or an important party? Imagine how great it would be to face getting dressed with confidence and excitement instead of anxiety or boredom. Well, you can, and you can also have a lot of fun while you're at it.

My sister Kim and me, both in Tuleh, at her thirtieth birthday party in Los Angeles, 2002.

EACH MORNING I INDULGED MY DEEPEST
FANTASIES IN GETTING DRESSED—THE REVLON
"CHARLIE" GIRL, A 70s YSL RUNWAY MODEL,
A MODERN-DAY VERONICA LAKE.

2002

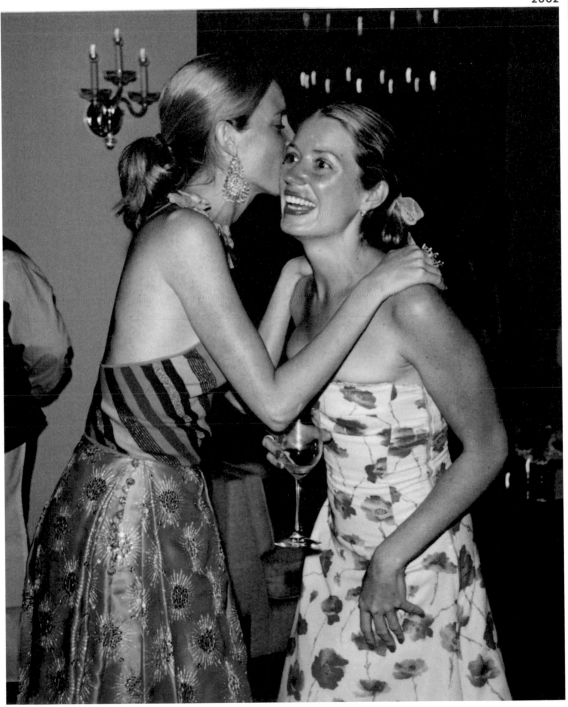

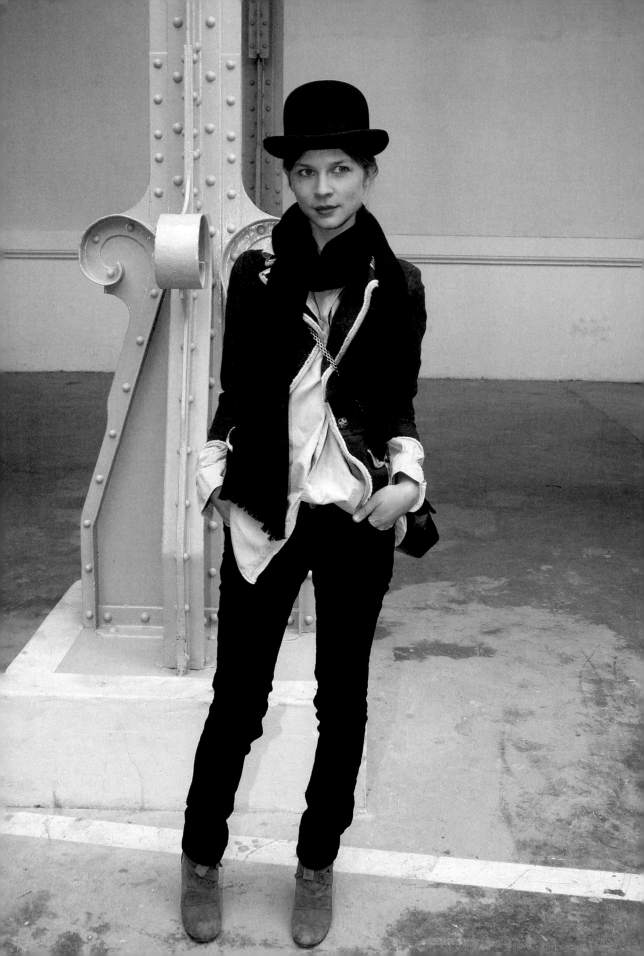

Getting Started

"INSIST ON YOURSELF. NEVER IMITATE."
—RALPH WALDO EMERSON

Let me begin by saying that finding your personal style is *really* about discovering yourself. There's lots of room for experimentation along the way, but arriving at a strong sense of style that suits you and makes you feel great every day and everywhere depends on confidently knowing who you are and what is important to you. Instead of blindly following a bunch of rules you heard from your friends or read in a magazine, personal style is about engaging in a constant creative process—one that evolves as you do. There are no rules to this, except the ones you make for yourself—and even those are made to be broken. When I am out and about, I constantly notice people trying their absolute best to look good. Many of them do look good, but I am always more impressed by those who look *different*. This is best accomplished not by wearing something that screams "Look at me!" but by subtly breaking a "rule" (she's wearing flat shoes with an evening dress), adding an unexpected accessory (fresh flowers in her hair), or establishing a signature touch (she always wears red lipstick).

Clémence Poésy, on her way to the Chanel show in Paris, 2007. I regularly look her up on the Internet to see what she's been wearing. She has great style.

INTRODUCTION
Getting Started

What is personal style and how do you find it? Trust me, you know it when you see it, but let me try to explain:

Personal style is a look that is all your own.
It is a way of putting yourself together that allows your own combination of tastes, desires, interests, inspirations, aspirations, lifestyle, and history to shine through. Many people today, especially in America, can no longer get dressed without the advice of advertising, celebrities, magazines, stylists, and designers. As a result, everyone looks the same! This book will give you the confidence to have fun with those trends that suit you without blindly buying into a cookie-cutter look that doesn't.

Embrace yourself and your history!
Even if you feel like you've had a pretty plain-vanilla life or just a downright unstylish one; you still have a story: where you grew up; what your parents were like; how you became interested in clothes; what kind of budget you had and have now; what your aspirations are; who or what you're trying to please, evoke, or run away from; and, most important, how your style has evolved over the years. Whenever I meet a girl with truly great style I immediately want to be her friend, because I can safely assume that she is confident and self-knowledgeable. It's impossible to overemphasize the importance of self-acceptance in this equation. Diane von Furstenberg once told me that she had struggled with her curly brown hair ever since her childhood in Belgium, where everyone's hair was blonde and straight. In the 1960s she ironed her hair every day, because that was the fashion, and then in the 1970s, she left it curly, because *that* was the fashion. After finding herself a slave to straightening again in the 1990s, she now says her hair is staying naturally curly for good. In her fifties she realized that those curls are really *her*, and she feels more herself in the world being true to her natural hair.

Self-confidence is good for both your soul and your style.
Finding your personal style means feeling exhilarated every day as you walk out your front door, knowing you look great before anybody tells you so (and, most important, not caring if they don't). By exposing yourself to all kinds of influences and dressing with an open mind, you will both discover new things that will inspire you to change and embrace the parts of yourself that you already love. I want to help you find the looks and moods that spark your imagination and encourage your inner personality to shine through.

Celebrate your creativity, express your different moods, and show off all facets of your personality.
If you've got personal style, you can change your look from day to day and always look like yourself. Take Kate Moss, for example. One moment she is chic and ladylike in a vintage dress while meeting the Queen of England, the next she is bohemian and grungy in a fur poncho at the Glastonbury Music Festival, and after that she is classic and feminine, wearing jeans with an Hermès Birkin bag and ballerina flats while doing errands. She can only pull this off because she knows who she is—and what suits her. Without that self-knowledge she would still be an astonishing beauty, but she wouldn't be one of the most widely admired and emulated clotheshorses in the world.

John Lennon and Yoko Ono in Battery Park, New York, 1970s. Her belt is so Alaia!

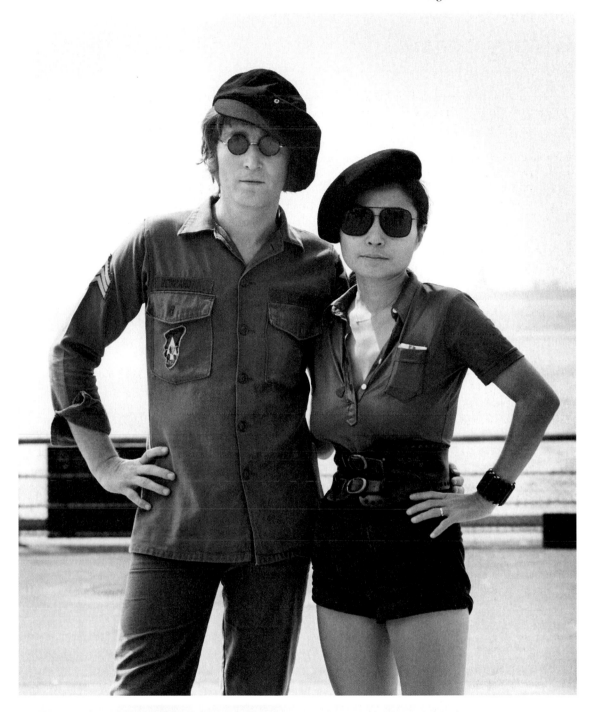

WHO ARE YOU GOING TO BE TODAY?

I once read a quote in a magazine from a woman who said, "Every morning I'm faced with the same problem: What should I wear? As a writer, model, avid equestrian, and mother of two, I'm trying constantly to find the right look to suit various aspects of my life." That always stuck in my head because her question is a good starting point for anyone getting dressed in the morning. What am I doing today? Where am I going? Who do I have to be today, and who do I want to be?

Amanda Brooks

INTRODUCTION
Getting Started

Make mistakes. It will be okay. Evolution depends on mutations, and you have to take the good with the bad. I never stop taking risks. At any given moment I can call to mind an outfit from the previous month that I have already filed under "What was I thinking?" If you leave the house in a mistake, grin and bear it. A smile will make you feel better and might even lead everyone else to suspect that your outfit is secretly brilliant.

My life hasn't been *entirely* full of style. Below are some of my more awkward moments.

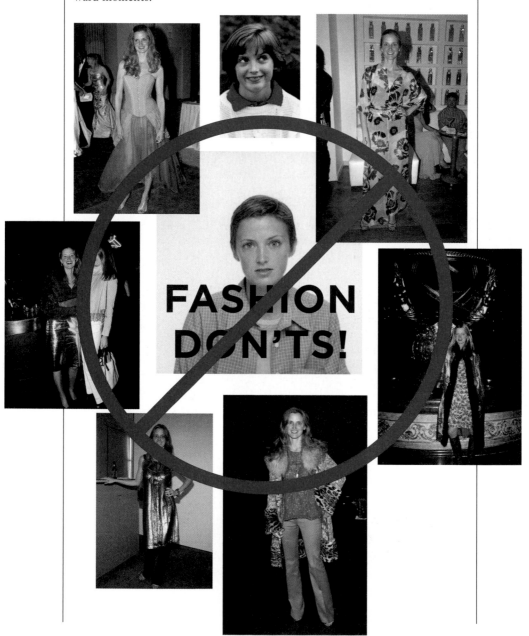

SIX WAYS TO
FIND YOUR STYLE

1. MAKE TEAR SHEETS

Read lots of magazines and books and tear out or make copies of things that resonate with you, whether they are whole outfits or just appealing color combinations, beautiful textiles, scenes that evoke a certain era or feeling, or anything at all that you think you want to express with your clothes. You can paste them into a style book, keep them in a folder, or even pin them up on an inspiration board. This is your style. Look everything over from time to time and observe what you still like months or even years later and what you have outgrown. Eventually your tear sheets will give you a better sense of yourself and the things that are classic for you as opposed to things you like only in passing.

2. WRITE DOWN YOUR STYLE HISTORY

Reflect on your life and take note of the things that have influenced you most. Your parents, your friends, your surroundings, your job, your lifestyle—or is your style a rebellion from one or all of those things? Which style memories make you happy, and which make you want to run a mile away?

3. TRY A LOT OF LOOKS

Experiment. Everything I know about my style and my taste has been the result of trying out every look in the book. If your budget is tight, go for thrift stores or cheap chic chain stores for your style experiments. When shopping, always try a lot of things on. Even the things that don't look good will educate you about what works and what doesn't.

4. CONSTANTLY ASK YOURSELF QUESTIONS

The more answers you have the more defined your style will be. What proportions flatter you? What fabrics and colors do you love? What kind of mood do you seek to create around yourself? What pieces in your closet do you come back to again and again?

5. FIND YOUR STYLE ICONS AND INSPIRATION

Identifying with someone whose style you admire is a great way to figure out whether something is "you." Whenever I'm not sure of an outfit I wonder, "Would Sofia Coppola like this?" It's like having your super-stylish best friend standing with you in your closet saying yea or nay. Find inspiration outside of fashion. Finding your own less obvious inspiration goes a long way toward making your style more unique. Museum shows, movies, cultural trends, travel, and personal experience all inspire fashion designers as they develop their collections. Why shouldn't they inspire you, too? Personal inspiration equals personal style.

6. MAKE AN EFFORT

Style will not appear in your life on its own. I always feel and look my best when I'm dressed in evening clothes because that is when I make the biggest effort. We can't go the whole nine yards every morning, but muster what energy you can and you'll feel better all day long.

> **"PEOPLE ASK ME HOW CAN I BE STYLISH, HOW CAN I BE ELEGANT AND WHAT CAN I WEAR? MY ONLY ANSWER IS STUDY! YOU HAVE TO LEARN."**
> —MIUCCIA PRADA

INTRODUCTION
Getting Started

A FEW THINGS
TO CONSIDER

YOUR BUDGET

I'm going to say something really important, so pay attention: You don't have to be rich to look good! *In fact, please don't spend a penny more than you have to. The time and thought you put into establishing your personal style will help you make smarter choices about how and where to grow your wardrobe. An unlimited budget is not necessarily a blessing when it comes to getting dressed; money can zap creativity. Some people think they look great just because they paid a lot for what they're wearing—and they're often wrong. At the same time, sometimes you just have to find room in a tiny budget for a single big-ticket item that you'll use a lot, something that will make a big impact on your look, rather than buying many inexpensive things that fall apart or go out of style too quickly.*

YOUR RULES

Giving yourself guidelines for getting dressed—dictated by taste, practicality, body type, mood—can simplify your life. Are there things you just know you wouldn't be able to carry off (sailor pants)? Are there things you oppose wearing under any circumstances (fur)? Is there something that works especially well for your body (bias-cut dresses)? What do you love, and what do you hate?

Here are some personal rules revealed to me by my more stylish friends:

"I only wear low-waisted pants."
"I always wear my hair up for evening."
"I do not wear high heels."
"I never wear fake jewelry."
"I always show off my legs."
"The color of my shoes and my handbag has to match."

YOUR BODY

You just won't look good in clothes if you consistently choose styles that don't suit your body. For instance, my skinny, curveless body looks fab in a secretary blouse, but my sister Kim's womanly curves do not. There is nothing better for Kim than a fitted, sexy strapless gown, but on me the same dress would look like an empty sack. You must get to know your body type and what flatters it. A wonderful resource is What Not to Wear *by Trinny Woodall and Susannah Constantine. It's the be-all and end-all guide to figuring out what suits your body.*

YOUR SIGNATURE

A signature is like a rule, but it's more permanent and noticeable. It is a part of your look so constant that it defines you, makes you stand out, and becomes part of your fashion identity. Anna Wintour's glossy bob is a famous example. Anne Slater, an Upper East Side society matriarch, always wears blue-tinted sunglasses—day/night, indoor/outdoor, casual/black tie—always. I have noticed that most women with distinct signatures are older than forty. To make such a commitment you have to really know yourself, I guess. Of course you can have loads of style without having a signature. It's just something to think about, or maybe to set as a long-term goal.

YOUR AGE

The word "appropriate" gives me the chills and has nothing to do with age when it comes to style. Women look best when they wear what they look and feel good in and what works for their budget and their lifestyle. Everybody's style evolves over time, but if you know what works for you and what you like you will never have to worry about dressing "appropriately" for your age.

AN UNLIMITED BUDGET IS NOT NECESSARILY A BLESSING WHEN IT COMES TO GETTING DRESSED; MONEY CAN ZAP CREATIVITY.

Chloë Sevigny
at a polo match
in New York,
2009. I have
always noticed
that polo
matches seem to
bring out the
best or worst in
people's style.
I suppose it
really comes
down to the
hat, which is
always a risk.
But Chloë's risk
was surely
worth taking.

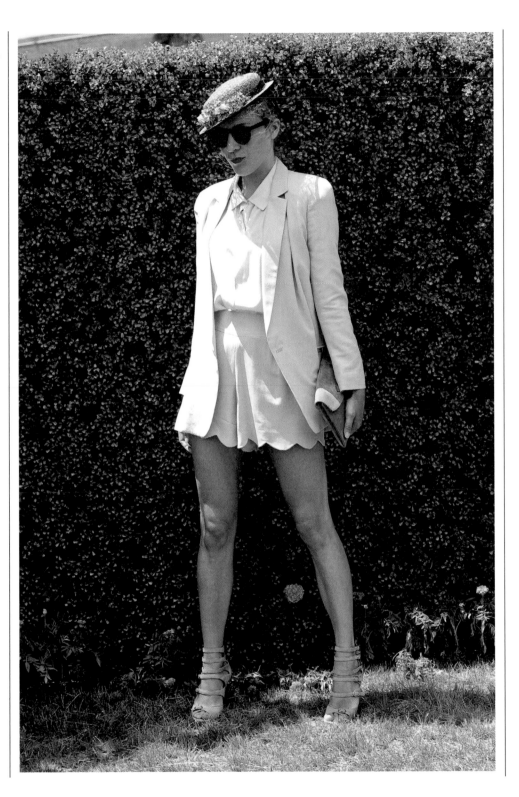

INTRODUCTION
Getting Started

You can't buy personal style, and you can't cook it up in a weekend. But if you want to, you can achieve it, and you can start playing with it today. There is a lot of fashion theory out there, but this book is about practice. I want to inspire the kind of self-reflection and adventure seeking that will set you on the path to dressing thoughtfully, with wit and originality and to great effect—be it elegant or laid-back, seductive or challenging, or something altogether more complicated (you will encounter the words "sexy lumberjack" before you turn the last page).

A NOTE ON THE PHOTOGRAPHS
You may wonder why there are so many vintage pictures included in the book. For me, there is a kind of validity given when the same item of clothing—say, a trench coat—is worn across decades. It just has more impact than seeing only a picture of one today. It announces that look as iconic by virtue of longevity and looking consistently good over time. Even something that could be considered non-classic, like a bohemian peasant blouse, becomes timeless by seeing one on Yvonne De Carlo in the 50s, Ali MacGraw in the 70s, and Sienna Miller today. That said, every picture in this book, whether taken in this century or last, looks relevant and current to me today.

Opposite, clockwise from top left:

Agyness Deyn (left) and her sister (right) with Karen Elson (middle) backstage at Anna Sui's fashion show, 2008.

Lauren Hutton, 1974.

Françoise Hardy, 1965.

Tina Chow, 1987.

It's okay to flip straight to the pictures. They're here to inspire you with limitless possibilities, and to help you begin to see which ideas might work for you and which won't. Every time I open a new issue of *Vogue*, I flip through the whole thing just looking at the glossy and instantly satisfying photos while folding down pages of articles I want to go back and read later. I encourage you to use this book the same way. Once you figure out what you like, you will gain the confidence to listen to yourself when you are getting dressed instead of the magazines, the designers, the advertisements—and even me! Until then, I am here to suggest and inspire by sharing my take on six distinct ways of dressing—classic, bohemian, minimal, high fashion, street, and eclectic—and four essential ways of shopping—basic, cheap chic, designer, and vintage.

Since it's somewhat easier to pin down consistent elements of classic, bohemian, and minimal styles, I call them "definable," even though there is a lot of room for interpretation in each one. In contrast—high fashion, street, and eclectic styles can be identified by a certain spirit, but their core elements are constantly changing. For that reason, I call them "indefinable." For each style I have gathered a bunch of great ideas and pictures to illustrate my take on that look, and I also describe key pieces and offer advice about how to get it right when you put everything together (so that you look like *you*—not like you in a costume). I've made lots of suggestions about the books and movies you can explore to deepen your understanding and love of the styles that appeal to you (yes—homework!). And I do believe that more than one style will appeal to you. As you develop a personal look, you'll find that devising surprising combinations of all kinds is half of the challenge—and the pleasure—of getting dressed.

Behind every woman with great personal style are some smart shopping strategies. I'll tell you everything I know about buying the basics, cheap chic clothes, designer labels, and vintage pieces. Each of these options is suitable for every style. If you have a good eye you can cobble together an elegant classic look from cheap chic chain stores, or you can pay through the nose for a designer outfit that makes you look like a homeless flower child. Just as I urge you to try new looks in your quest for personal style, I also suggest you explore new ways of shopping. Whether you're a student dreaming big at Neiman Marcus or a label snob checking out the latest high-low line at Target, you can learn a lot in the dressing room even if you don't end up buying a thing.

No less an authority than Yves Saint Laurent said, "To have style, you must believe in yourself." Start today—plunge into this book, take a little fashion risk, pull pages from your magazines, get used to being creative—and before you know it, *I Love Your Style* is something you'll hear wherever you go.

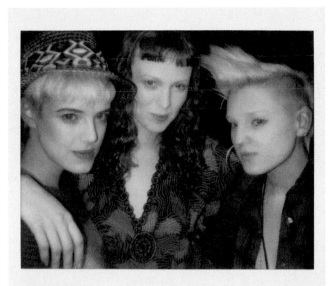

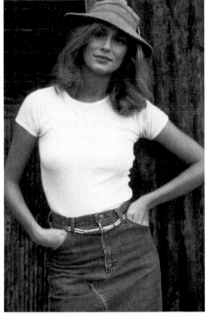

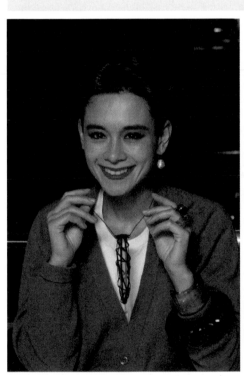

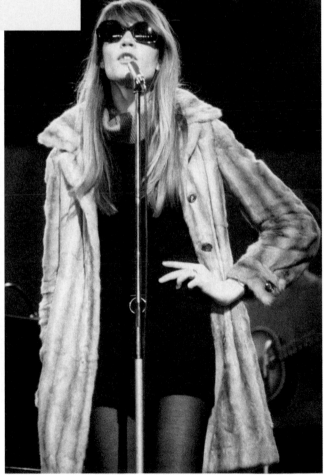

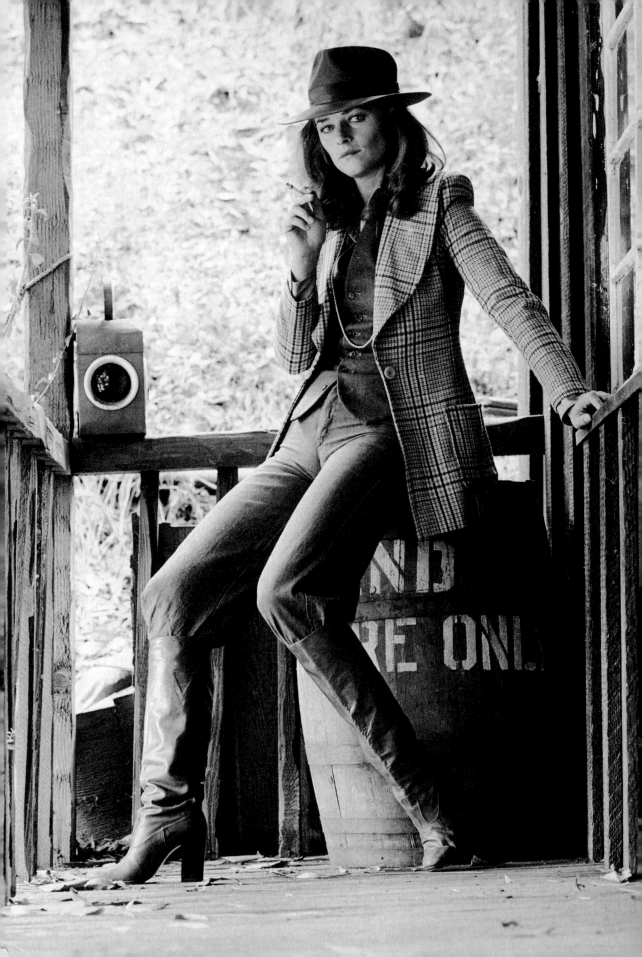

classic

INNOVATION! ONE CANNOT BE FOREVER INNOVATING. I WANT TO CREATE CLASSICS."
—COCO CHANEL

Whether the words "classic style" evoke the image of a smiling, windswept woman wearing aviator glasses and a striped French sailor sweater on the beach or an impeccably coiffed midcentury society lady wearing a graphic sheath and ballet flats to lunch, chances are you already have a good (and quite personal) idea of what this chapter is all about. As clothing trends relentlessly recycle every sartorial idea the twentieth century had to offer, certain pieces never stop speaking to a certain kind of woman: a boyish blazer, a family locket, a crisp white shirt, a precisely cut trench coat. Their appeal is not hard to see. Done right, classic clothes can lend an air of good taste and timelessness to their wearer without overwhelming her personality.

Everybody has a few classic pieces in her closet, except perhaps Björk (and, you know, even she might surprise us with one or two). Since we all rely to some extent on these longstanding staples, it's important to know when classic is chic and when it is boring. Classic style is chic when it is pared down (beautifully cut men's tailored trousers), simple (a perfectly fitting cream silk blouse), and elegant (a well-loved cashmere overcoat). But it is a big snore when it is derivative (the reinvention of Lilly Pulitzer),

Charlotte Rampling, 1976. I wish I could buy her blazer now. It's perfect.

overly gimmicky (whales on your pants), or just too conservative (sweater sets worn without irony).

Having classic style does not mean ignoring fashion trends, or wearing the same brown penny loafers for twenty years. I do advise, however, that you stick to pieces you know you will like for a long time, and also that you recognize when to give a familiar silhouette your own personal twist. Doing this requires that you know yourself and your closet inside and out, so you can look chic without putting a lot of energy into composing a successful outfit every morning because you already have a dozen tried-and-true combinations to rely on. That appearance of effortlessness is the result of a great deal of discipline and cultivated foresight. Think of Carolina Herrera. She has consistently worn a white shirt as a key element of her look throughout her life.

Classic dressing should feel authentic, not theatrical. It's about making smart shopping choices and keeping the clothes you buy for a long time; whether you have been or not, it's always chic to look as if you've been wearing the same pieces for years. There's nothing better than a pair of worn-in boots, a time-softened cotton blouse, or khaki pants that have molded to your shape. It's not com-

CLASSIC
My Classic Style

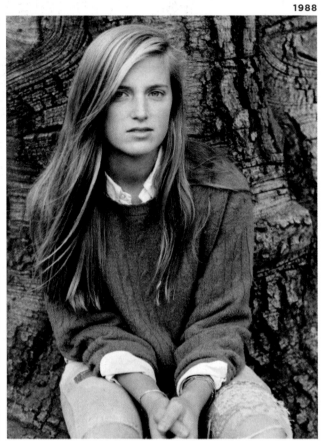

1988

**I WAS
DIFFERENT. BUT
I LIKED IT. AND I
THRIVED ON
THE SENSE OF
INDIVIDUALITY.**

1982

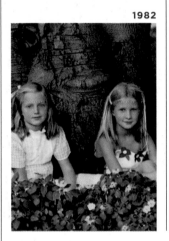

*This page:
(Far left)
My friend
Alexandra and
me in our
favorite
Florence
Eiseman
dresses, sitting
in front of the
old beechnut
tree in
Bronxville,
New York,
1982.*

*(Left)
Here I am six
years later in
front of the
same tree. This
was the year
before I went to
boarding school,
but I was
clearly already
channeling the
prep school look,
1988.*

*Opposite:
(Top left)
My sister's college
graduation—
a sea of tasteful
navy, 1995.*

*(Bottom left)
Spring break in
Boca Grande,
Florida, with
all my boarding
school buddies,
1992.*

*(Right)
I got this
vintage Lanvin
blazer at a
thrift store in
London for
$100. It's one of
my best finds,
2009.*

Growing up, I was immersed in standard-issue preppiness. Lacoste and Laura Ashley were coveted designer labels. As a teenager I emerged from this sea of pastel to attend the Horace Mann School. Instead of madras-clad Episcopalians with ribbon belts and lockjaw accents, Horace Mann was populated by rich city kids from Manhattan in tie-dyed leggings dotted with rhinestones. Nobody looked like me, nobody talked like me, and nobody dressed like me. I wasn't even allowed to wear black or shave my legs at that age. I was different. But I liked it. I thrived on my sense of individuality, and the confidence I gained from being accepted and befriended by my peers despite our differences.

I lost my spark a bit when I left the city for boarding school and encountered 550 other students who dressed and had grown up pretty much exactly as I did. Every day was a parade of J.Crew barn jackets, Ann Taylor tweed, and Joan and David loafers. Not that I wasn't wearing those things—believe me I was—it was just that I missed feeling different as opposed to of the masses. The seeds of my rebellion against classic style had been planted—as a freshman in college I decided to leave most of my clothes at home and start over.

By my twenties, I was no longer on speaking terms with my staid, predictable roots. I turned up my nose at anything classic and embraced futuristic green suede Prada Sport sneakers instead. By day I was an assistant in a chic downtown art gallery, but at night I went home to my parents' chintz-and-antique-filled Upper East Side apartment. To prove to my new world that I was

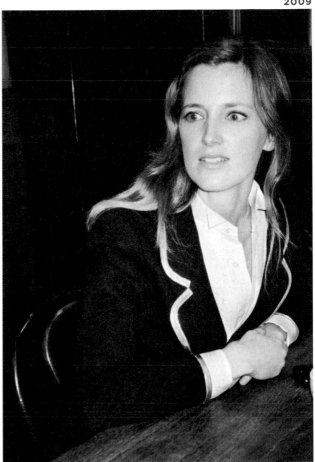

2009

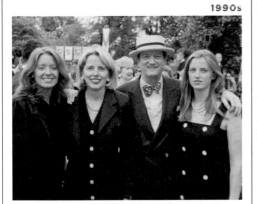

1990s

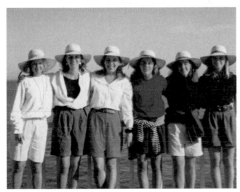

not a Muffy, I wore Dries van Noten blouses with frayed edges, Joseph pleather pants, and chunky Freelance boots.

Now, ten years later—having spent my twenties experimenting with trends, high fashion, and vintage inspiration, trying (rather desperately) not to look preppy—I have come full circle to embrace the traditional, conservative influences of my formative years. I can no longer deny that classic guidelines inform the way I dress: I like symmetry. I like matching. I like a classical sense of proportion. But, I've finally come to realize that classic doesn't have to mean predictable or boring impec-

I LOST MY SPARK A BIT WHEN I ENCOUNTERED 550 OTHER STUDENTS WHO DRESSED AND HAD GROWN UP PRETTY MUCH EXACTLY AS I DID.

cable American prep. There's French classic, movie star classic, tomboy classic. The list goes on. And when I experiment with trends and outrageous designer clothes, I incorporate classic pieces to keep me from looking like I'm wearing a costume. The undercurrent of classic keeps me looking like myself.

My goal with classic dressing today is to look back ten years from now and not be mortified by pictures of myself. Because I certainly am mortified now by pictures of me taken ten years ago. I am so impressed with the photographs of women who *always* look inspiring, no matter the trends. Their style holds up over time. That is what I want for myself for the future, and that is what I look for in classic clothes.

CLASSIC
My Favorite Things

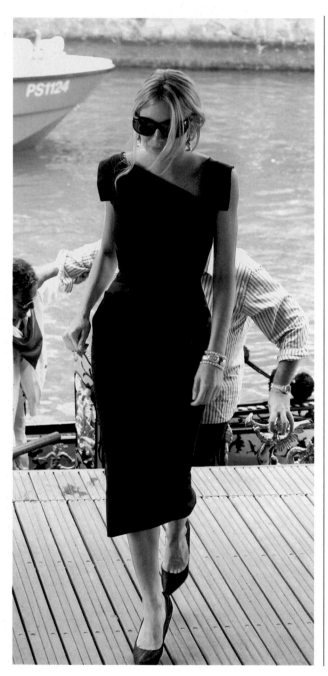

I know. I know. Everyone loves to talk about how great the **LITTLE BLACK DRESS** is, but I didn't really understand it until I found the right one. With the exception of a few very special lace ones that I have borrowed from Chanel, the black dresses that have passed through my life have lingered unworn in the back of my closet. Usually when I pick a dress for an event I anticipate wearing it with great excitement. I never got that feeling about a black dress. But then a designer friend gave me a black dress with a matching short jacket that excited me even before I tried it on. The shape was super simple: Sleeveless with a slight boat neckline, it skimmed my body perfectly down to the hem, just below the knee. Nothing has ever fit me better or flattered my body more (I confess I wear my silicone bra liners to amp up the boob a bit). Because the hem is on the longer side for me I like to wear it with obscenely high Miu Miu platform pumps. This amazing dress is simple enough to wear with a belt, or a chubby fur bolero, or some serious costume jewelry, but I actually think it looks the prettiest on its own, showing off its beautiful cut, precise fit, and rich, textured wool fabric. I am converted.

I have always had a love/hate relationship with a **SUIT**. The "corporate" and "appropriate" look of a suit has always turned me off. But I have learned over the years that a great suit can be one of the most stylish and useful things in your closet. My mom always told me to buy all the available pieces (the skirt, the jacket, and the pants) at once; even if I never wear them all together I can mix and match them with the same blouse and accessories, making it easier and faster to get dressed in the morning. This rule has served me well.

*Twiggy,
1971. I don't
know what
decade this
suit wouldn't
look good in—
it's completely
timeless.*

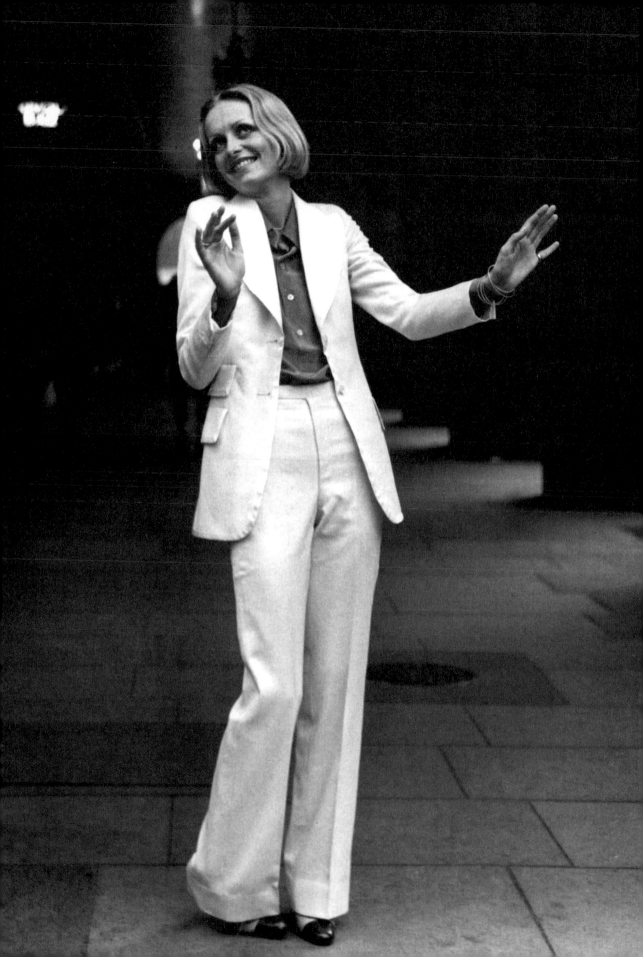

CLASSIC
My Favorite Things

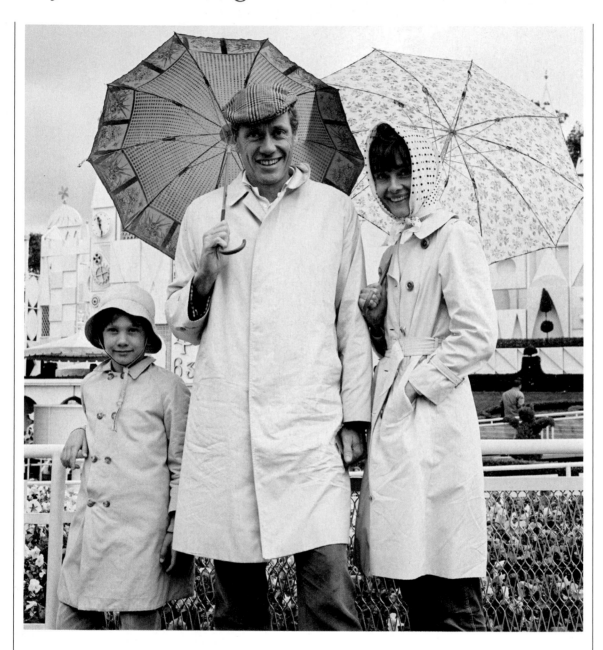

The **TRENCH COAT** is my favorite classic piece. It is a must-have in any wardrobe. Trench coats look good with everything (pants, skirts, even ball gowns), and they look good with nothing. If I'm running out to, say, a movie screening and don't have time to come up with an outfit, I can throw on a trench coat and go, confident that I look pulled together. Actually, you might say I collect trench coats: classic beige, waterproof black, leopard silk faille, vintage white, navy satin, and so on. The wonderful thing is that you can find them everywhere at every price.

Audrey Hepburn and family at Disneyland. I wish people at Disneyland looked this chic today.

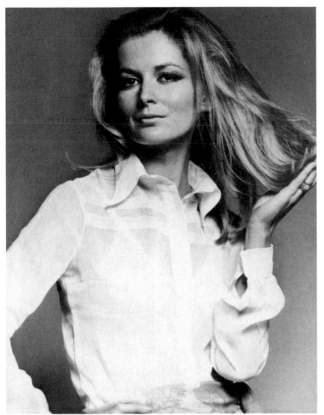

Sixties model Sandra Paul, 1969.

The key to the wearing a **WHITE BUTTON-DOWN SHIRT** (left) is *how* you wear it. You have to give it your own attitude to make it intriguing. My mom's white shirt is always dramatic and formal: fitted in the body, cuffs folded back, collar up. But the French actress Charlotte Gainsbourg wears hers slightly rumpled and loose, looking almost as if she slept in it and didn't bother to change in the morning. This is a younger, more casual look, but it suits her perfectly. I wear my white shirt pressed, with the collar down, and I roll up my sleeves two rolls past my elbows, so it almost looks short sleeved. You can't really go wrong with how you wear your white shirt, as long as you feel comfortable and the look works with your style.

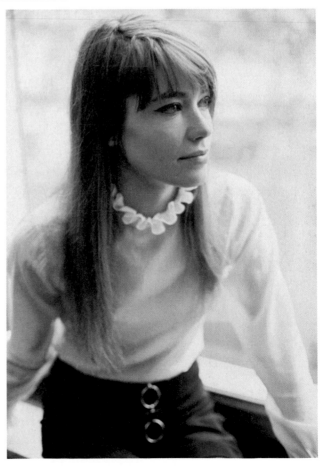

A **CREAM SILK BLOUSE** (right) is one of the most useful and enduring things you can have in your closet. There are dozens of shapes that work beautifully in cream silk, from feminine peasant blouses to traditional masculine tailoring. The choice of shape depends on what suits your body and works with the rest of your clothes.

French singer and actress Françoise Hardy, 1970. Perfect French chic.

My Favorite Things

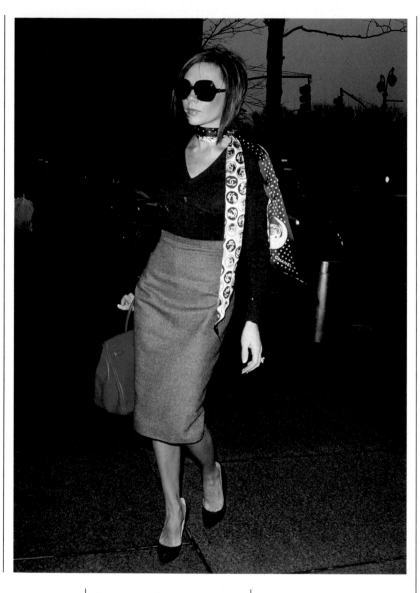

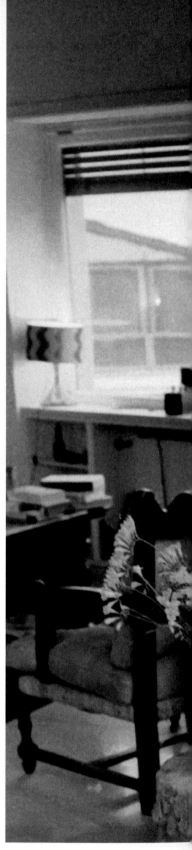

Sometimes I am tempted to get an office job as an excuse to wear a **PENCIL SKIRT** more often. I find them so sexy. That said, of course, fit is everything. It should be snug over your hips so that it comes in under your butt, but not so tight that it gathers on your front side. When in doubt, visit a tailor.

This page: Victoria Beckham keeps on getting chic–er—the more ladylike her look, the better, 2008.

Opposite: Italian movie star Monica Vitti shows how stylish a boy's blazer can look on a girl, 1965.

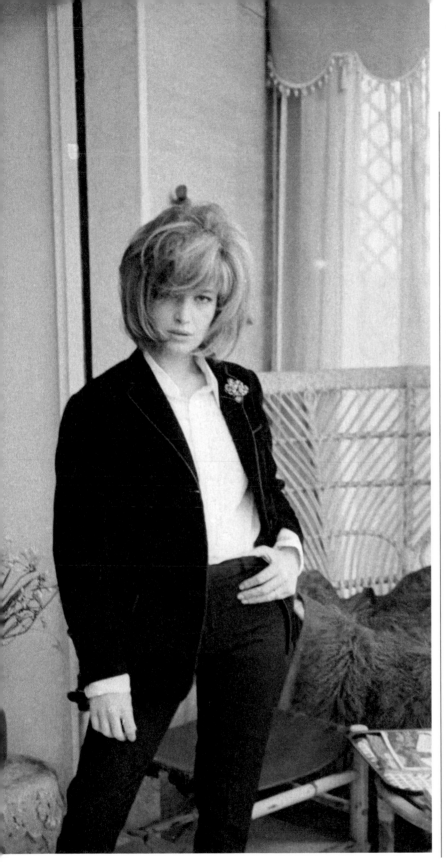

A beautifully **TAILORED JACKET** or **BLAZER** in a classic color (black, brown, gray) can anchor your entire wardrobe. It provides the perfect bit of contrast to feminine, soft, romantic clothing, yet when worn more literally with tailored clothes it can create a perfect tomboy look. I have a collection of classically tailored jackets that I wear most every day over jeans, sneakers, and a few layered T-shirts, but they also look great buttoned up over an evening gown or cocktail dress. I have recently become interested in buying men's tailoring in a small size. I love the truly classic old-school cut and styling of stores like Brooks Brothers and Ralph Lauren.

I HAVE RECENTLY BECOME INTERESTED IN BUYING MEN'S TAILORING IN A SMALL SIZE. I LOVE THE TRULY CLASSIC OLD-SCHOOL CUT AND STYLING OF STORES LIKE BROOKS BROTHERS AND RALPH LAUREN.

Amanda Brooks

CLASSIC
My Favorite Things

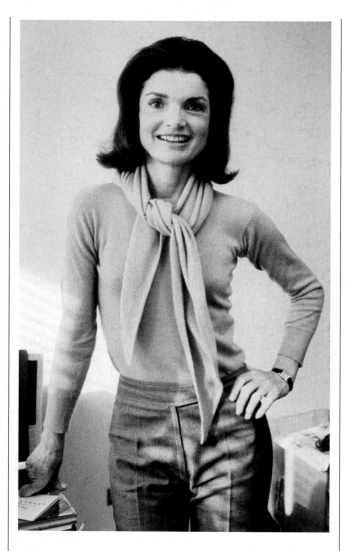

*Jacqueline
Kennedy
Onassis, 1977.*

"I LOVE SWEATER SETS. ESPECIALLY VINTAGE ONES. THEY'RE THE CRUCIAL PART OF MY SEXY SECRETARY LOOK. I WEAR THEM WITH A REALLY TIGHT PENCIL SKIRT, HIGH-HEELED SHOES, AND MY SEXY/NERDY GLASSES. OH! AND RED LIPSTICK—THAT'S KEY."
—LIZ GOLDWYN

I have two favorite shapes for **CASHMERE SWEATERS**. The first one is the **PULLOVER**, either a crewneck, a turtle-neck, or a V-neck. This looks sexy with nothing underneath, sporty over a T-shirt, and just plain chic over a blouse or men's tailored shirt. Then there is a long fitted **V-NECK CARDIGAN**. For day this is one of the most important things in my closet; I love it because you can still see the pretty blouse or shirt you are wearing underneath and it's easy to pull on and off.

A **FISHERMAN'S SWEATER** is almost so preppy it's camp, but when worn simply (with, say, black trousers and flats) it can be chic and timeless.

I have a confession. *There are a lot of classic sweaters I do love, but I am not a fan of the* **SWEATER SET***. I think it looks uptight and boring. I really, really don't like it. That said, after I took this definitive and slightly aggressive stand, I called my girlfriend Liz Goldwyn—a jewelry designer and documentary filmmaker who has enviable style—because I suspected she would see things differently. "I love sweater sets," she said. "Especially vintage ones. They're the crucial part of my sexy secretary look. I wear them with a really tight pencil skirt, high-heeled shoes, and my sexy/nerdy glasses. Oh! and red lipstick—that's key." There you go. That's the amazing thing about style. There may be things that are not right for you, but it's almost impossible to rule anything out for everybody. Even if you can't pull something off, chances are someone else can.*

The **BRETON SAILING TOP** (below) is named after the seaside town in France where the style originated, but it's also known as a "Picasso sweater" because Pablo himself wore them so often. This is a boatneck off-white sweater or shirt with dark navy or red stripes, sometimes with buttons on the shoulder on one side. I love, love, love this shirt. It represents all that is cool about old-school classic. It's been around forever and never goes out of style.

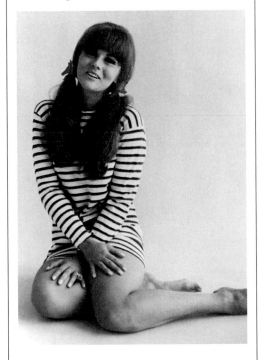

I would feel too preppy in a **FAIR ISLE SWEATER** (right), but I've seen friends look great in them. To pull it off you must, must, must add an ironic twist—nerdy preppy, sexy preppy, tomboy preppy—anything but straightforward preppy.

Above:
Ann-Margret,
1960s.

Right:
Mia Farrow,
1965.
Adorable.

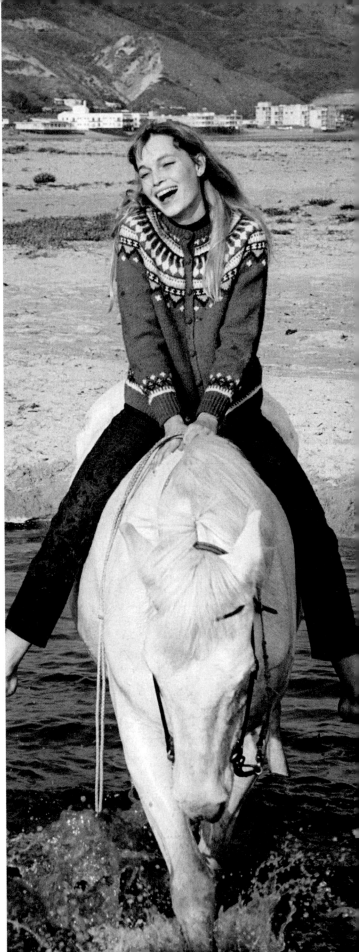

My Favorite Things

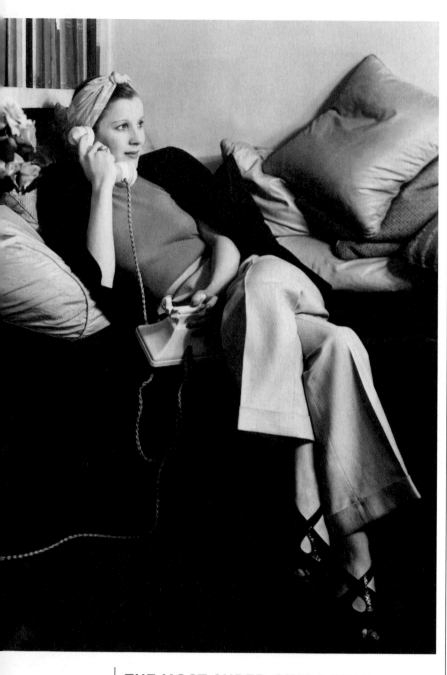

Diana Wynyard, 1932. It's hard to believe this photo was taken in the 30s. She would be equally chic in her neatly pressed pants today.

THE MOST SUPER-CHIC DETAIL ON A FORMAL TROUSER IS A PRESSED CREASE DOWN THE FRONT OF THE LEG.

I am a devoted fan of classically **TAILORED TROUSERS**. I like them best with a bit of masculinity in them: the tab closure, the belt loops, the back pockets. For casual purposes I even like them to have a men's fit, but for evening, fewer details and a slimmer fit work best.

The most super-chic detail on a formal trouser is a pressed crease down the front of the leg. But you have to make sure the pants fit well, and not too tight. There's nothing worse than a pressed pleat that doesn't hang straight because the pant is pulling.

Tastes and trends in fur come and go, but a **MINK COAT** is always chic.

Whether or not you choose to wear fur is an intensely personal decision. While I am clearly okay about wearing it, I am not here to suggest that you should. However, if you believe it's all right to wear fur, then I am thrilled to help you pick the best styles. All that said, I'm not into faux fur. Yuck. It looks (and feels!) dreadful. Don't go there.

Sofia Coppola's ankle boots make her mink coat look younger and more modern. 2008.

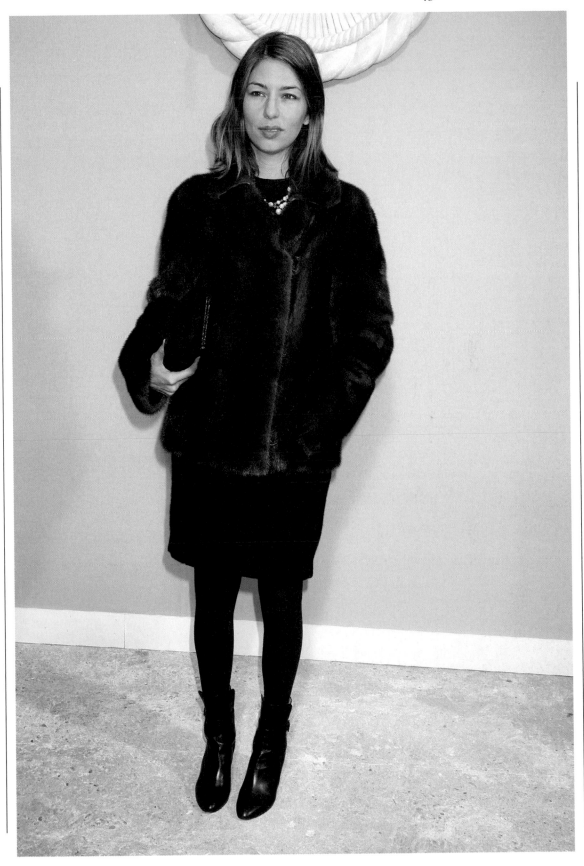

Amanda Brooks

CLASSIC
My Favorite Things

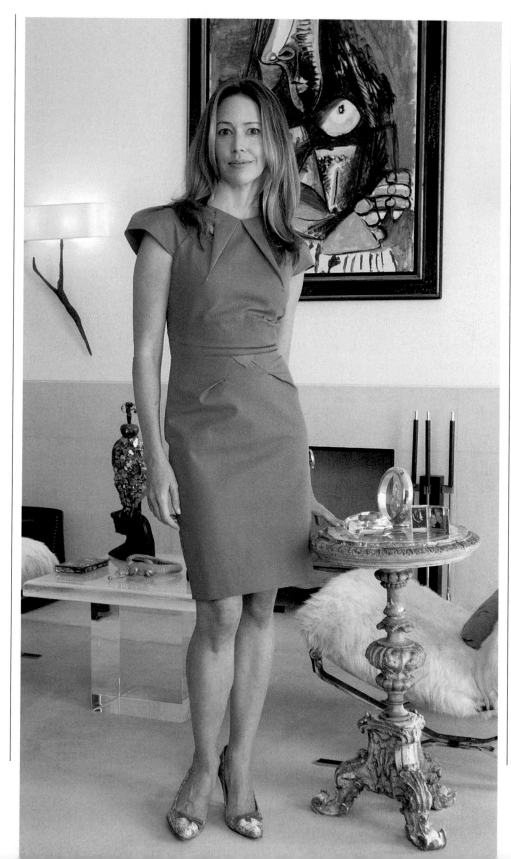

Samantha Boardman (in her NYC bedroom, 2008) shows us that shift dresses don't have to look as conservative as they once did.

I Love Your Style

I have spent much of my life being terrified of the **SHIFT DRESS** (opposite). To me it signaled "lady-like" in a way that seemed more relevant to my mom's generation than to my own. But recently I have started to see the enormous potential for chic in shift dresses. I don't know if it's my age or the fact that my friends and I are not locked into ladylike orbits, but shift dresses no longer seem threatening to me. They look great in the day with flats, sandals, even flip-flops, and they easily dress up for evening with heels and some sexy eyeliner. Dresses in the 60s had great simple shape and styling, so that's where to look for inspiration. Remember this: When it comes to accessorizing a shift dress, less is more.

There is a part of me that wants to yawn when I think of **HOUNDSTOOTH**, **TWEED**, and **PLAID**. They have all been used and overused as a classic material, not only in clothes but in interiors too. But then I look at pictures of the 40s, 50s, and 60s when women were expected to be more feminine and formal, and suddenly these geometric prints look fresh and new and exciting to me. Just when I thought I could never be a houndstooth person, a houndstooth wool tulip skirt took me by surprise. I bought it and have been wearing it ever since. There are so many ways to go right and wrong with these fabrics that it might be best to go a little wrong on purpose; some plaid, tweed, or houndstooth can add just the right retro element to a look when you are verging on being too tasteful.

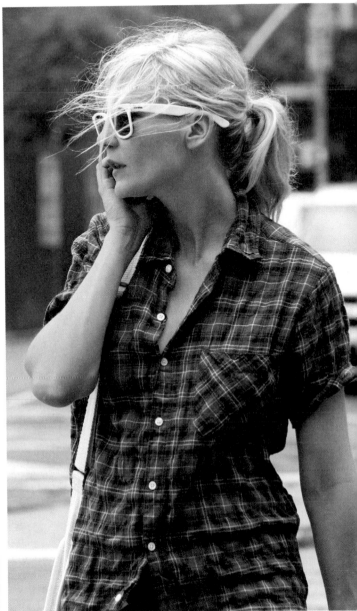

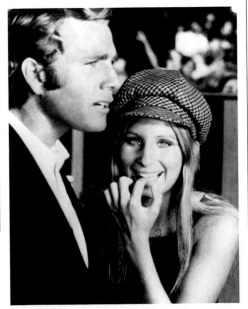

*Above:
I like how
Kirsten Dunst's
white
sunglasses give
her plaid shirt
an updated
look, 2008.*

*Left:
Barbra
Streisand
with
Ryan O'Neal,
1972.*

JUST WHEN I THOUGHT I COULD NEVER BE A HOUNDSTOOTH PERSON, A HOUNDSTOOTH WOOL TULIP SKIRT TOOK ME BY SURPRISE.

CLASSIC
Accessories

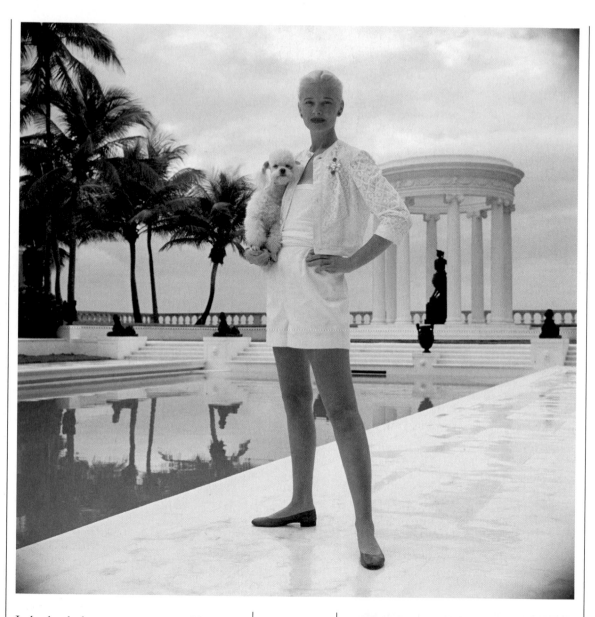

I absolutely love **BALLET FLATS**. The most luxurious classic ballet flat is the Chanel cap toe. If you're going to buy anything from Chanel, this shoe probably gives you the biggest impact for the least money, especially if you choose a classic color like beige, black, or navy. But there are also great options at other (lower!) prices. You just need to keep a few things in mind to find the best pair.

C. Z. Guest at her home in Palm Beach, Florida, 1962.

TIPS Shopping for ballet flats:

- *Find the shoe with the lowest, thinnest heel possible. The chicest ballet flats are literally flat!*

- *Make sure the toe isn't too round. A very round toe looks cheap and shortens your legs.*

- *Make sure they are low cut on the top of the shoe (but avoid too much toe cleavage!).*

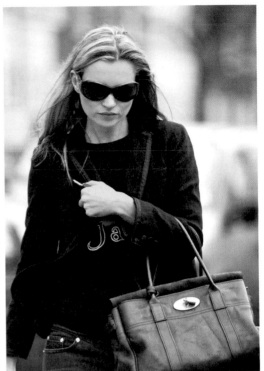

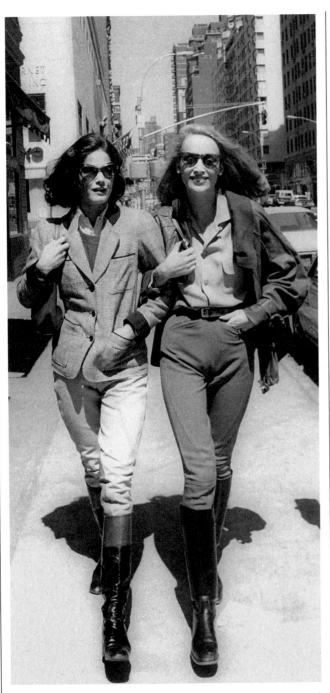

Some people are really into collecting handbags these days. I am personally not so into it. It's ridiculously expensive and a great way to ensure that you never know where your wallet, keys, and phone are hiding. Trust me. If you are a classic dresser, or like the simplicity of consistently carrying one bag like I do, a **BLACK** and a **BROWN HANDBAG** are all you really need. Choose carefully and spend as much as you can—or even a little more! Avoid excessive hardware; you'll get sick of it over time, and it will often interfere with your jewelry or your outfit. If you usually wear gold jewelry, buy a bag with gold hardware and vice versa if you're a silver/platinum jewelry wearer. That might be the matchy-matchy side of me speaking, but I suspect that most of you classic dressers are pretty matchy-matchy too.

Left:
Jerry Hall,
strutting in her
chic Gucci
riding boots,
with a friend,
1978.

Top:
Kate Moss
doing errands
in London with
a Mulberry
bag, 2004.

What could be more timeless and chic than **RIDING BOOTS**? And the greatest thing about them is that they last a lifetime, and the more worn-in they look the better.

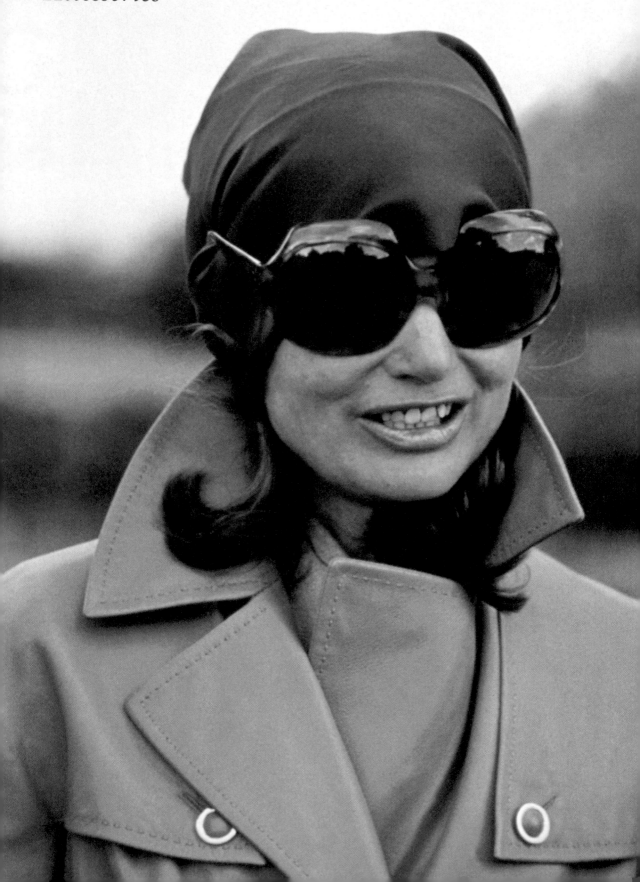

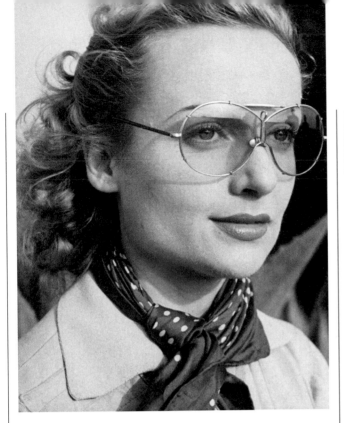

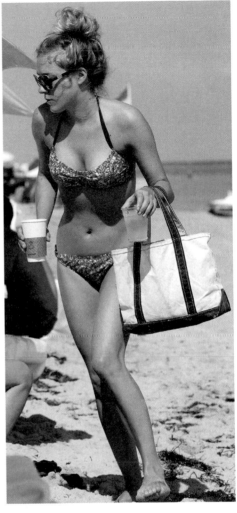

OVERSIZED SUNGLASSES (left), as popularized by Jackie O, still look great. I don't care how many people try to imitate this look; I still love them. But the size overwhelms some faces, and for others they're too much of a statement.

I lived in Ray-Ban **AVIATORS** (above) from ages thirteen through seventeen, and I see people wearing them now who still look so chic. A great option for those who don't feel right in the Jackie O look, aviators are more streamlined and subtle—perfect for the elegant understatement.

Above:
Carole
Lombard in
early aviator
sunglasses,
1938.

An **L.L.BEAN CANVAS TOTE** is an inexpensive, functional, old-school classic.

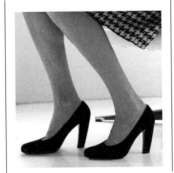

Opposite:
Jackie O, 1976.
I love this more
eccentric side
of her—
reminds me of
Grey Gardens.

Right:
My favorite
Prada pumps,
2009.

The ideal classic **PUMPS** change slightly from year to year depending on the trends. Just take a look at a pair of pumps you thought were classic ten years ago, and you'll see what I mean. Look for something without overt decoration (a stitching detail or leather/suede combination is fine, but no grommets or jewels or highly contrasting colors) and a restrained shape (no asymmetrical toes or weirdly angled heels here).

Above:
As much as
Chloë Sevigny
loves high
fashion, it's
her love of
simple, classic
things—like
an L.L. Bean
tote—that
makes me
appreciate her
style most,
2008.

CLASSIC
Accessories

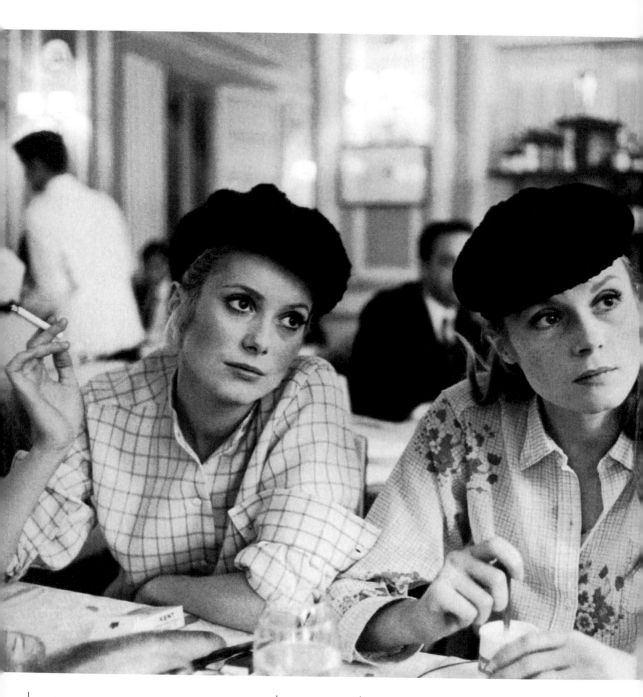

A **BERET** looks great on anyone who has the confidence to carry it off. The key to wearing a beret is not to try too hard. Standing in

Catherine Deneuve and her sister, Françoise Dorléac, 1966.

front of the mirror for hours trying to angle it in just the right way might crush your spirit. Just throw it on and go.

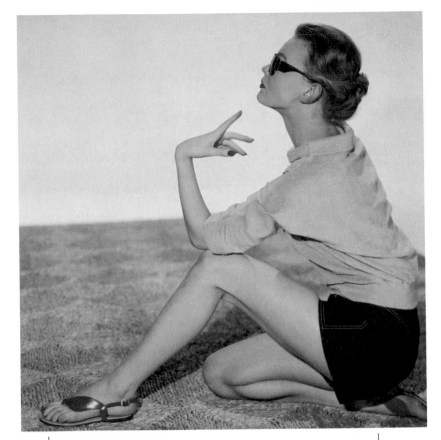

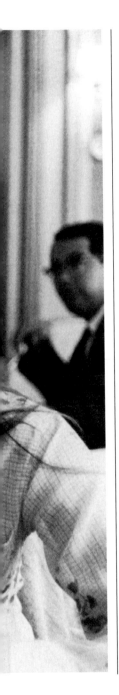

The perfect red sandals, 1955.

If you're a classic girl, the best **SANDALS** are the simplest ones. A plain thong and a Grecian-inspired gladiator sandal both look simple and chic in leather or suede. If you're craving novelty go for color, not decoration. My favorite place to buy sandals is Atelier Rondini in St. Tropez. You have to go there—or check them out online at www.nova.fr/rondini/. I've also bought leather sandals on my travels through Mexico, Greece, and Turkey. I always keep an eye out for sandals while traveling.

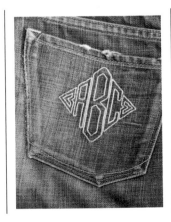

You can get your monogram sewn on your jeans pocket at Earnest Sewn, New York City.

You can put a **MONOGRAM** on just about anything—shirts, handbags, wallets, belts, even embroidered on the back pocket of your jeans—and it will give your outfit a classic look.

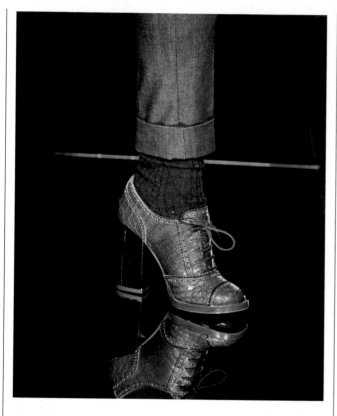

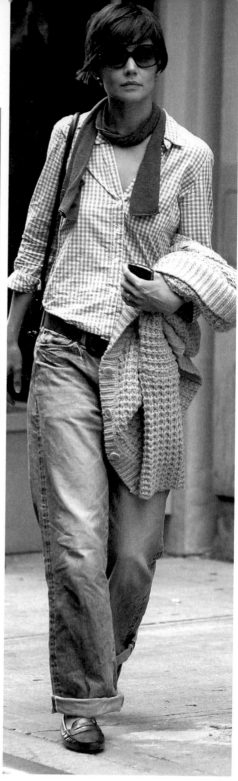

ANIMAL SKIN—such as crocodile, alligator, leopard, lizard, or ostrich—lends accessories an air of luxury, timelessness, and long-lasting quality. My mom bought a chocolate brown ostrich Gucci handbag with a bamboo handle when she was twenty-five and wore it steadily for fifteen years. When it fell apart she had the same exact bag custom remade by Gucci, and she still wears it today, almost twenty years later.

Above:
I wish I'd seen
these Dolce and
Gabbana shoes
when they were
in the store.
I would have
bought them
instantly.

Opposite:
Jackie O
wearing a
Cartier Tank
watch, 1969.

Right:
Katie Holmes
in New York
City, 2008. An
old-school
preppy look
really suits her.

LOAFERS have evolved over the years both in function and in style. The penny loafer comes to mind first, but in the last decade the **DRIVING SHOE** has evolved into the new millennium version of the loafer. Softer, more comfortable, and distinctly more casual in feel, the driving shoe has become a new icon of classic style.

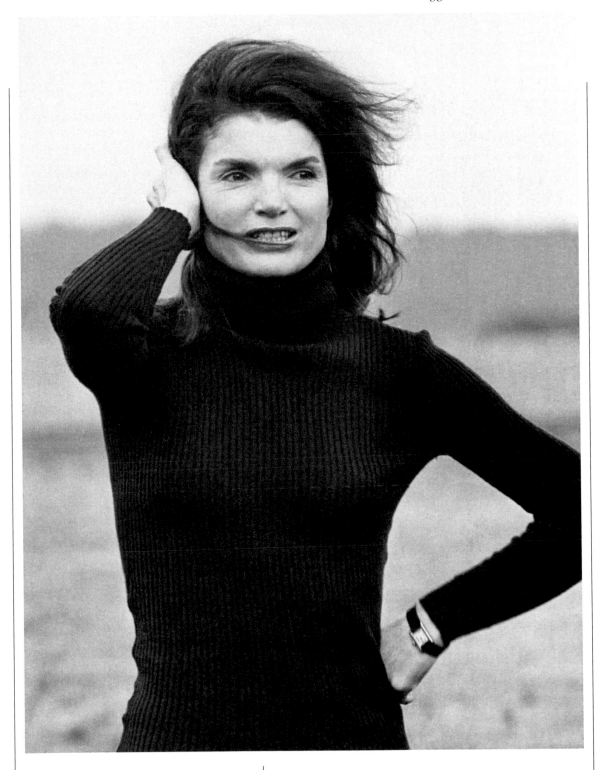

"THE ONLY ROUTINE WITH ME IS NO ROUTINE AT ALL."
—JACQUELINE KENNEDY ONASSIS

One of the best investments you can make is a timeless **WATCH**. I've been wearing a stainless steel Cartier Pasha with a lizard band for ten years and still can't imagine growing tired of it.

CLASSIC
Accessories

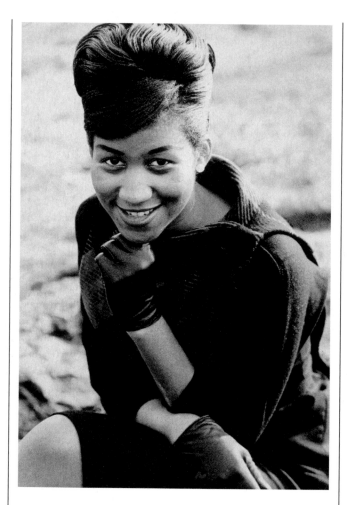

LEATHER GLOVES can add *a lot* of style to any look. Long kid gloves for evening, sporty mesh driving gloves for the weekend, and cashmere-lined leather gloves for a cold wintery day all look amazing.

Above: Aretha Franklin in chic black leather gloves, 1961.

Right: The bracelets my grandfather had custom-made for my grandmother.

Opposite: Coco Chanel, in her signature pearls, on a beach at the Lido, 1930.

One way to create a signature in your style while exhibiting classic consistency is to invest in a **PIECE OF JEWELRY** (opposite) that you love and wear every single day. My husband gave me a walnut wood and gold link chain bracelet from the fancy Park Avenue jeweler Seaman Schepps when my son was born. It pulls every outfit I wear together, and I know I will love it forever.

There is something that really touches me about **PERSONALIZED JEWELRY**. No matter how specific the design, wearing something you love and hold close to your heart is definitely classic.

MY FAVORITE Personalized jewelry:

- *My friend Nathalie's pendant necklace with her mother's thumbprint engraved on it.*
- *My grandmother's gold ID bracelet with her name written on the name plate in my grandfather's handwriting—in diamonds!*
- *My mother's gold bracelet with "I love you Liz with all my heart" engraved in my step-father's handwriting.*
- *My gold-and-glass heart locket with a lock of my dad's hair tucked inside.*
- *My friend Zandy's gold heart stent pendant necklace (a stent is a medical cure for a "bro-ken" heart).*

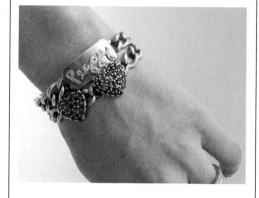

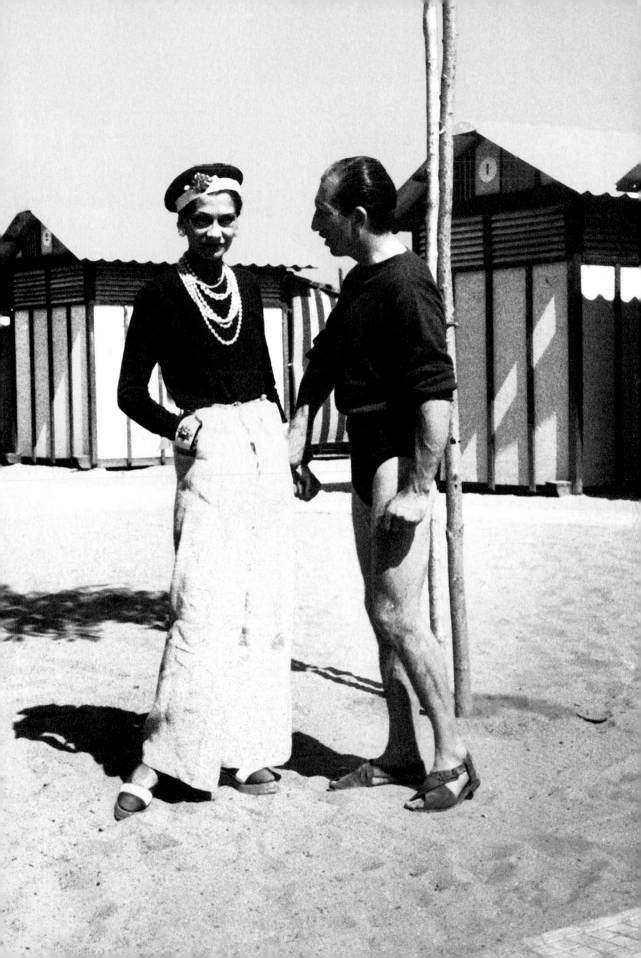

CLASSIC
Mixing It Up

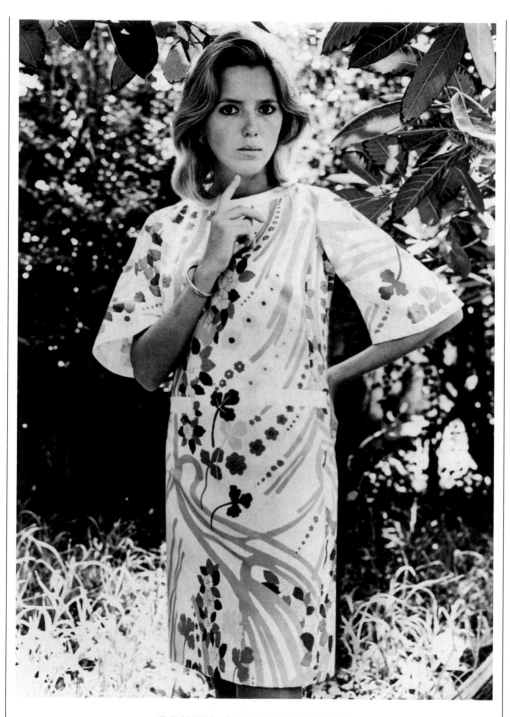

**PRINTS CAN BE TRICKY
BECAUSE THEY ARE SO PERSONAL,
BUT THAT'S JUST IT.
THEY ARE SO PERSONAL!**

*This page:
My mother
modeling a
Lilly Pulitzer
print dress in
Palm Beach,
c.1960s.*

*Opposite:
(Left)
Nonni Phipps,
Palm Beach,
1959.*

*(Right)
Lou Doillon,
in a cowboy-
inspired tomboy
outfit, 2005.*

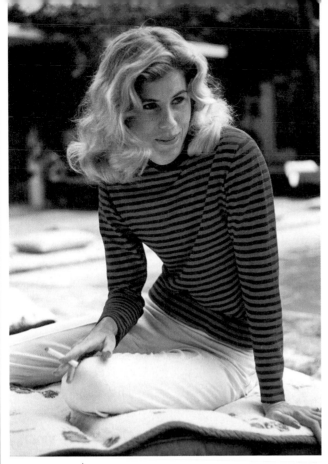

The graphic effect of **CLASSIC STRIPES** adds intrigue to an otherwise basic look.

If you want to keep a classic look from being too straight up, a **BOLD PATTERN** or **PRINT** (opposite) can make a big impact. Prints can be tricky because they are so personal, but that's just it. They are so personal! Some people don't like prints and never will. But if you would like to try, the box below contains some guidelines.

TIPS Shopping for prints:

- *Start with a print that is small in scale. Choose one that has either tonal colors or very few colors.*

- *If you are confused about what color shoe to wear, pick any color that is in the print and it will probably work.*

- *Try a printed dress. Then you don't have to figure out what pants/skirt/blouse to wear with it.*

- *Prints look modern when worn with neutrals (gray, black, brown, or white), especially when the print itself has a lot of color in it. Sure, my grandmother looked great in a printed floral blouse with matching lavender pants, but that was the 60s. Somehow it doesn't translate so successfully to today.*

SAFARI JACKETS and **ARMY JACKETS** are highly stylized, but they have a certain romantic chic that has made them staples. Easy to wear for women of any age and virtually any figure, these jackets come in a vast variety of prices and materials. Their neutral colors combine well with most casual outfits.

The formality of classic clothes, like a tailored jacket or a cashmere sweater looks less expected when worn with **LAID-BACK DENIM**. A mini is always youthful and cute, but you must take a good hard look at your legs before you try it. If you don't like what you see, a longer denim skirt is more forgiving and can do the same trick. For more on jeans, see the basics shopping chapter.

A touch of **COWBOY INFLUENCE** (below) enlivens otherwise straightforward pieces. Thrift stores are full of classic pearl button cotton shirts, Western belt buckles, and worn-in cowboy boots. Just don't wear them all at once! Literal cowgirl is not a good look.

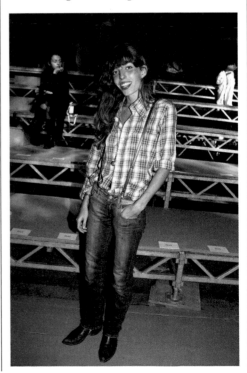

CLASSIC
High Risk, High Reward

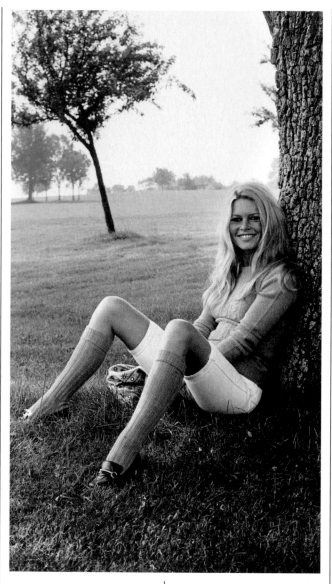

Near right: I could never imagine thinking these shorts with knee socks (and Gucci loafers no less!) would make a good outfit, but on Brigitte Bardot it's inspiring, 1965.

Right: Diane Keaton in a scene from Annie Hall, 1977.

Opposite: I often think of Mick Jagger's irreverent take on classic clothes when getting dressed, 1973.

A **PANAMA HAT** (opposite) can create a similar classic yet excitingly androgynous effect.

The **FEDORA** is not for everyone but on the right girl it is sensational. Confidence is key, so if you put the hat on and it doesn't seem to click, you should probably take it off.

SPECTATOR SHOES (opposite) can be truly horrid on a woman: too contrived, too masculine, all wrong. However, I have seen the occasional spectator shoe that adds just the right amount of high fashion tomboy charm to an outfit.

A girl in a **HEAD SCARF** can channel Twiggy, Jackie O, or Grace Kelly at the height of their chic. Unfortunately she can just as easily channel a 50s housewife or the Queen of England protecting her hair from the wind—not so cute. Head scarves are best with casual, thrown-together looks, tied on in a way that looks spur-of-the-moment, not studied and contrived.

It's pretty simple: Your legs make or break the way you look in **SHORTS**. If you do have the legs, shorts can create a silhouette that is classic but unexpected, and they aren't only for recreation. A feminine blouse looks great with fitted tailored shorts, with flats for the day or high heels for the evening.

Diane Keaton's **TIE** peeking out from under a black vest in *Annie Hall* is one of the quintessential fashion moments of the 70s, and it still looks fearless and inspiring today. But this is a highly stylized look, and only women with a certain confidence and innate tomboy instinct can pull off wearing a tie.

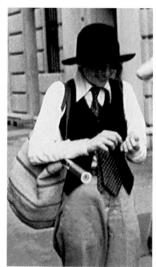

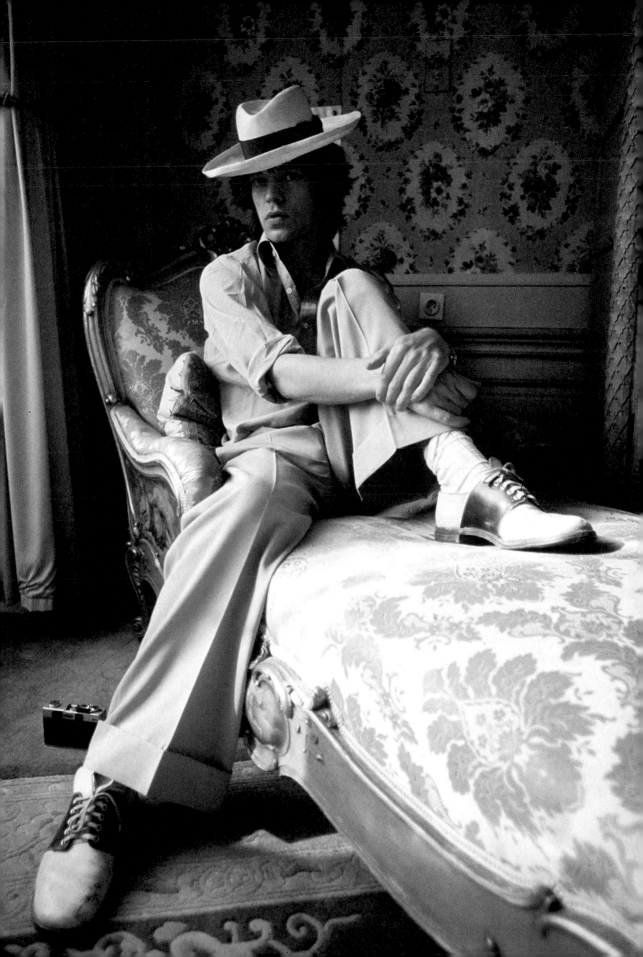

CLASSIC
Evening

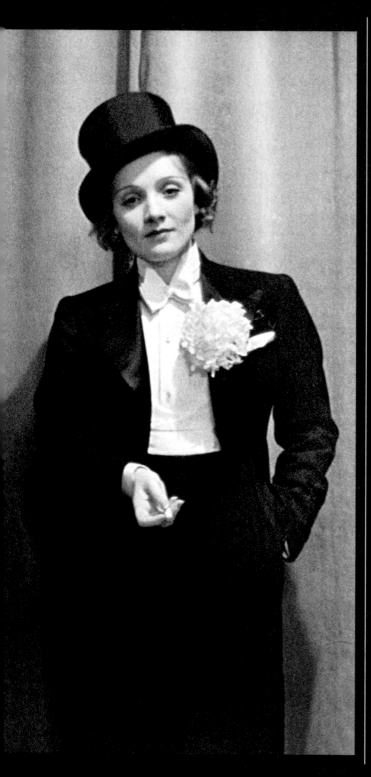

Evening clothes are often so expensive that it makes a lot of sense to buy classic evening pieces that you can mix with different accessories to wear over and over again.

A CLASSIC BLACK TUXEDO (left) has to fit you perfectly. Buy the most expensive one you can afford and have it tailored to fit you if necessary. If price is prohibitive try the boys' department at a men's store like Polo Ralph Lauren or Brooks Brothers.

If you're feeling sexy wear it without a blouse underneath. You can pin the lapel shut if you're scared of flashing people. A vintage jeweled pin or a fresh flower tucked into the lapel is a great way of adding some softness to an otherwise severe look. Hair could be down and full or tucked neatly into a low sleek bun.

I also like a tuxedo with a white tuxedo shirt. You can either go Patti Smith and wear messy hair and little makeup or you can go Brigitte Bardot and do big loosely curled hair and 60s black eyeliner.

The jacket of a tuxedo worn alone is useful for evening as well. Once I was wearing a Gucci chiffon baby-doll minidress and needed a coat to wear over it. My Viktor and Rolf for H&M tuxedo jacket was perfect, with the hem of the dress just sticking out below it. The tailoring of the jacket was a great contrast to the softness of the chiffon dress.

A BLACK LACE DRESS (opposite, left) is seasonless, feminine, and sophisticated. It is also versatile: edgy with white pumps, messy hair, and strong makeup; schoolgirl chic with black flats, mascara, lip gloss, and a ponytail with a black bow in it; 60s chic with black patent leather pumps, bouffant hair, and dramatic eyeliner.

The great thing about a LONG EVENING SKIRT (opposite, right) is that you can wear virtually anything dressy on top to reinvent the look over and over again.

Marlene Dietrich is the original and probably all-time chicest tomboy, 1929.

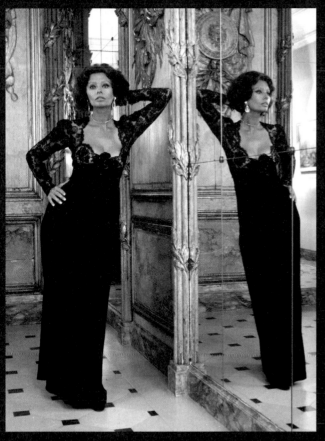

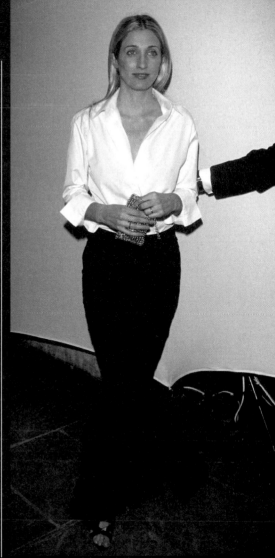

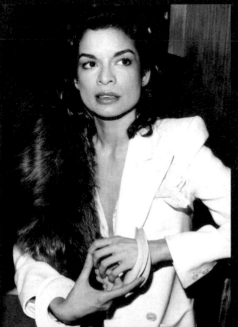

"THE MOST IMPORTANT
THING IS TO ENJOY
YOURSELF AND HAVE
A GOOD TIME."
—C. Z. GUEST

A touch of FUR (left) is a great way to jack up an evening outfit. A fur wrap, stole, scarf, vest, or bolero just instantly makes you look glamorous. Fox, lynx, mink, and chinchilla are all dressy-looking skins that have a strong impact, and black and white are the best colors for evening. Natural-colored skins are more casual looking and suitable for daytime.

Clockwise from top left: Sophia Loren, 1979.

Carolyn Bessette Kennedy was so good at making modern clothes look classic and classic clothes look modern, 1999.

Bianca Jagger, 1980.

Amanda Brooks

CLASSIC
Getting It Right

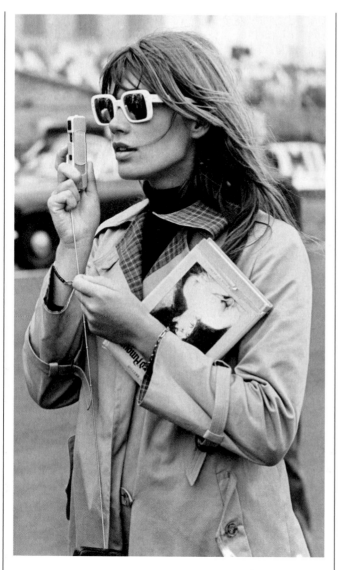

Try adding a touch of **SOMETHING TACKY**. Chanel is a wonderful source of inspiration because it repeatedly takes a piece that epitomizes classic style (the two-piece suit, the quilted bag, the ballet flat) and reinvents it with irony—usually by adding a well-considered dash of tackiness: a plastic fringe, a beaded sleeve, shiny fabrics, patent leather, oversized sunglasses, and so on. This is the heart of Karl Lagerfeld's genius, and the strong foundation of classic style at Chanel allows him to experiment in a way that other designers simply cannot.

Styling yourself with **MESSINESS** is another way to avoid looking like a cliché. Lauren Santo Domingo, a stylist for *Vogue*, has classic looks and classic style, but she gets away with it (and she really does get away with it—she always looks great!) thanks to her messy hair. Whether dressed for day or night, office or fun, she either wears her hair in a messy bun or lets it hang disheveled about her shoulders.

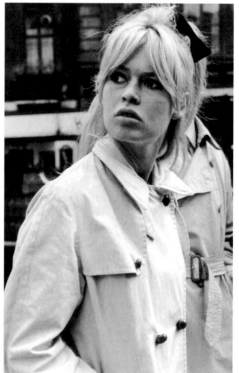

The way you wear classic clothes is particularly important. Because the clothes themselves are on the whole simple and recognizably part of a specific style, you must be vigilant about wearing them in a way that telegraphs your personality. Remember, classic does not have to be boring, but it can be. It is most successful today when it includes a touch of the unexpected.

If, like me, you feel like a caricature in a cashmere sweater and charm bracelet, here are some ways to subvert a classic look:

*Above:
Françoise
Hardy, 1966.*

*Right:
Brigitte
Bardot, 1963.
I love the bow
in her
messy hair.*

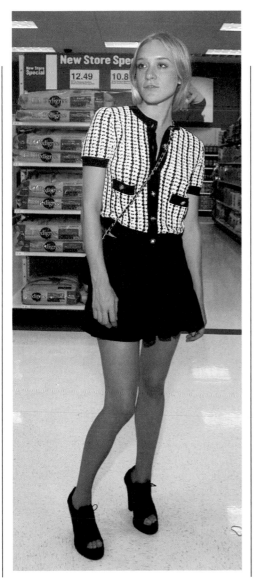

Because **PROPORTION** is an essential component of looking put together in a classic way, one of the easiest ways to achieve subversive contrast within your outfit is to play with proportion and scale. Classic skirts and dresses typically hit right below the knee, and classic shirts, blouses, and sweaters are generally modest. Skirts and pants hit the waist or sit squarely above the hips. Replace one of these staple items with something shorter, longer, more revealing, tighter, or looser to make your look interesting. You can also use accessories to throw off the symmetry of a classic outfit. A wide belt, oversized bag, or printed scarf can easily change your look from "I work in an office" to "I'm totally channeling Charlotte Rampling."

FAIL-SAFE CLASSIC PROPORTIONS
- Trousers with a silk blouse (tucked in, of course)
- Oxford shirt with a pencil skirt and cardigan (and a little heel)
- Little black dress with a strappy high heel and a boxy jacket
- Boot cut jeans with a tucked-in white shirt and riding boots
- Belted trench and stiletto heels

IRONIC CLASSIC PROPORTIONS
- A shrunken fisherman's sweater worn over a flared miniskirt
- An oversized men's shirt with a tight pencil skirt
- A low-cut blouse with a wide-legged trouser
- A men's blazer (with the sleeves rolled up) with skinny jeans

One of the most distinguishing features of a classic wardrobe is the use of classic **FABRICS** such as wool, cotton, cashmere, linen, and silk. There is something about a piece of clothing made in a 100 percent natural fiber that gives it a wonderful, authentic, old-school feeling.

TIPS on trends:

If you have classic style, you probably like to hold on to things for a long time. Sometimes one of those things becomes suddenly trendy, and you fear that people will think you—gasp!—ran out and bought the latest thing (so unlike you!). Let's talk about T. Anthony luggage. These canvas bags with leather trim come in four different colors. They've been around forever and have always been a kind of WASP secret. But recently they became really trendy. Kate Moss has them. So does Gwyneth. What do you do? You hold on. You get through. You keep going. You keep it and you wear it through the trend and you wear it years after the trend. If you get rid of something you love just because it becomes trendy then you are the fashion victim!

A WIDE BELT, OVERSIZED BAG, OR PRINTED SCARF CAN EASILY CHANGE YOUR LOOK FROM "I WORK IN AN OFFICE" TO "I'M TOTALLY CHANNELING CHARLOTTE RAMPLING."

Chloë Sevigny makes a Chanel suit look years younger by changing the proportion to a shorter skirt, a smaller jacket and a chunkier shoe, 2004.

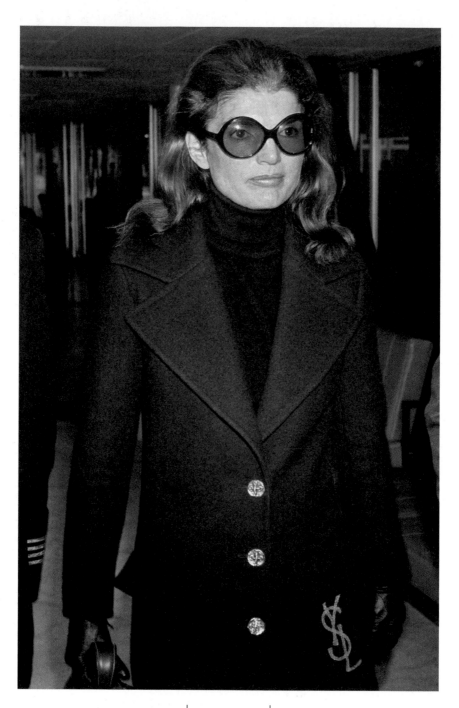

Arguably our most famous fashion icon, **JACQUELINE KENNEDY ONASSIS** defined the concept of American style for her generation and beyond. She may be most famous for her

I know there are a lot of Jackie O photos in this book, but this one is my favorite, 1970.

pink tailored suit and pillbox hat, but it is her more casual and "unofficial" outfits that inspire me most.

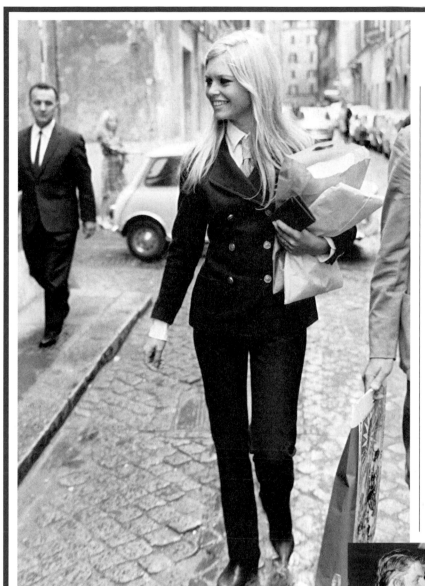

Left:
Brigitte Bardot
in Rome, 1967.

There's no one like **BRIGITTE BARDOT**, never has been, and never will be. In her heyday she was the most beautiful woman in the world, and she is still regarded as one of the most intriguing actresses and iconic sex symbols of all time. Bardot's clothes were chosen to emphasize her delicious hourglass physique, and everything she put on became instantly sexy. She loved thigh-grazing dresses, tall boots, pencil skirts, and skinny belts that highlighted her tiny waist. She is a great reference point for anyone looking to add a dash of sex appeal to her wardrobe, and she proves that classic does not equal prudish or matronly.

"I ABSOLUTELY LOATHE LUXURY. IT IS THE ONE THING I CANNOT STAND."
—BRIGITTE BARDOT

Right:
With her
husband,
Gunther Sachs,
in London,
1967.

CLASSIC
Icons

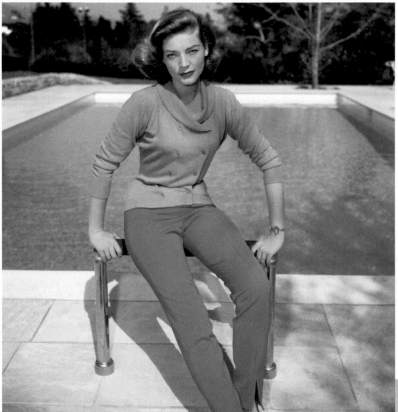

*Lauren Bacall,
1955, 1972,
and 1943.*

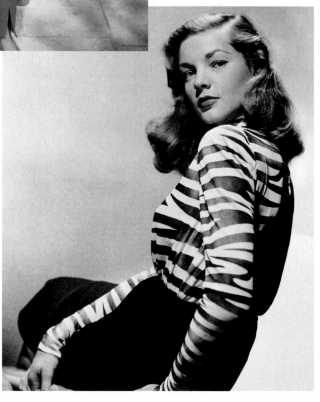

The thing I love most about **LAUREN BACALL**'s style is how easy and casual it looks. She looks like she just chose a simple shirt and pants or a skirt from her closet and went about her day—nothing fussy about the process or its effect. Besides being one of the all-time best actresses, she's also a true pioneer of the American "sportswear" look.

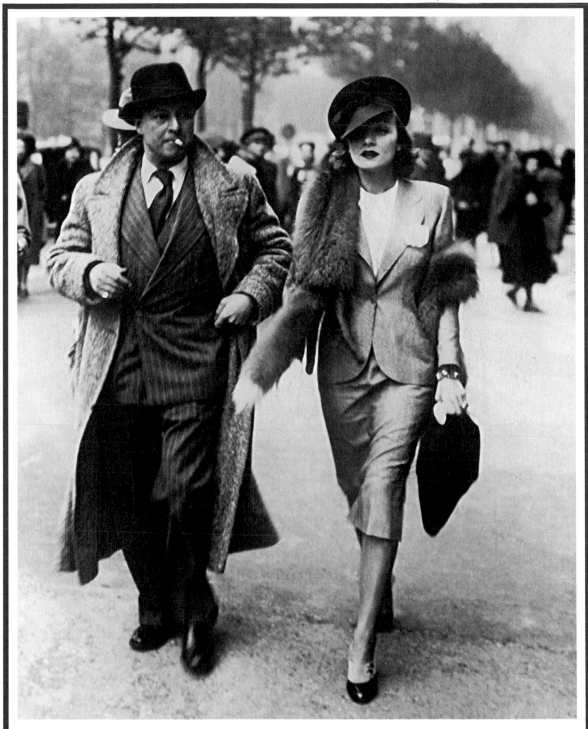

Marlene Dietrich with her husband Rudolph Sieber in Paris, 1938.

"I DRESS FOR THE IMAGE. NOT FOR MYSELF, NOT FOR THE PUBLIC, NOT FOR FASHION, NOT FOR MEN."
—MARLENE DIETRICH

MARLENE DIETRICH's ability to switch between masculine and feminine with such convincing ease is fascinating. She was clearly partial to men's-inspired tailoring and styling, but the end result was always glamorous and without a doubt womanly.

Amanda Brooks

CLASSIC
Icons

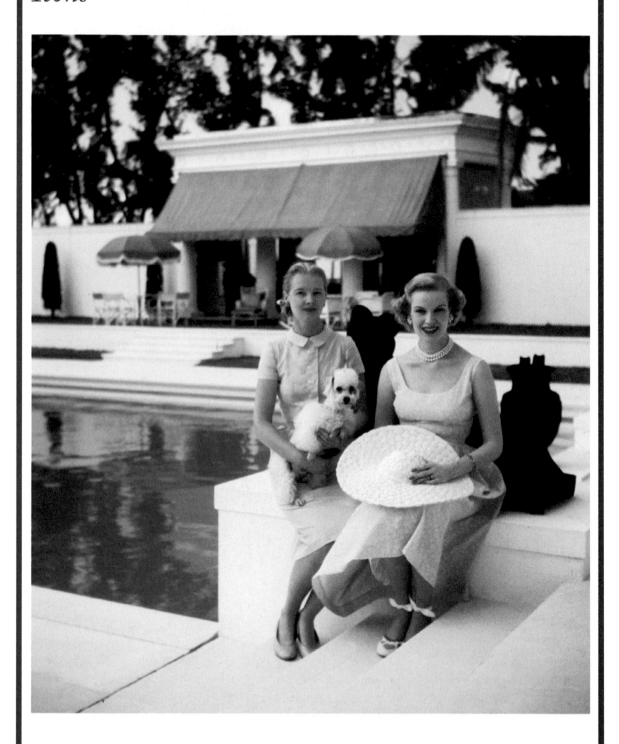

Society queen **C. Z. GUEST** is the quintessential icon of supremely tasteful uptown style, *C. Z. Guest (left) sitting with a friend in Palm Beach, 1955.* pearls and all. She was the chicest blonde on Park Avenue.

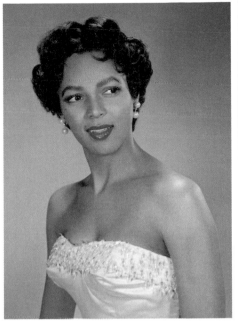

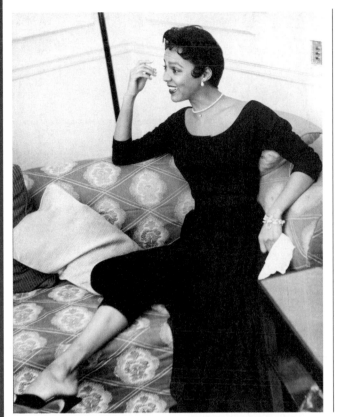

In addition to being the first African-American actress in a leading role to be nominated for an Oscar, **DOROTHY DANDRIDGE** also epitomized classic 50s style. It's amazing how dated some women from the 50s look today—with their poodle skirts, saddle shoes, and scarves around their ponytails. Yet Ms. Dandridge knew just the right, more refined pieces that would keep her look relevant all the way to today and beyond.

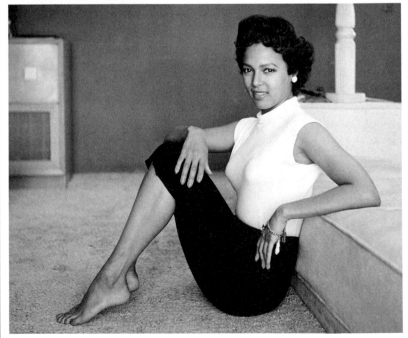

Dorothy Dandridge (clockwise from left), 1956, 1955, and 1954.

CLASSIC
Icons

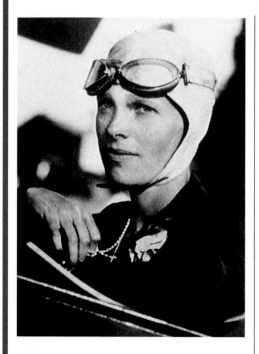

With her fitted leather jackets, men's ties, and cropped hair, **AMELIA EARHART** was the original dashing tomboy. She looks like she walked straight out of a Ralph Lauren ad. Her beauty mixed with her masculine/feminine style blows me away.

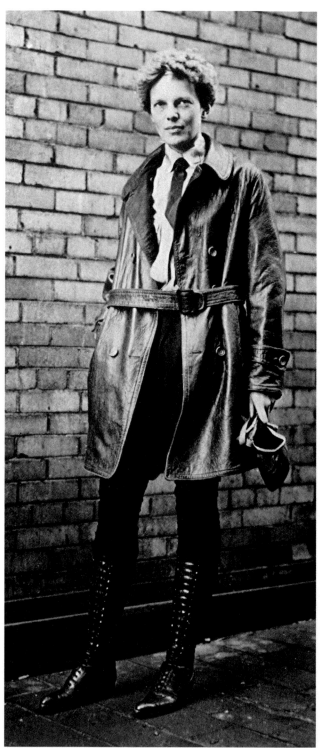

Amelia Earhart's sporty yet feminine style was way ahead of its time, 1925 and 1928.

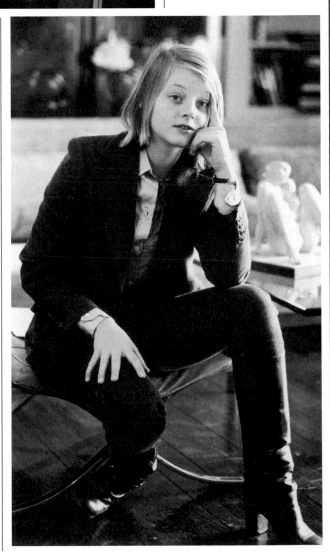

Jodie Foster (clockwise from left), 1976, 1979, and 1976.

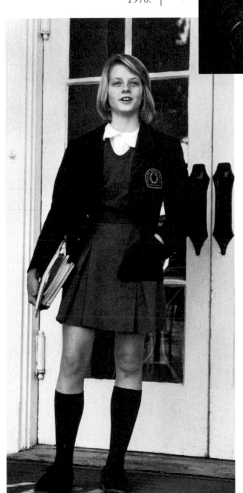

Of all the pictures I've looked through in search of a classic look that is young and speaks to today, these—taken in the 70s!—of **JODIE FOSTER**'s informal take on classic clothes seem completely of-the-moment in this first decade of the twenty-first century.

Amanda Brooks

CLASSIC
The New Originals

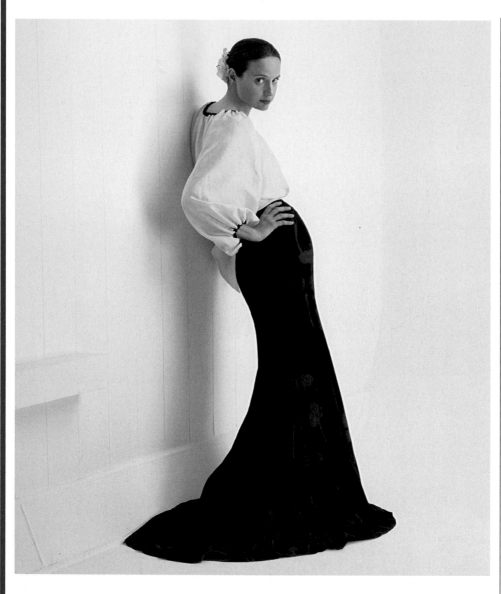

This page: Alexandra Kotur, 2006. Photograph by Jonathan Becker.

Opposite: (Top) Bonnie Morrison makes a vintage Adolfo suit look new with chunky jewelry and non-traditional shoes, 2008.

(Bottom) Tory Burch in a vintage shirt. I especially like the military-inspired epaulets on the shoulders, 2007.

ALEXANDRA KOTUR style director at *Vogue*
Alexandra is one of the most highly disciplined and focused dressers you will ever see. For the office, she has devised a uniform that changes only in subtle ways. She wears a men's tailored shirt (sometimes cream, sometimes off white), a pair of custom tailored trousers (always in a dark color, always the same cut), and flat shoes (could be ballet flats, could be a loafer). Her hair is always parted in the middle and pulled into a low bun. No makeup. None. And just when you think this might become a bit bland, she transforms into a peacock for evening: dangling jeweled chandelier earrings, brightly colored silk taffeta ball skirts, fresh flowers tucked in to her bun, and even the slightest hint of lip color. After the restraint of her daytime look, she really goes for it in the evening. She is one of the most successful (in look) and fascinating (in theory) dressers I know.

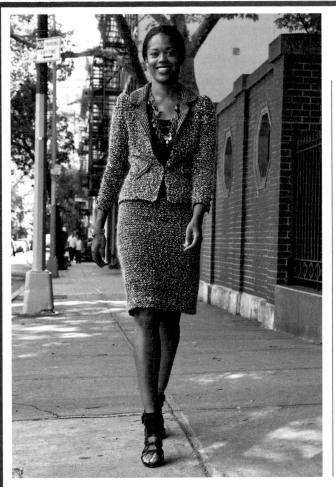

BONNIE MORRISON
fashion public relations executive

Banana Republic cable knit sweaters, flat-front khakis, and ballet flats—this is what Bonnie wore when I met her my sophomore year at Brown. Her style never changed in college, and that discipline—at that age—was very impressive to me. Most of our friends (myself included) were so busy trying out new looks that Bonnie's dedication to her look stood out.

After I graduated I didn't see Bonnie for a few years. Then I saw her at a fashion show: my old friend, but incredibly chic and infinitely more sophisticated. We started seeing each other regularly and her style transformation was unbelievable. She wore beautifully tailored classic black dresses, ballet flats, and trench coats carefully mixed with trendier pieces like neo-hippie embroidered sweaters, a voluminous tulip skirt, or a platform pump. Bonnie still doesn't stand out too far from the crowd, but the grace and elegance of her look command my attention every time I see her.

TORY BURCH fashion designer

Tory Burch is a New York fashion designer who has skillfully packaged her youthful uptown style in the wildly successful clothing brand that carries her name. It's great, but it's not the whole Tory. I especially love the more eccentric, specialized, personal, *and* unbranded Tory. She has the biggest and most stylish collection of *real* jewelry of anyone I know in my generation. She is an avid vintage collector and will fearlessly wear a hot pink silk vintage Dior gown with a gigantic bow at the neckline, or a 50s Chanel dress covered in large-scale polka dots. Her style is tasteful, sophisticated, classic—and ballsy!

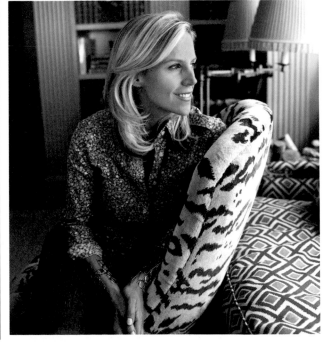

Amanda Brooks

CLASSIC
Refining Your Style

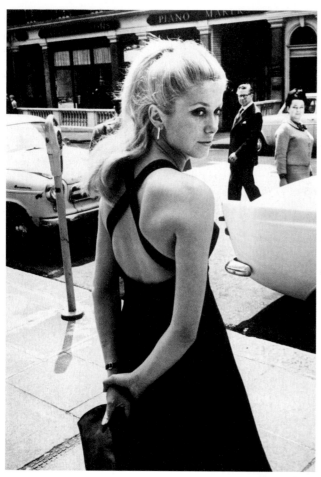

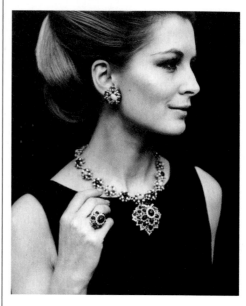

LADYLIKE CLASSIC
A suit, a shift dress, sling-back heels, loafers, crisp pants, pearls, classic gold jewelry, evening gowns.

FRENCH CLASSIC
Black dress, trench coat, leopard print, a headband, pussycat bow blouse, couture fashion.

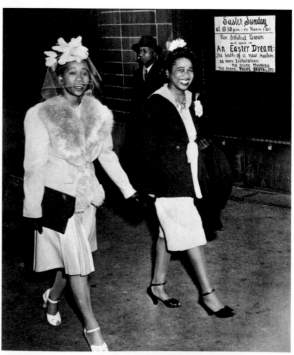

SUNDAY BEST CLASSIC
Classic suit, coordinated accessories, a festive hat, impeccable hair and makeup, conservative jewelry (pearls).

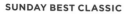

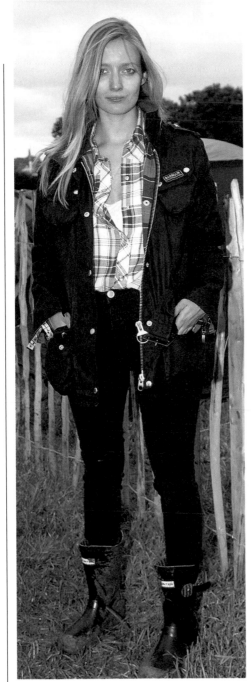

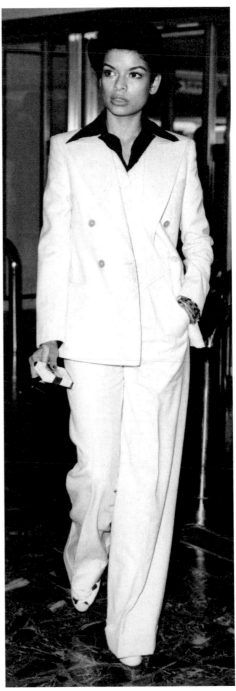

Opposite:
(Clockwise
from left)
Catherine
Deneuve, 1964.

Sandra Paul,
1969.

Easter Sunday,
1943.

This page:
(Left)
Vogue UK
market editor
Emma Elwick at
the Glastonbury
Music Festival,
England, 2008.

(Right)
Bianca Jagger,
1972.

ENGLISH CLASSIC
Barbour coats, plaid, tweed, Wellington boots, wool sweaters with holes in them, fancy hats.

MEN'S WEAR CLASSIC
Oversized tailored shirts, suspenders, blazers, V-neck sweaters, tailored trousers, newsboy caps, even ties.

CLASSIC
Refining Your Style

CLASSIC SPORTS are also a great inspiration for classic dressing as they inspired many of the signature pieces that characterize American sportswear today.

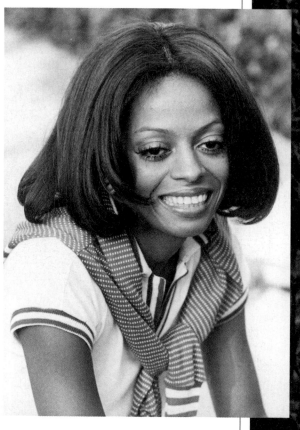

TENNIS
White tennis shirts, pleated miniskirts, sneakers, and pompom socks.

RIDING
Knee-high leather boots, horse-bit hardware, riding jackets, jodhpurs, braided hair.

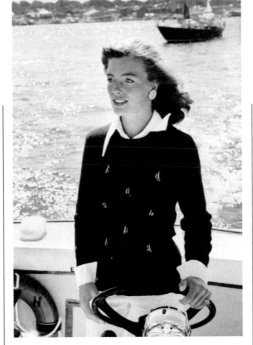

SAILING
Primary colors, sailor pants, striped sweaters, the rope motif, boatneck collars, white trousers.

Opposite:
(Left)
Diana Ross,
1973.

(Right)
My mom, getting
ready to go riding
at the Hunt Club
in Gates Mills,
Ohio, 1961.

This page:
(Clockwise
from top)
Susannah
Wassaman,
boating in
Newport, Rhode
Island, 1974.

Nan Kempner on
the slopes, 1970.

Harold
Gillingham in
Sussex, England,
wearing his
touring blazer
for the 1929–30
cricket tour of
New Zealand
and Australia,
1929.

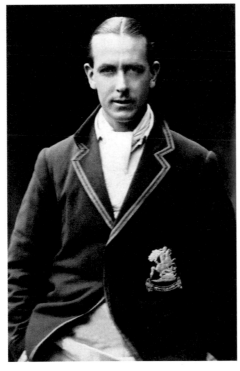

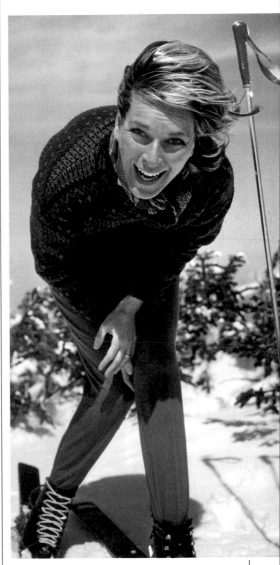

CRICKET
White shirt and trousers, cricket sweater (white cable knit sweater with stripe accents around the V-shaped neckline, sleeves, and waist).

SKIING
Parkas, stretch pants, furry après-ski boots, vintage striped racing sweaters, knit caps.

CLASSIC
Inspiration

BOOKS

A Wonderful Time
by Slim Aarons
Fashion people love this book for its iconic images of wealthy society types—WASPs, royalty, and rich Europeans—in the comfort of their own environment. They are not styled, except for the way they have styled themselves. Lucky for everyone who doesn't already own this book (the original now costs a fortune), Slim Aarons republished a newly edited version of it in 2003 called *Slim Aarons: Once Upon a Time* and another one in 2005, just before his death, called *Slim Aarons: A Place in the Sun*. They are all worth having. They show classic style in a more personal way than any other book I've seen.

Jackie: A Life in Pictures
by Yann-Brice Dherbier and Pierre-Henri Verlhac
This is just the best coffee table book about Jackie O. It presents her life in a series of photographs, arranged chronologically from her birth to her death, showing intimate, inspiring moments.

Seaman Schepps:
A Century of New York
Jewelry Design
by Amanda Vaill and Janet Zapata
A big coffee table book with beautiful pictures about legendary New York jewelry designer Seaman Schepps. My favorite piece of jewelry *ever* is on page 98: a cuff bracelet with a gigantic cabochon amethyst surrounded by emeralds and diamonds and a love poem by William Cartwright engraved in platinum all around the cuff. So chic.

Happy Times
by Lee Radziwill
Lee Radziwill has style for miles and miles and this book does justice to her impeccable taste. It features tons of amazing photos from her personal archives as well as some delightful illustrations created by Radziwill and her equally stylish sister Jackie O. The photo of Radziwill standing in front of her Francis Bacon in a hot pink caftan gets me especially excited.

The Little Black Dress:
Vintage Treasure
by Didier Ludot
This book features photos of the author's impressive collection of vintage little black dresses, including designs by Chanel and Balmain. The accompanying photos of LBD-clad starlets such as Jeanne Moreau and Sofia Loren are equally lovely.

Hitchcock Style
by Jean-Pierre Dufreigne
This book is worth buying for the cover photo of Tippi Hedren alone, but it also includes incredible stills of Hitchcock heroines Grace Kelly, Kim Novak, and Eva Marie Saint (among others), and their amazing costumes.

Dolce Vita Style
by Jean-Pierre Dufreigne
An in-depth look at one of the quintessential fashion films, with a wealth of lovely stills and pictures of the costumes.

American Ingenuity:
Sportswear 1930s–1970s
by Richard Martin
Written by the head of the Costume Institute at the Metropolitan Museum of Art in New York, this is a historical look at American designers defining sportswear in the last century. It shows how the concept of classic American clothes came to be defined. I am completely taken by the Claire McCardell gown on page 32.

Malick Sidibé
by Alexis Schwarzenbach (Author), Malick Sidibé (Photographer)
Malick Sidibé photographed people who lived in his hometown in Mali, Africa, during the 50s, 60s, and 70s. He focused on informal life and clothing worn in the local nightclubs and during the day. The way Malians interpreted tailored, Western world clothes (likely influenced by British occupation of parts of Africa) is fantastic. So, so chic. It's one of my favorite books. I get excited every time I look at it.

FILMS

Philadelphia Story
Katharine Hepburn radiates elegant 40s charm. Think sleek evening gowns and wide-legged trousers.

Belle De Jour
As the most stylish call girl ever, Catherine Deneuve wears supremely tasteful Yves Saint Laurent ensembles and Roger Vivier buckle shoes.

La Dolce Vita
This Federico Fellini classic has influenced fashion designers for decades. Incredible classic evening clothes.

Chinatown
Faye Dunaway exudes magnetic 30s style in glamorous dresses, precise red lipstick, long strands of pearls, and chic little hats.

Chariots of Fire
Watching this movie reminds me of the timelessness of menswear. The central characters look polished and fashionable in three-piece suits, cable knit sweaters, and fedoras.

L'Avventura
A jet-setting Italian aristocrat's casual yet elegant approach to classic style is refreshingly practical.

Bonnie and Clyde
Faye Dunaway again. She sparked a craze for berets and maxiskirts when it was initially released and has inspired dozens of fashion shoots since.

Out of Africa
Meryl Streep is the ultimate Ralph Lauren muse in *Out of Africa* with her 1910s safari clothes, equestrian chic, and irrepressible femininity. There are endless costume changes, so you will be constantly amused.

The Talented Mr. Ripley
This is 50s American classic with a hint of jet-setting European chic. The way Gwyneth Paltrow knots her white shirts on her waist looks particularly stylish.

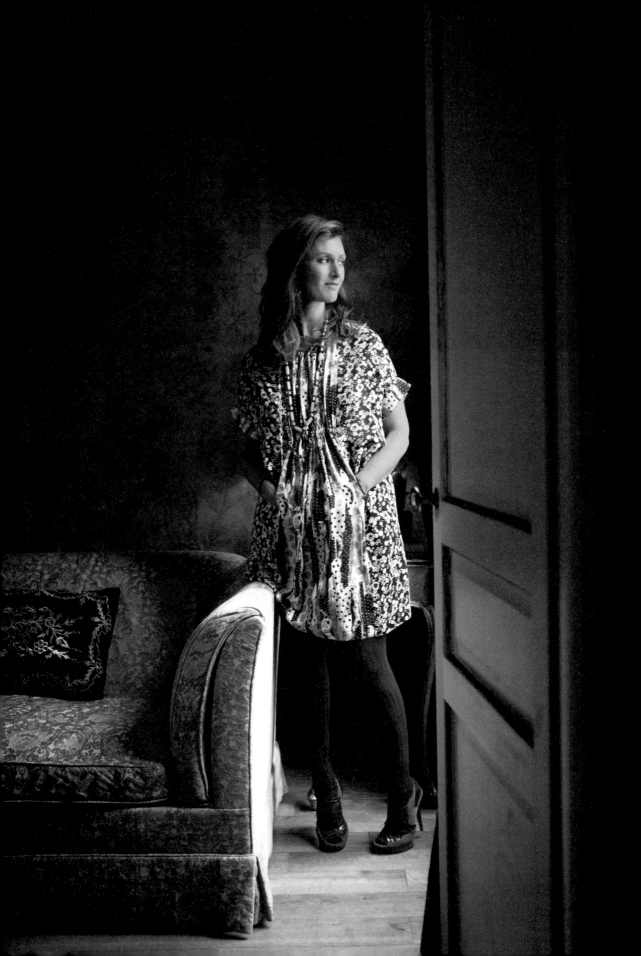

Bohemian

"YOU CAN'T BE A BOHEMIAN IN TIGHT CLOTHES, IT JUST DOESN'T WORK. YOU HAVE TO BE ABLE TO MOVE AND DANCE AND CLIMB."
—DIANE VON FURSTENBERG

Something about bohemian style always reminds me of the way little girls play dress up: they like things that float and twirl, they aren't afraid of color and sparkle, they want to look pretty, be comfortable, and have a good time! Bohemian style is laid-back, comfortable, and—most important—self-expressive. It is never, never about pouring yourself into the clothes someone else thinks you should wear, whether that someone is your mother, your boss, your boyfriend, or your favorite magazine.

In the United States, we turn to the hippie movement for bohemian style—blue jeans, flowers, beads, fringe, peasant blouses, peace, love, and rock 'n' roll—but every society has had its free-spirited outsiders who dress to please themselves instead of conforming. Today there are many variations of bohemian fashion from all over the world, and these continue to evolve as the mainstream greedily incorporates exciting elements of "outsider" style.

Now successful, even bourgeois women have taken to dressing in a bohemian way. Plenty of designers are happy to oblige them with counter-culture-inspired items whose price tags are right at home on Madison Avenue and Rodeo Drive. In post-Olsen

Sally Singer, wearing a Duro Olowu dress at a friend's apartment in Paris, 2009.

twins New York, you can see a grungy young "bag lady" walking down the street only to notice she is carrying a $2,000 handbag. In North London, wealthy young women wear layers and artful tatter—seemingly engaged in a posh scarecrow look-alike competition. Classic dressing often provides security for those who desire to look polished, but many women today relish the challenge of putting together a more free-spirited wardrobe.

But we haven't lost all the bourgeois-bashing bohos. In my neighborhood I see loads of students, artists, and freelancers who don't live the nine-to-five life, and many of them express themselves through their clothes in a more traditionally rebellious way. They can often look more sloppy than stylish, but every now and then a true old-school bohemian saunters by looking pretty damn good.

Bohemian style suits individualistic, creative, and unconventional lifestyles. You don't have to be a rebellious person to dress like a bohemian, but this may not be the right weekday look for you if you work in an office with a strict dress code. In a more laid-back workplace or on the weekend, however, anyone can incorporate bohemian elements into her look. And if you work at home or in the arts, why not play dress up every day?

BOHEMIAN
My Bohemian Style

DAD WOULD MIX A MEXICAN TUNIC AND BIRKEN-STOCKS WITH CHIC, CENTER-PLEATED KHAKI PANTS AND A GOLD ROLEX.

1960s

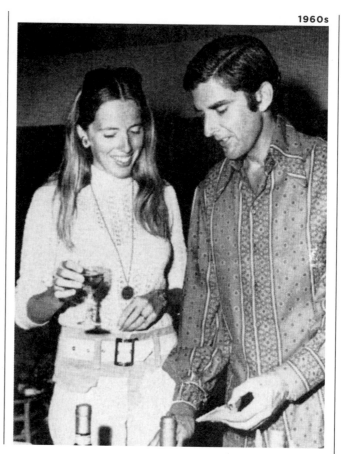

1925

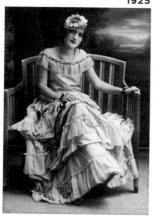

Far left: I have always been inspired by this photo of my step-grandmother Peggy Stewart, 1925.

Left: My mom and dad, Palm Beach, late 1960s.

There is always a small element of bohemian lurking in my style. I never brush my hair, and I wash it only once a week; no matter where I'm going, I always pack a peasant blouse, and I sometimes love to pile on the jewelry. However, I've also been through a couple of full-on bohemian phases as well.

When I was at boarding school in the early 90s, I was madly in love with a Dead Head—yes, a follower of the Grateful Dead. Dead Heads spend vacations and summers following the band around the country, sometimes dropping out of school completely in order to attend all their concerts. It was kind of a hippie hangover from the 60s and 70s—people who couldn't let go—and I joined in to be with my boyfriend. The long floral Putamayo skirts appeared, as did the Indian beads and the hand-block-printed T-shirts. I bought almost everything from Indian stores. My hair was actually the same as it is now—long, wavy, and messy. My sister got into the hippie thing too. She even stopped shaving her legs for a while. I didn't go quite that far, but I did feel very romantic at the time. Part clothes, part love, I'd say.

I had another bohemian moment in 2005. It was partially inspired by the large peasant skirts going down the fashion runways and Kate Moss's public embrace of fringed boots and fur ponchos (I'm always a sucker for a trend if it suits me), but also I was driven by a desire to feel comfortable in my clothes. Before then I had been working as the creative director at Tuleh, and it was my job to be fashionably inspiring. I'd trot over there every day in sky-high Manolo Blahnik stilettos, unforgiving tailored trousers, elaborately tied blouses—

1989

2005

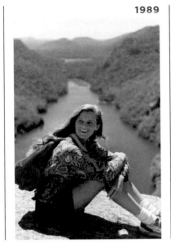

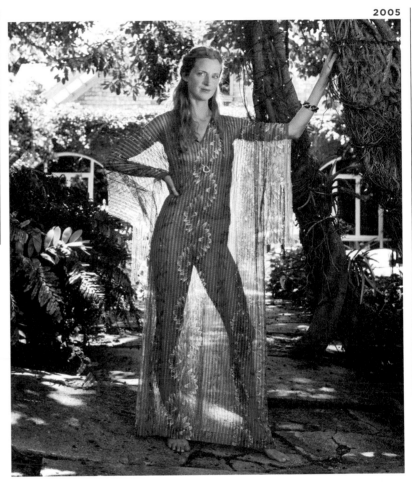

THERE IS ALWAYS A SMALL ELEMENT OF BOHEMIAN LURKING IN MY STYLE.

*Left:
Me, hiking in
the Adirondacks
in my "crunchy"
phase, 1989.*

*Me, wearing
my great-aunt
Molly's vintage
Giorgio
Sant'Angelo
painted lace
caftan, 2005.
It's one of my
most coveted
vintage pieces.
Photograph by
Jonathan
Becker.*

basically doing whatever it took to look good. (Being a muse is harder than it looks!) But now I was at home most of the day working on this book and hanging out with my two young kids. I *do* have to look good to feel inspired to write, but I can't concentrate if my pants, however stylish, are suffocating me. Happily I rediscovered the bohemian thing, which allowed me to spend comfortable hours at my desk without looking like a slob.

This time, though, my take on bohemian was decidedly different. I was inspired by my mother and father's Palm Beach version of hippie in the 60s and 70s: part classic, part luxury, part flower child. My dad would mix a Mexican tunic and Birkenstocks with chic, center-pleated khaki pants and a gold Rolex. My mom had

many memorable outfits, among them these green silk bell-bottom trousers with silk patches of fruit sewn up the side of one leg, which she wore with a gold Lurex knit turtleneck sweater. Even though I probably never would have worn the pants, I am devastated that she didn't keep them for me. So as a nod to that memory of comfortable yet spirited luxury, I'd wear a crocheted peasant top with real gold jewelry (including my Dad's gold St. Christopher medallion), skinny jeans (with a little stretch), and Miu Miu platform sandals that I bought on eBay for $40 (they're comfortable, I swear). It was a simpler, less over-the-top bohemian look with a luxurious twist, and it suited my age and my life at the time.

BOHEMIAN
My Favorite Things

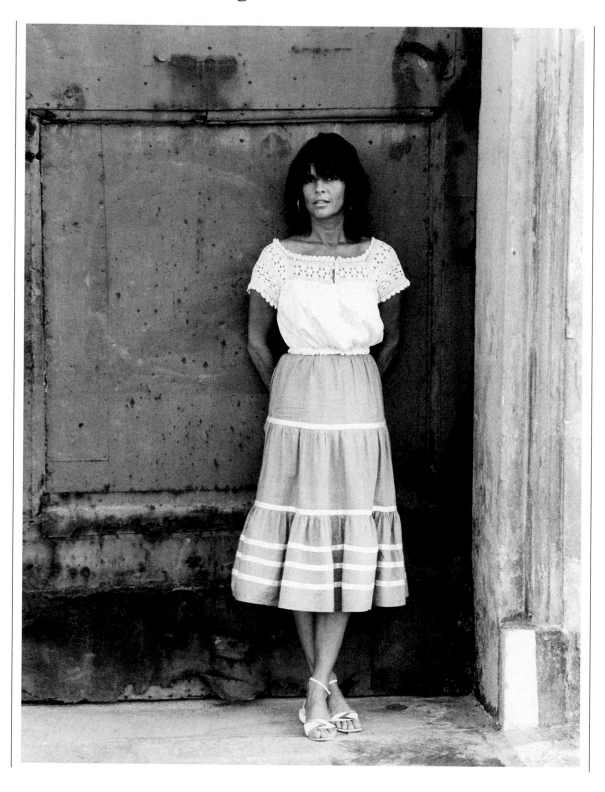

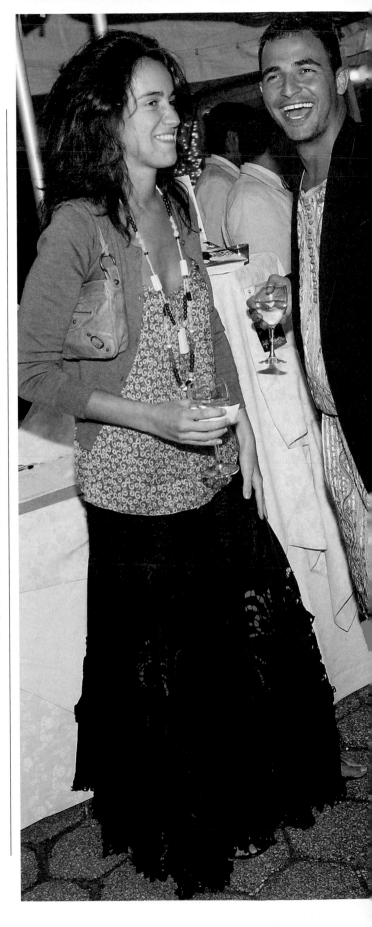

Opposite:
Ali MacGraw,
1970s.

Right:
Coco Brandolini
in a black lace
Oscar de la
Renta skirt,
with Zac Posen,
2005.

The **PEASANT BLOUSE** (left) can take many shapes, usually defined by volume either in the sleeve or in the bodice, and is adorned with romantic and decorative details (lace, crochet, embroidery). My two favorite peasant blouses are very different from each other. One is very simple but luxurious: vintage Cacharel in cream silk with beautiful billowy sleeves and a square neckline. The other is completely casual: cotton with short sleeves and colorful crochet trimming. Although I bought it in a vintage store in London, it looks like it originally came from a Mexican market. It's the real deal.

When looking for a peasant blouse, you may find that fabric can be as effective in creating a bohemian look as shape. Cotton gauze, matte silk, and embroidered cotton come to mind.

The most obvious **HIPPIE SKIRT** is loose and fluid and flows all the way to the ground. A long skirt is a very personal thing. Either you're a long-skirt person or you're not.

WHEN LOOKING FOR A PEASANT BLOUSE, YOU MAY FIND THAT FABRIC CAN BE AS EFFECTIVE IN CREATING A BOHEMIAN LOOK AS SHAPE.

Amanda Brooks

BOHEMIAN
My Favorite Things

FUR can add endless glamour to a bohemian look. Wilder-looking pelts like coyote, raccoon, lynx, or fox are the most obviously bohemian-looking.

A **FUR VEST** (opposite) is one of the most useful fur pieces you can own. I wear them everywhere with everything, for most of the year. Over an evening gown or cocktail dress, a fur vest keeps me much more glamorously warm than a wrap or a shawl. It also works over a blouse with jeans or trousers, dressing that look up a bit—an easy way to go from the office to dinner. And when I am dressed down on the weekends and want to go out to dinner and the movies with my husband without changing my comfortable clothes (usually jeans and a sweater), I throw on a fur vest. It's cozy, it dresses up my casual clothes, and it makes my husband think I've made an effort to look cute.

I love suede cropped **JACKETS TRIMMED WITH FUR** (below), and I find that they work for most occasions—dressy or casual. The same variety of jacket is also good in a longer belted version, if you prefer that proportion. The most important factor in buying one of these jackets is fit. It's okay if the sleeves are kind of short, because they almost always are and it's actually cute, but the shoulders and the waist *must* be fitted.

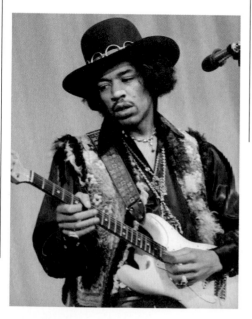

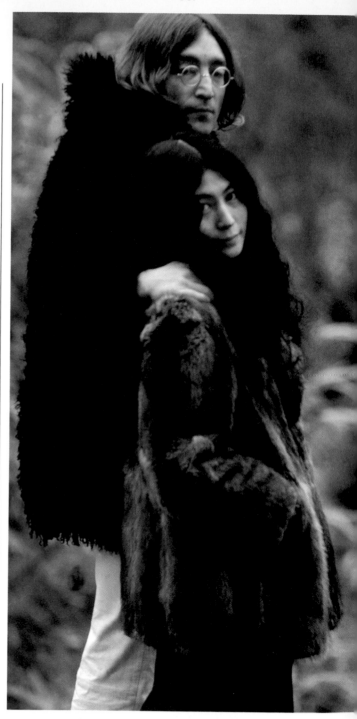

If you want a **FULL FUR COAT** (above), short or long, that looks bohemian, remember to go for the wilder-looking furs. Raccoon and coyote look great and cost less than many other furs. If you want something more luxurious, Finn raccoon is wonderful but really expensive and hard to come by.

RACCOON AND COYOTE LOOK GREAT
AND COST LESS THAN MANY OTHER FURS.

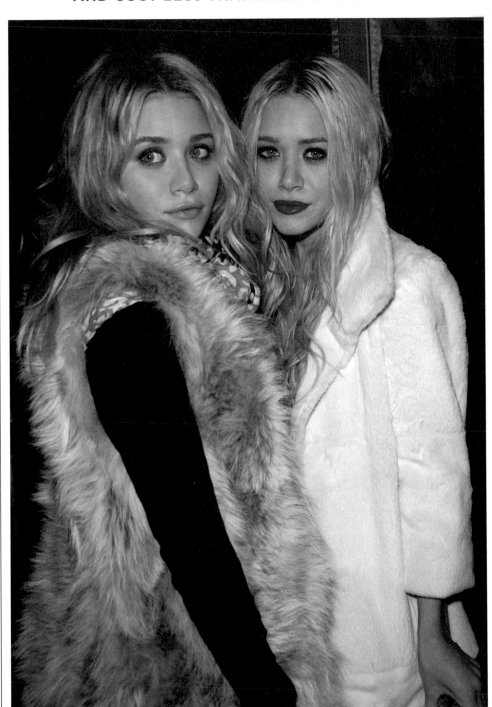

*Opposite:
(Far left)
Jimi Hendrix,
1960. I love his
embroidered
vest with
Mongolian
lamb fur trim.*

*(Left)
John Lennon
and Yoko Ono,
1968.*

*This page:
Mary Kate and
Ashley Olsen,
2007. Ashley's
fur vest would
look great with
virtually any
style of clothing.*

BOHEMIAN
My Favorite Things

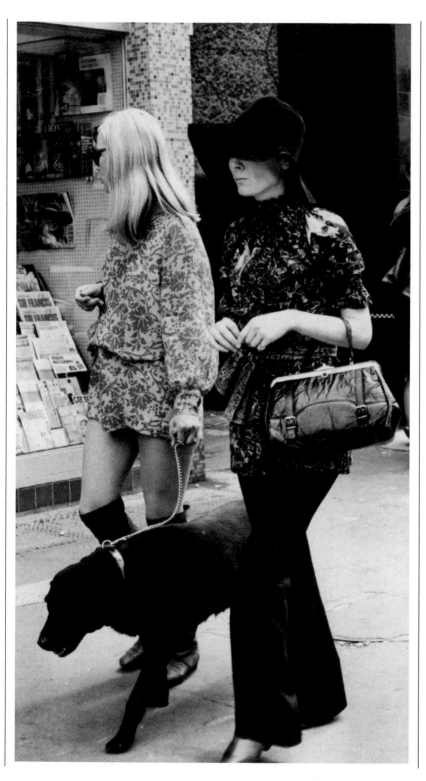

A **TUNIC** (left) is a short version of a caftan, usually falling just over your hips. Some people can make a tunic work as a minidress, but when in doubt a tunic is most chic and flattering worn over long tailored trousers, capri pants, or jeans.

I know I'm not alone when I say that a **CAFTAN** (right) makes me think of Talitha Getty standing on a rooftop in Morocco in the 60s—an iconic fashion image. Amazingly she transformed the caftan from something only your grandmother would wear into something chic and glamorous. Thank goodness—it is an incredibly useful piece of clothing.

Caftans are for warm resort locations only. They do not look good in the city (unless maybe you're pregnant and have nothing else to wear). If they work for you, you can wear them all the time: in cotton by the pool, at lunch, even to bed; in silk or chiffon, with a flat sandal, for evening. You can also belt a caftan to define your waist and wear it with a high-heeled sandal for a dressier/sexier look.

A TUNIC IS MOST CHIC AND FLATTERING WORN OVER LONG TAILORED TROUSERS, CAPRI PANTS, OR JEANS.

Women shopping in Chelsea, London, 1967.

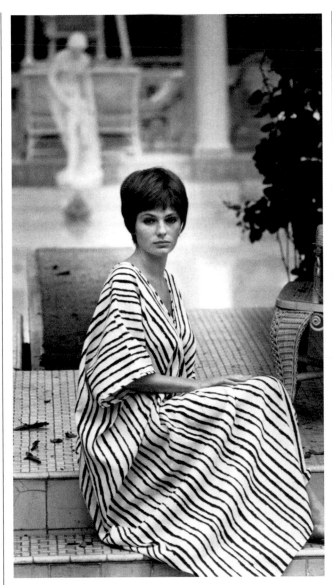

The defining factor of a **ROMANTIC BOHEMIAN DRESS** (below) is a feeling of fluidity and volume, usually in the sleeve and in the skirt. Sometimes there is a fitted bodice, or an empire waist. Often a dress can have a bohemian feeling by way of the print or pattern of the fabric. Or sometimes it can be a solid color—even black—but have a very loose, untailored construction. When you get the feeling there is a lot going on in a dress (as is often the case with bohemian ones) you might want to "chic it up" by wearing simple classic accessories. Ballet flats or simple pumps, gold hoop earrings, a chic bun, and simple makeup will all work to tone it down and make your dress feel modern, as opposed to overly nostalgic.

I have a weakness for vintage designer hippie dresses. I especially like those by Ossie Clark, Biba, Thea Porter, Holly Harp, Missoni, and Yves Saint Laurent.

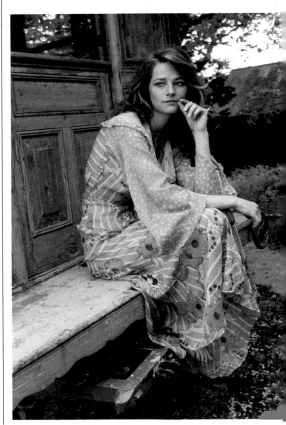

BOHEMIAN PRINTS have achieved classic status, as far as I'm concerned. I'm thinking of paisley, tapestry, romantic florals, basically anything that makes you think of the 60s or 70s (but forget the psychedelics). A modern way to wear a colorful bohemian print dress or blouse is to accessorize it with one solid color—I prefer black but gray or brown could work as well. So you'd wear your colorful printed dress with black tights, black shoes, black bag, black scarf, and so on.

Above: Jacqueline Bisset, 1968. While her caftan is decidedly bohemian, the stripes add a nice classic contrast.

Right: Charlotte Rampling sitting on a gypsy caravan, 1971.

BOHEMIAN
Accessories

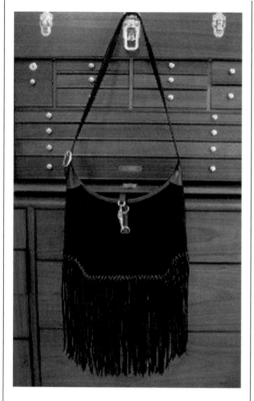

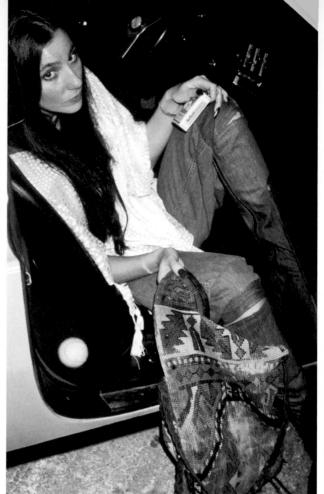

I *love* **BOHEMIAN HANDBAGS**. Everyone should have one, even if bohemian is not your thing. They just add so much personality to your look. A chic tailored jacket with jeans is vastly more interesting with a fringed slouchy bag than it is with a predictable "ladylike" bag. Even better, these bags generally improve with wear, so you don't have to treat them like precious objects. Go ahead and chuck your boho bag down on the floor and jam pack it full of stuff. That's how it's meant to be used.

The chicest of the chic **SLOUCHY BAG** is made by Hermès (above). I can't afford one but if I could it would be mine. I want it so badly! Until then, thrift stores also offer up a chic hobo bag every now and then. The 70s produced some very plain bags that look cool now because of their relaxed shape and simple vintage hardware. There is a caramel-colored leather that was very popular in the 70s, and it looks great all old and worn in. In fact it looks good with everything.

You may notice in the pages to come that I have a thing for **Cher***'s bohemian style. What I like about it is that it possesses all the originality and personality of her more outlandish 80s looks without the "look at me" drama. First of all, she was stunningly beautiful in her boho phase, but also there's an ease and casualness about the way she takes a risk or adds something unusual to her look while keeping the rest of her outfit laid back, feminine, and flattering.*

Designers have adorned hobo bags with everything under the sun: studs, fringe, grommets, rhinestones, feathers, buckles, straps, you name it. Some work. Some don't. If you're going to go for a trendy hobo bag, go high or go low. Buy a beautifully crafted one made by an expensive designer, making sure you love it (and that it's *you*) before you blow all that cash; or buy a super cheap one so you're not bummed out when you grow bored of it (almost always sooner than you think). Super cheap bags can be kind of "tongue-in-chic"; they're tacky and fun and show that you're not taking yourself too seriously with a silly bag.

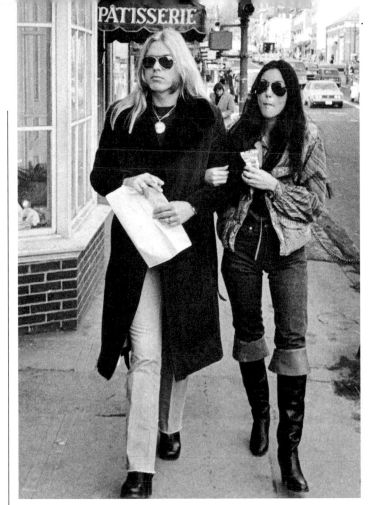

Opposite:
(Far left)
The fringed
Hermès bag
that I covet.

(Left)
Cher, with her
tapestry hobo
bag, 1970.

This page:
Cher, on the
street with
Gregg Allman,
1977. Her
boots are
fantastic!

A **CRAFTY BAG** (opposite) is any shape of bag with a lot of embellishment—particularly signature "hippie" decorations like fringe, tooled leather, embroidery, and patchwork—and it will definitely give you a bohemian feel. The shape of the bag can contrast with the decoration, making for a little personal irony in your look. My favorite example of this is a bag a friend of mine found at a thrift store. It is a copy of a very classic ladylike Gucci bag from the 60s—brown leather, very stiff construction—but then it has all this long fringe hanging off of it. We're talking two feet! This bag cracks me up—it is a daring combination of seemingly disparate ideas, but it actually works. People went nuts decorating bags in the 60s and 70s, so for me, once again, the thrift store is the place to find your crafty bag. There are a few good designer versions of them now but they often feel contrived to me.

Because bohemian style is all about casual comfort, **BOOTS** are a must-have item.

FRYE BOOTS are very authentically 70s college coed. You have to be kind of a tomboy to pull these off. They're not the most feminine shape.

Vintage stores sell **SLOUCHY BOOTS** from the 70s and 80s, but if you like this style of boot, you're better off getting a new pair with a cleaner, simpler heel shape. And in most cases, unless you are very tall and thin, you should opt for high heels here. Flat slouchy boots are very hard to pull off.

CHEAP BAGS CAN BE KIND OF "TONGUE-IN-CHIC"; THEY'RE TACKY AND FUN AND SHOW THAT YOU'RE NOT TAKING YOURSELF TOO SERIOUSLY WITH A SILLY BAG.

BOHEMIAN
Accessories

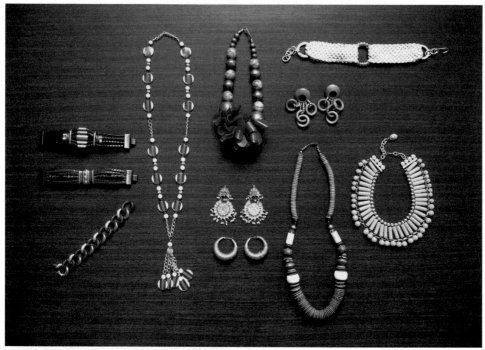

This page:
(Left)
Some of my favorite bohemian jewelry.

(Bottom)
As Veruschka shows us, the key to piling on lots of jewelry is to wear it with something really simple, 1969.

Opposite:
I'm not sure I would have thought to put a belt over a baggy sweater like Julie Christie does here, but she makes it look great, 1970.

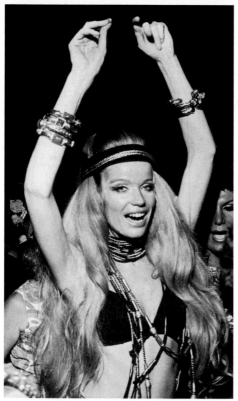

Whatever else you're wearing, adding a few **LONG NECKLACES, CHUNKY RINGS, DANGLY EARRINGS,** or **BANGLE BRACELETS** will give you an instant bohemian feeling and they can be made of almost anything—**AFRICAN BEADS** or **PRECIOUS STONES, CRYSTALS** or **WOOD, PEARLS, METAL CHAINS, LEATHER, ROPE,** etc.

SILK SCARVES (opposite) are incredibly versatile. Wrap one around your waist as a belt, or around your head like a do-rag, around your neck, on your handbag, in your ponytail. There are so many possibilities.

A **WIDE BELT** (opposite) can be functional and/or decorative, worn at the waist or on the hips. In its functional moments a wide belt gives you a waist when you are wearing something loose (like a caftan, a tunic blouse, or a loose dress); accentuating the waist is a more classic look and a good solution for women who don't want to emphasize their hips. Accentuating the hips is groovier, younger, and trendier, and generally for women with small hips. As decoration a belt can simply enrich your look. Wear a wide belt over the belt loops of jeans (it doesn't have to fit through!) or again over a dress or a long blouse.

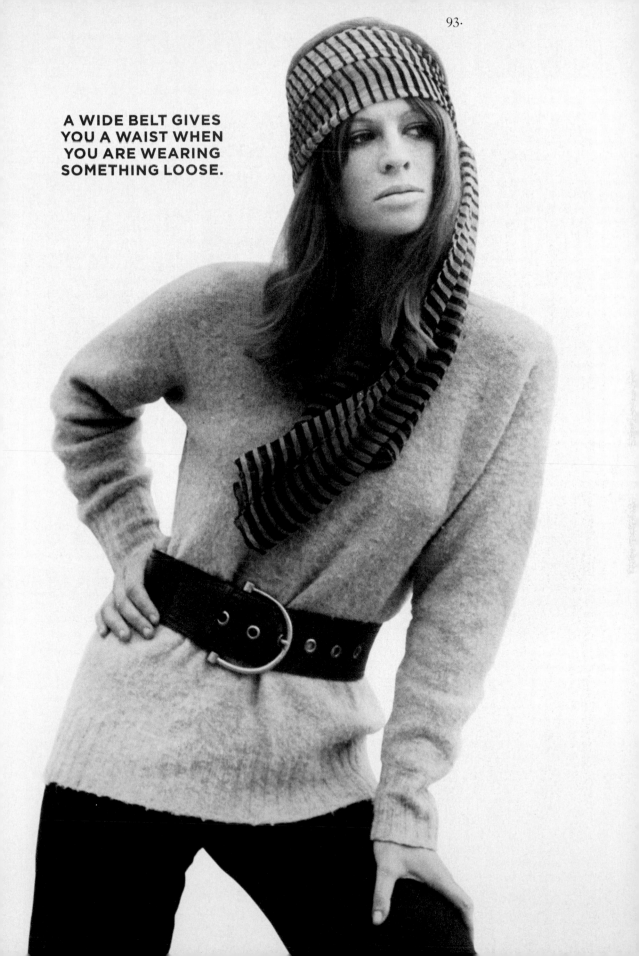

A WIDE BELT GIVES
YOU A WAIST WHEN
YOU ARE WEARING
SOMETHING LOOSE.

BOHEMIAN
Mixing It Up

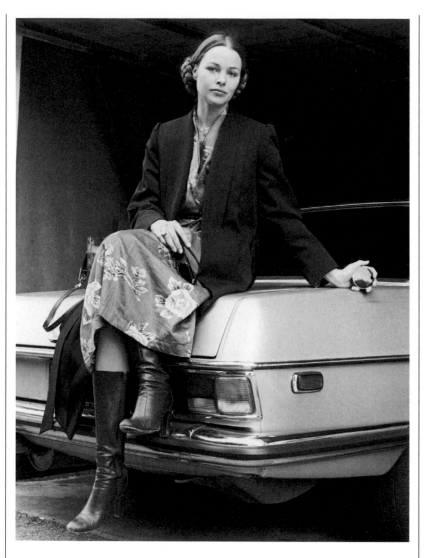

Michelle Phillips's tailored jacket adds a clean contrast to her otherwise romantic outfit, 1970.

A BIT OF UPTOWN LUXURY COMPLIMENTS BOHEMIAN STYLING.

ANYTHING WITH STRUCTURE—a tailored blazer, a pleated skirt, a 60s-style shift dress—will contrast nicely with your bohemian look.

I really love the strictness of **TAILORED TROUSERS** with a feminine peasant blouse and frivolous dangly earrings.

CRISP DENIM (no fading, no holes, no other artificial wear) can add a feeling of modernity to an otherwise straight-forward bohemian look. You can find great "stiff" jeans that have a bit of stretch for comfort.

I am obsessed with ribbed **SILK TANK TOPS**. They aren't cheap, but they're infinitely functional. With very dressy, elaborate items like an embroidered, beaded peasant skirt, they make the entire outfit feel younger and less formal. They also make a great first layer under a sweater or a chiffon blouse. Sometimes I'll wear one tank top on top of another in two different colors with a fringed scarf and a chic pair of pants. If the luxury of silk wife beaters is not in the cards for you, you can get almost the same effect with cotton tanks from Old Navy, Fruit of the Loom, or the Gap.

A **MINISKIRT** forms a definitively unbohemian silhouette. If you're a miniskirt girl, incorporate something short into a younger, sexier bohemian look.

A bit of uptown luxury complements bohemian styling. **CLASSIC JEWELRY**—gold, diamonds, lockets, charm bracelets, pearls—is great here.

CLASSIC SHOES look great with long, flowing skirts or dresses. A ballet flat is cute with an Indian print wrap skirt. And a high heel—even a pump—can be a great show of personality when worn with a romantic dress.

BOHEMIAN
Getting It Right

You can achieve a great bohemian look on a limited budget. If any style is not weighed down by expensive must-have status pieces, it's this one. But even this theoretically relaxed style demands that your clothes fit, if you want to look good, and that you keep that editorial eye open, if you want to avoid looking like you're wearing a costume.

If you want to make bohemian look modern instead of romantic, try sticking to **COLORLESS COLORS**: gray, brown, black, white, and so on. It puts the decorative quality of the clothes in a new context.

Another way to play with color is **COLOR BLOCKING**. For example, a peasant-shape dress that is broken up into a different solid color on each tier gives the dress a whole other graphic modern reference. However, when mixing bold colors, make sure one is neutral, like white or gray.

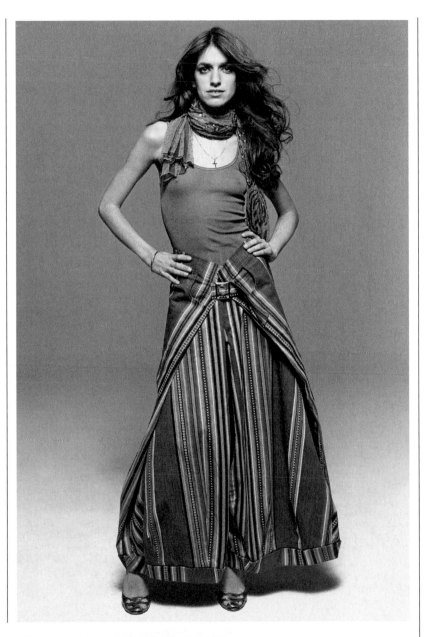

I love the simplicity of Joana Preiss's tank top worn with those insane gaucho pants and the metallic-laced scarf.

Here are some of my favorite **BOHEMIAN PROPORTIONS**:
- *A short dress with high boots*
- *A big belted peasant blouse/tunic over tight pants or leggings tucked into high boots*
- *A tank top with a peasant skirt and a tailored jacket*
- *A soft, full skirt with a vest*
- *A peasant blouse with dark tailored jeans and a stiletto or wedge-heel sandal*
- *A peasant blouse with a long skirt (the waist must be defined)*

BOHEMIAN
High Risk, High Reward

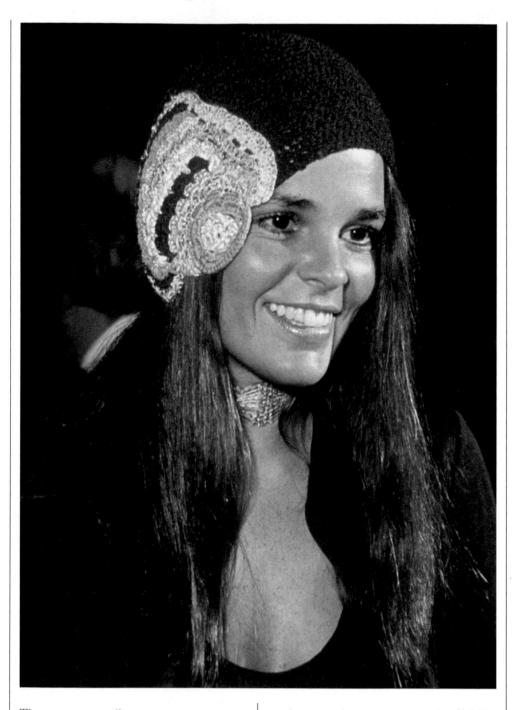

*This page:
I don't know
if anyone can
succeed at this
look as well as
Ali MacGraw
does, but it's
worth a try.
She looks
adorable, 1971.*

*Opposite;
Arden Wohl's
style signature is
her headband.
You almost never
see her without
one, 2008.*

There are some really great **BOHEMIAN HATS**: floppy felt ones with big brims, Russian fur peasant hats, crocheted skull caps. But—and this seems to be a recurring theme with hats— you just gotta have guts to carry it off. I like hats best on straight or slightly wavy hair. Super curly hair is its own decoration. Adding a hat is overkill.

The safest way to approach anything "crafty," such as **PATCHWORK**, **CROCHET**, and **FRINGE**, is to do it in moderation: a patchwork belt, a cotton dress with crochet trim, or a macramé bracelet. And fringe works really well on accessories: a suede fringe on a handbag or boots, or a silk fringe on a shawl.

I know for certain that I never could nor would wear a **BOHEMIAN HEADBAND** (meaning, around your forehead as opposed to sitting on top of your head). But every now and then I see Nicole Richie or artist Arden Wohl wearing one, and I think it suits her style and looks pretty great. If you think this might be the look for you, proceed with extreme caution and a large dose of self-esteem.

A **PONCHO**'s success depends on its proportion to your body. The last thing you want is to see more of the poncho than of you. And this can happen. The trick is to make sure the poncho is neither too wide nor too long. It should probably never hang below your knees. If it does, belt it to show where your waist is. In fact, I like ponchos belted, period. I have seen people look good in unbelted ponchos, but even when it works it's a little Pocahontas.

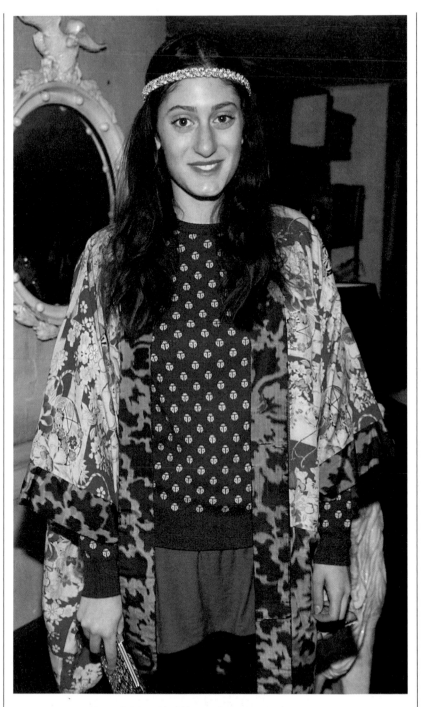

IF YOU THINK THIS MIGHT BE THE LOOK FOR YOU, PROCEED WITH EXTREME CAUTION AND A LARGE DOSE OF SELF-ESTEEM.

Evening

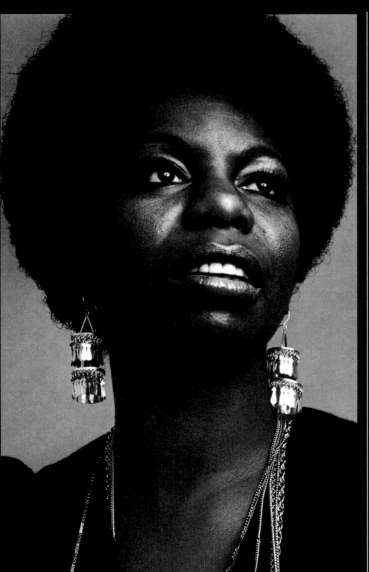

Don't be afraid of **PRINTED GOWNS** (right). The right print can make any gown feel bohemian. I personally love Missoni gowns but if you are on a budget look for a pretty printed chiffon dress from a vintage store and wear it with a great rhinestone belt.

Try **LAYERING**. Just because you're wearing a fancy dress doesn't mean you can't add a few things on. A fur vest, a lace wrap, or a fringed shawl can all give personality to your look.

Look for something with **ETHNIC EMBROIDERY**. I love the combination of bohemian designs with luxurious materials. Look out for Chinese embroidered capes, Mexican embroidered skirts, and vintage embroidered shawls.

Wear a **DRESS WITH LOTS OF MOVEMENT** (below). Fringe, ruffles, tiers, and draping are all free-spirited. Think of Spanish flamenco dancers, Greek goddesses, elaborately layered gypsies, or Frida Kahlo.

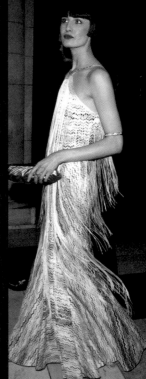

The unconventional comfort of "bohemian" can indeed mingle with the formality and conventional demands of "evening dress."

Wear **CHANDELIER EARRINGS** (above). Chandelier earrings give even the simplest dress a bohemian feel. Wear your hair short or pulled back to fully display your statement earrings.

Above: Nina Simone, 1969.

Left: Erin O'Connor reminds me that you always have to move in an evening dress to really see how it's going to look. Don't be afraid to do a little runway walk (even if it makes you blush) before you settle on a gown for a big event.

Opposite: Ashley Olsen and Arden Wohl, 2008.

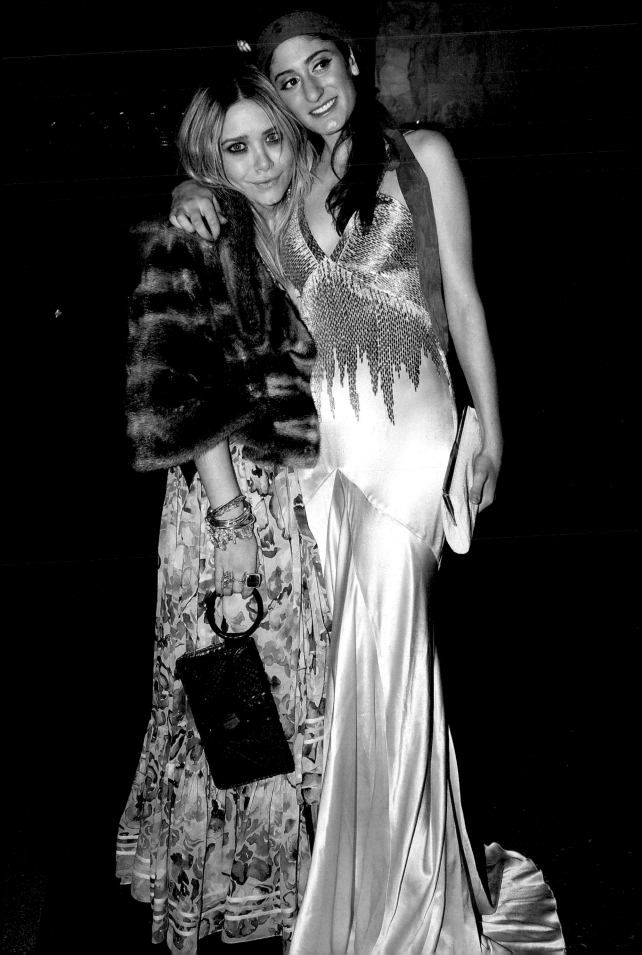

BOHEMIAN
Icons

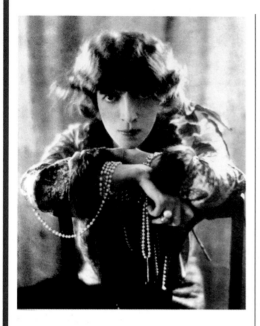

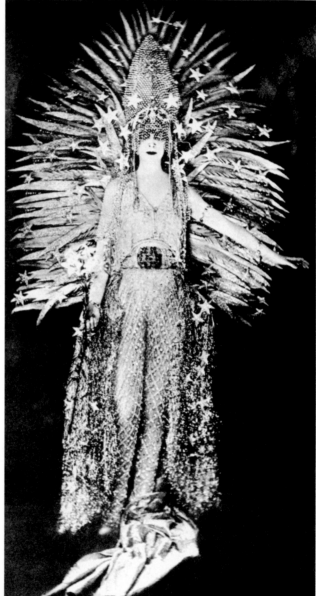

MARCHESA CASATI was the original "bobo" (*bo*urgeois *bo*hemian) muse. Born in 1881, she was soon left an orphan—and the wealthiest heiress in Italy at the time. Instead of conforming to aristocratic Italian society, she became one of the most eccentric, scandalous, and inspiring women of the twentieth century. She wore live snakes as jewelry. She took her pet boa constrictors to stay with her at the Ritz in Paris. She had nude male servants—complete with gilded skin. And she was known to take late-night strolls, naked beneath her furs, parading her pet cheetahs on diamond-studded leashes. Her love of domesticated "wild" animals inspired Cartier's famed Panther design. If you can't find some inspiration in her life, I don't know where you will.

Top left: Marchesa Casati by Baron Adolph de Meyer, Venice, 1912.

Right: Marchesa Casati wears a costume symbolizing light to a fancy dress party in Paris, 1922. The costume, designed by Worth, is made of a net of diamonds, incorporates a gold feather sun against a diamond tiara, and has a glittering silver fringe.

But she was perhaps best known for tirelessly commissioning a vast variety of artists to paint her portrait, supporting and nurturing their careers all the while. People say she is the most artistically rendered woman of all time, after Cleopatra and the Virgin Mary. She pursued the cutting edge in everything she did, becoming the most avant-garde of aristocrats. On her grave are Shakespeare's words: "Age cannot wither her, nor custom stale her infinite variety." I love that.

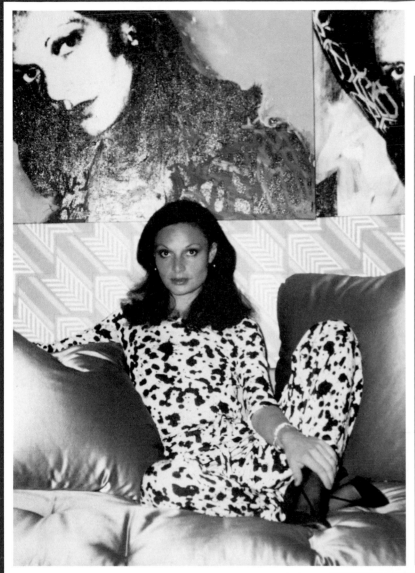

I am inspired by some women whose lifestyles are as bohemian as their wardrobes. **DIANE VON FURSTENBERG** is a great example. She has the fabulous curly hair, the flowing printed dresses, and the occasional fur vest—but, much more important, she is just a genuine free spirit. She does everything her own way and doesn't live by anyone else's rules. She is devoted to yoga, and she travels constantly, never staying in one place for more than a few days. She is also a patron of the arts, hosting young artists, writers, and musicians in her studio.

In terms of style, what is most remarkable about Diane is how well she knows who she is and what works for her. Check out these portraits taken throughout her life. They all feature her lounging in her trademark printed clothing, her famously sexy legs in the foreground, and her iconic portraits by Andy Warhol behind her. Talk about signature style.

"I AM A GYPSY AT HEART. AND I'VE ALWAYS BEEN A GYPSY AT HEART."
—DIANE VON FURSTENBERG

Diane von Furstenberg, 1976 and 1998.

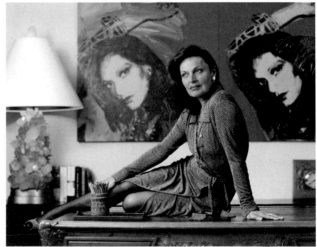

BOHEMIAN
Icons

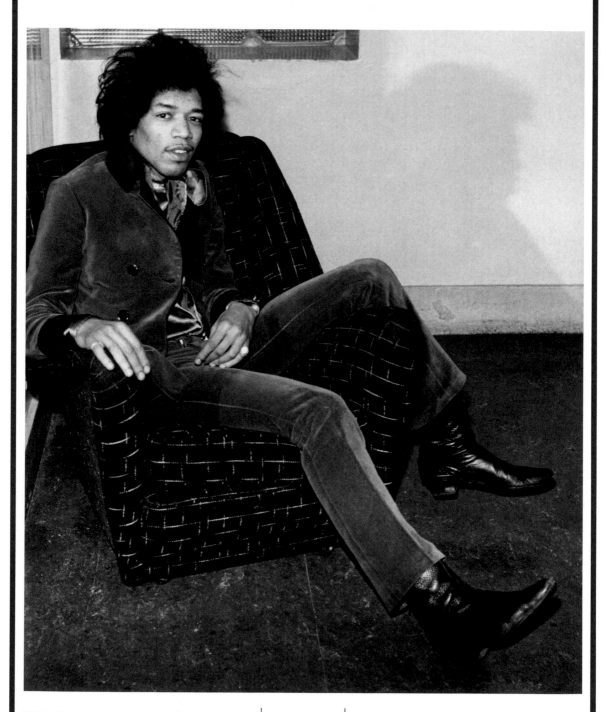

If I had to choose a famous bohemian style to emulate, it would be the boho dandy looks of **JIMI HENDRIX**. I love his use of neck scarves, his disheveled hair, his black satin pantsuits, and his

Jimi Hendrix, 1966.

affinity for prints, whether on a floral blazer or a head scarf tied round a fedora. No matter how far out, there is something in almost every Jimi Hendrix look that gets me going.

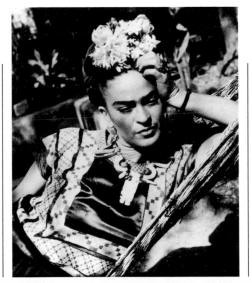

I often think of the Mexican artist **FRIDA KAHLO** when I get dressed to go out in the evening. She understood decoration better than anyone, so I refer to her when adding jewelry, flowers, fringe, shawls, or braids to my look. I can't do them all at once as she did, but even one of the elements can make a big impact. She was also one of the twentieth century's best self-portrait artists, and so gives food for thought to any woman thinking about self-presentation. It's worth a trip to Mexico just to see her paintings.

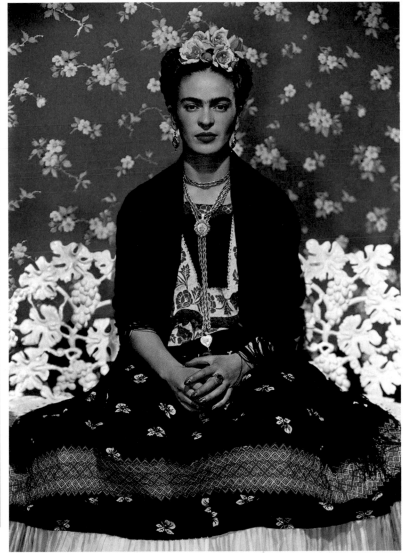

Frida Kahlo, 1950 and 1939.

Amanda Brooks

BOHEMIAN
The New Originals

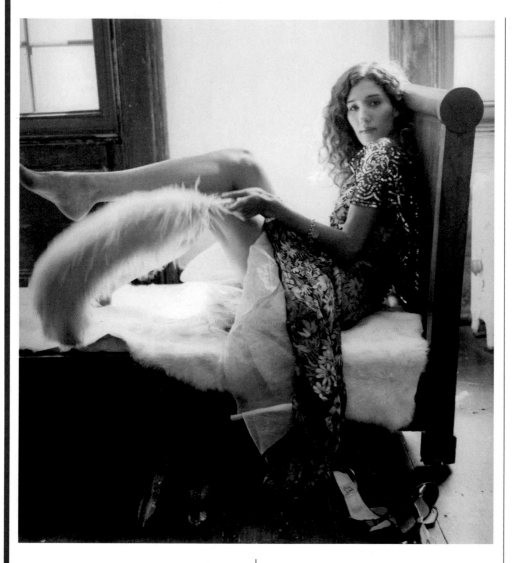

LEAH FORESTER L.A.-based fashion stylist Leah is like a young Marisa Berenson. Her wild, big, curly hair and long, dangly, skinny legs look irrepressibly bohemian no matter what she puts on her body. When she was a little girl she lived alone with her mother, and they had very little money. Nevertheless her mother always looked great, thanks to flea markets and thrift stores. She had an innate sense of style. She also saved money diligently in order to send Leah to private school in Beverly Hills. So Leah grew up surrounded by rich girls wearing 80s teen fashion like Benet-ton, Camp Beverly Hills, and Fiorucci, but—inspired by her mother's taste and style—she spent more time at the flea market than the mall. When Leah was a teenager her mother married a man with a lot of money and enjoyed being given fabulous diamond jewelry and designer clothing. Sadly Leah's mother passed away a few years ago, but she left Leah with great taste, a high/low approach to dressing, and her fabulous diamonds. And now Leah's life story is right there in her style—a mix of cheap chic, 80s fashion, Mexican ethnic bohemian, and amazing diamonds. So chic!

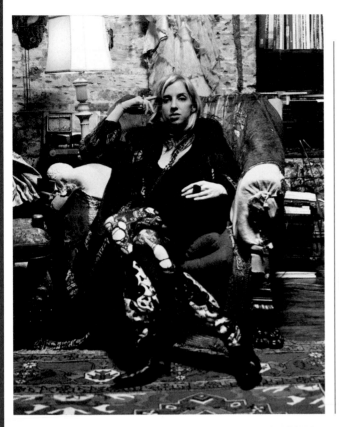

HOPE ATHERTON artist

Hope Atherton has an incredibly complex sense of style. Everything she wears, and the way she wears it, has deep symbolic meaning to her. She is at once bohemian, gothic, deconstructionist, and vintage-inspired. She allows her moods, whims, feelings, and fantasies to drive the way she dresses—buying, making, altering, and scavenging if necessary to suit her needs on any given day. She is a renowned painter and a sculptor (check out her work at www.BortolamiGallery.com) who thinks as carefully about getting dressed as she does about making her art. And it is absolutely apparent. She is one of a kind.

I admire Hope's style (as does *Vogue*—she is constantly featured in their pages) because it is so deeply personal. She absolutely refuses to look like anyone else, combining a trunk of her grandmother's old threadbare lace dresses, leather scraps she uses to make both sculptures and skirts, the odd piece of discarded designer clothing (old samples, sale items, or vintage pieces), and an obsessive relationship with H&M and the flea market to assemble her signature look.

SALLY SINGER fashion news/ features director at *Vogue*

Sally is intriguing because she doesn't fit the *Vogue* stereotype of being overtly fashion conscious, yet I always love what she is wearing. She looks real. Although she spends her days deliberating on matters of style, she is remarkably relaxed about her appearance and looks truly comfortable in her own skin. She knows herself. She embraces her upbringing in the hippie 60s and 70s in California (long, dangly jewelry, messy hair). She knows that a 50s-style dress best flatters her busty, curvy figure (vintage "Italian countess" dresses). She also accepts the cravings she naturally goes through (the "dress and pump" phase, the "neutral color" phase, the "wide skirt and cardigan" phase). What is most bohemian about her is her attitude toward dressing. She never looks predictable or definable. So even if she's wears something iconic, like a white shirt, she'll add layers of sweaters, jewelry, and scarves so that no one can pin her down into any cliché. She always looks original.

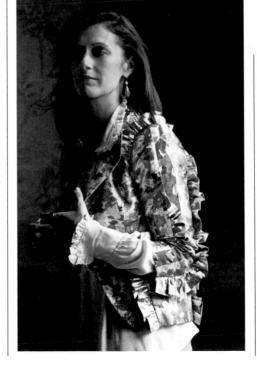

Top:
Hope Atherton
in her studio,
2006.

Left:
Sally Singer
in a Duro
Olowu jacket,
2009.

BOHEMIAN
Refining Your Style

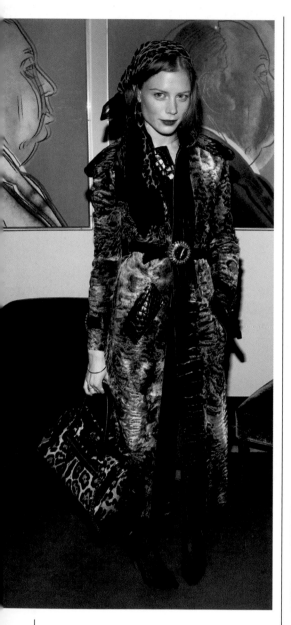

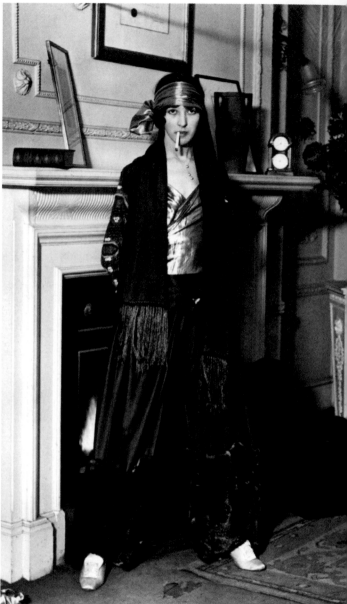

BOURGEOIS BOHEMIAN
Silk caftans, bold statement jewelry, designer handbags and scarves, embellished tunics, animal prints, fur coats, turbans.

VINTAGE BOHEMIAN
Armloads of bangles, tangled necklaces, battered leather sandals, crocheted dresses, well-worn denim, tooled leather, hippie skirts.

*Left:
Jessica Joffe,
2007.*

*Right:
A woman
wearing a
"smoking suit,"
1922.*

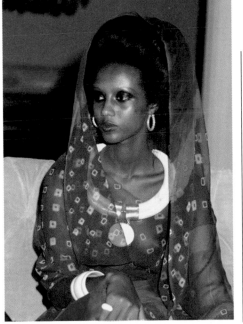

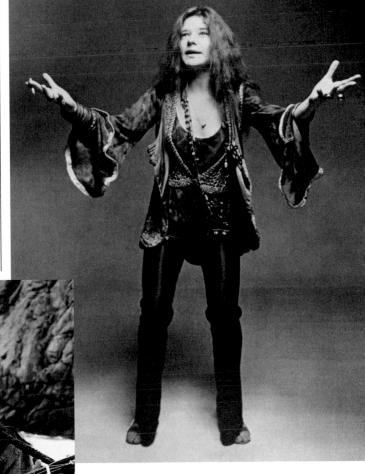

ROCK GODDESS BOHEMIAN
Fur-trimmed vests, velvet blazer (think Brian Jones), skinny scarves, tall leather boots, sequined tunic dress, hip-huggers, embellished belts.

ETHNIC BOHEMIAN
Embroidered dashikis, wood jewelry, ethnic sandals, saris, bold prints, head scarves, crafty bag.

PARED-DOWN BOHEMIAN
Solid tunics, Grecian sandals, classic leather hobo bag, layered tank tops, denim skirt, simple printed dresses.

Top:
Iman, 1975.

Above:
Joan Baez,
1962.

Right:
Janis Joplin,
1970.

BOHEMIAN
Refining Your Style / *Rock Goddess Bohemian*

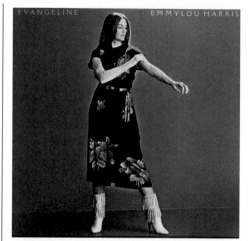
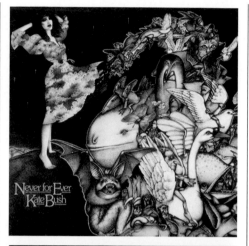
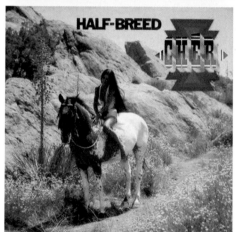
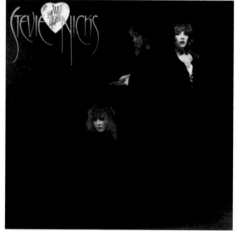
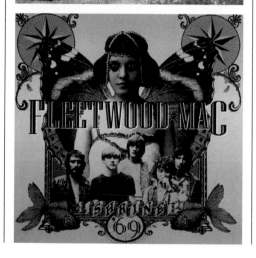
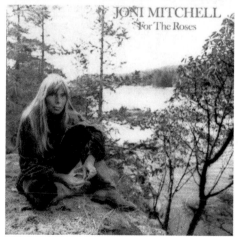

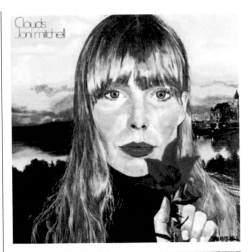

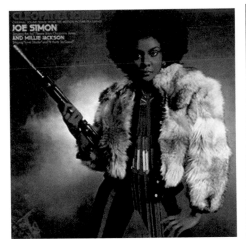

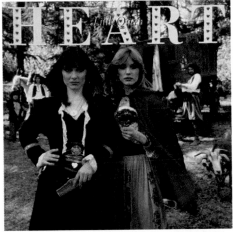

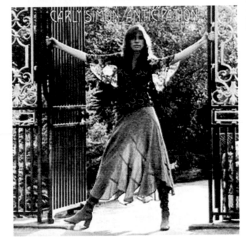

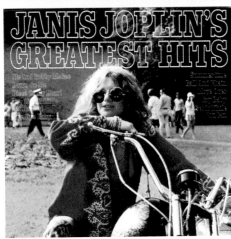

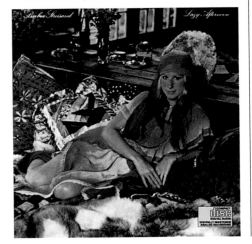

Amanda Brooks

BOHEMIAN
Inspiration

BOOKS

**Bohemians:
The Glamorous Outcasts**
by Elizabeth Wilson
A heavily footnoted, extremely informative history for those who are seriously interested in bohemian culture. Wilson traces it from its nineteenth-century roots to the Beatniks of the 60s.

Infinite Variety: The Life and Legend of Marchesa Casati
by Scot D. Ryersson
I am hard-pressed to think of anyone cooler than Marchesa Casati (she wore live snakes as jewelry, for goodness sake!). It's hard to imagine a biography that does justice to her incredible life, but this one does.

Native Funk and Flash
by Alexandra Jacopetti
This cult favorite focuses on the craft-work movement that flourished in the Bay Area during the 60s and 70s. It features the work of such less-well-known designers as Kaisik Wong, whose patchwork vest famously inspired Nicholas Ghesquière.

Hippie
by Barry Miles
A photo-heavy scrapbook of sorts that documents the counterculture that flourished from 1965 to 1971. The psychedelic posters and album covers are a fantastic bonus.

Biba: The Biba Experience
by Alwyn W. Turner
This gorgeous book includes everything you ever wanted to know about Barbara Hulanicki's Biba label and famous London boutique.

FILMS

Performance
If you love bohemian style, this is a must-rent. Anita Pallenberg looks amazing in her caftans and billowy dresses.

Cabaret
Liza Minnelli gives us bohemian meets glamour queen meets circus performer (but in the best possible taste). Her brightly colored nails and bold eye makeup add the perfect punch to her over-the-top looks.

Klute
Some of the best examples of 70s fashion captured on film. Jane Fonda has a very cool shag hairstyle and wears a casual mix of tall boots, miniskirts, and a particularly fabulous leather-trimmed trench coat.

Woodstock
The frequent crowd shots in this documentary give you an amazingly direct picture of Woodstock's iconic hippie style.

The Rose
As Janis Joplin in this 1979 rock-musical biopic, Bette Midler wears ripped T-shirts, sequin dresses, and piled-on accessories, all to a grungy boho chic effect.

Last Tango in Paris
I love Maria Schneider's carefree Parisian look here. She wears relaxed suits and fur coats, and her wild curly hair gives everything she wears an instant bohemian feel.

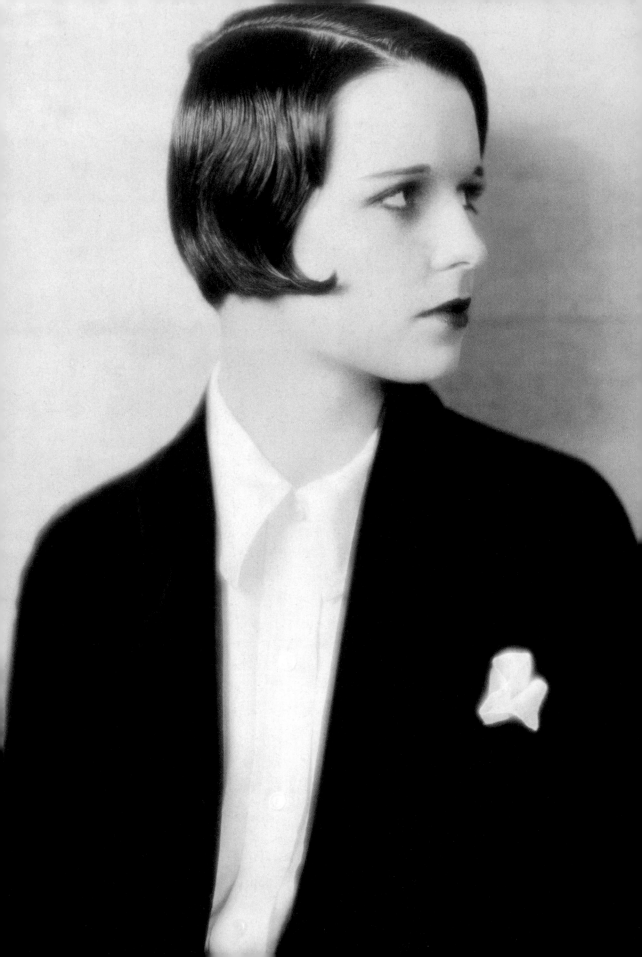

Minimal

"

MINIMALISM IS NOT ABOUT ABANDONING PATTERN OR PRINT. I SEE MINIMALISM TO BE A PHILOSOPHY THAT INVOLVES AN OVERALL SENSE OF BALANCE, KNOWING WHEN TO TAKE AWAY, SUBTRACT. IT'S AN INDULGENCE IN SUPERBLY EXECUTED CUT, QUIET PLAYS OF COLOR TONES AND CLEAN STRONG SHAPES."
—CALVIN KLEIN

"Minimalism is not defined by what is not there," John Pawson writes, "but by the rightness of what is, and the richness with which this is experienced. Novelty as an end in itself is overrated.... Originality is something you have to find inside yourself, within the ordinary rather than the extraordinary." As the famous minimalist architect who designed the Calvin Klein flagship store on Madison Avenue, Pawson should know. Minimalism is an entire life philosophy. The more you read about it, the more the whole concept starts to sound pretty spiritual. It's about having less and enjoying the things you have more—it's about cutting through the excess to discover what is essential.

Minimalist style requires discipline, consistency, and attention to quality. Most minimalists—Sofia Coppola is my favorite example—are methodical about getting dressed and have a heightened sense of self-awareness. They are often devoted to certain brands for their guarantee of good cut, fabric quality, and reliability in design. Because there isn't much to distract the eye, everything they wear must be of great quality; it must fit perfectly; the color and shape must flatter.

Louise Brooks's whole look is amazingly contemporary, c.1920s.

As a fashion concept, minimalism is ripe for thoughtful reinterpretation. The strict lines, stark simplicity, and downright severity of its 1990s incarnation aren't really relevant anymore. They are too harsh for today's less contrived aesthetic. But the idea is strong. Who isn't attracted to simplicity and purity? Today's minimalism, as I've witnessed in the work of design houses such as Calvin Klein and Jil Sander, abandons high-minded ambition and concerns itself with the reality of how women want to dress. There is still room for black (or monochromatic) clothes, and starkness still has some relevance, although now it is softer, more organic, and more feminine—less cartoonishly austere. On the whole, minimalism today revolves around simplicity, period.

Minimalism is a challenging style to carry off with success. It takes a great deal of self-knowledge and discipline to get it right. It's one thing to forego pattern and ornament and look perfectly chic in an understated look; it's another to look like you just haven't made an effort or are thinking of entering a religious order. However, there is nothing more stylish than a woman who knows the simplest, most refined pieces of clothing that suit her best, so it's worth getting it right.

MINIMAL
My Minimal Style

When I started this chapter I had to do a lot of research. I am not a natural minimalist. And I wanted to understand the ideas behind minimalism as a philosophy not only for fashion, but also for music, art, film, and architecture. Once I had absorbed these principles through reading a pile of books delivered from Amazon, I decided that I couldn't write about minimalism without trying out at least the fashion part for myself. So I began to pare back when I dressed, sticking with what was essential instead of piling on lots of extras.

Taking Pawson's words to heart, I concentrated on making an impact with my outfit by getting it right—achieving a careful balance of color, texture, and shape—instead of frivolously pushing the envelope. I kept the prints and ruffles in my closet, but I willed my eye to rest on the simpler things: a vintage black silk blouse with a very plain shape, an H&M tuxedo jacket, white shirts from the boys' department at Brooks Brothers, black suede over-the-knee boots, leggings, a slew of well-worn J.Crew T-shirts in white, gray, and black; I even resurrected an old black leather Gucci bag from the 90s that has no hardware whatsoever on it. I was surprised by how many looks these pieces could create, and by the sense of relief I felt thanks to my newly limited choices. A closet chock full of clothing in every different style can overwhelm a girl.

After a month of trying the look on at the office and at home, my new style was ready for its public debut. My lovely friend Francisco Costa, the designer of Calvin Klein, invited me to be his guest at a benefit dinner. I wore a black silk jersey dress, long to the floor. There was asymmetrical pleating below the knee on one side, and, apart from a few structural seams, that was it. Very plain, very simple. For shine and glamour, I added a trifecta of black patent leather accessories: narrow belt on the waist, platform "bondage" shoes by Yves Saint Laurent, and an astonishingly chic Calvin Klein box clutch. I slicked my hair back in a tight bun like a Robert Palmer girl from the 80s and wore lots of black mascara and eyeliner. I faced the mirror: sleek, chic,

modern, but maybe a little too severe. I scanned my jewelry box for something that might soften the outfit, knowing already that any jewelry would spoil the simplicity of the look. And then a bouquet of flowers in my bedroom caught my eye. I cut two white roses out of the arrangement and pinned them to one side of my bun. I wear fresh flowers in my hair often, so that addition made me feel like myself, even though I was officially a minimalist for the night.

Though I received many compliments on my newly simple look, nobody seemed to think I had undergone a complete transformation. And for me that's always the goal—to try out new things, new looks, new inspirations, but not to sacrifice that certain something that makes me feel and look like myself. I may not be a born-again minimalist, but my experiments with minimalism inform the way I think about getting dressed now.

Since that night I have looked forward to each Calvin Klein show as a further exploration of minimalism and also as the inspiration for keeping a greater deal of simplicity in my wardrobe. From what I have learned there are two versions of minimalism in fashion. There is the heady, more conceptual idea of inventing new shapes, proportions, and silhouettes as a way to create interest in the absence of decoration. And then there is the idea of taking more classic shapes and proportions and stripping them down to their barest essentials. I definitely relate way more to the latter of the two. Putting on a precisely constructed double-breasted blazer—in the most subtle yet becoming shade of gray tweed with matching Katharine Hepburn–style wide-legged trousers and a soft T-shirt—makes me feel that it would be a crime to add anything to this perfectly simple, yet timelessly chic look. It doesn't need a belt or a bracelet to make it interesting. It hardly even requires hair and makeup. I just put it on and I go, and I feel great. What more could I ask for?

Me, having a fitting with Francisco Costa, at the Calvin Klein showroom, 2008.

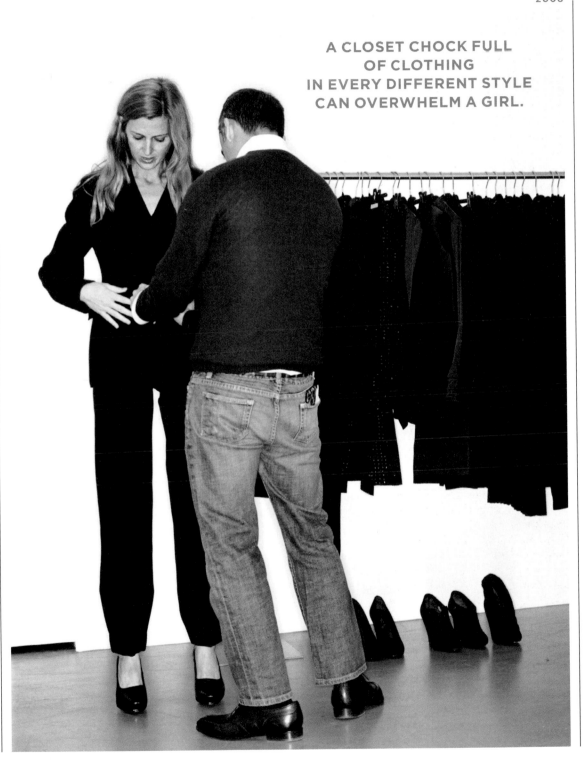

2008

A CLOSET CHOCK FULL
OF CLOTHING
IN EVERY DIFFERENT STYLE
CAN OVERWHELM A GIRL.

Amanda Brooks

MINIMAL
My Favorite Things

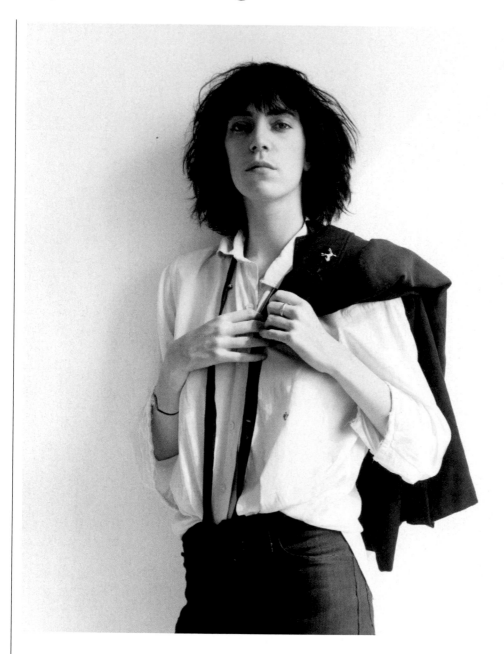

BUTTON-DOWN COTTON SHIRTS are a minimal staple. If you are an extreme minimalist you might appreciate a shirt that lacks many traditional details like a breast pocket, princess seams, or collar buttons. The *Vogue* writer Marina Rust has an aversion to buttons. They completely freak her out. So her local tailor copies an old favorite Isaac Mizrahi shirt of hers that has a placket covering the buttons down the front. This kind of attention to detail and refinement defines minimalist style.

For a softer more feminine look, the same style shirt looks great in **SILK**.

Patti Smith, 1975. I'm not sure a white shirt could look any cooler than that.

The quest for **PERFECT BLACK PANTS** (below) is truly endless, since there isn't just *one* perfect pair out there. I have three pairs of perfect black pants that serve different purposes. My *most* perfect pair are black viscose (a high-end version of rayon) straight-leg classic trousers from Tuleh. The magic of viscose is that it is flattering and comfortable even as it maintains its shape, working effortlessly for day or for evening. I have worn these pants with a T-shirt and flats to visit a friend in the hospital, and I have worn them to a black tie party with an embroidered bolero. My second favorite pair are very skinny, a wool/silk blend from Helmut Lang in 2001. I love that the leg is skinny yet the top has men's tailoring details like a button-fly and belt loops. Because they are super long I wear these only at night, with stilettos. And in third place are Marc by Marc Jacobs wool pants (they're lined so they're not itchy) with flapped pockets. They're super comfortable, and the length is perfect for flats or sneakers in the daytime. They also really flatter my butt. So when you are looking for your perfect black pants, ask yourself what purpose they need to serve and how you intend to wear them.

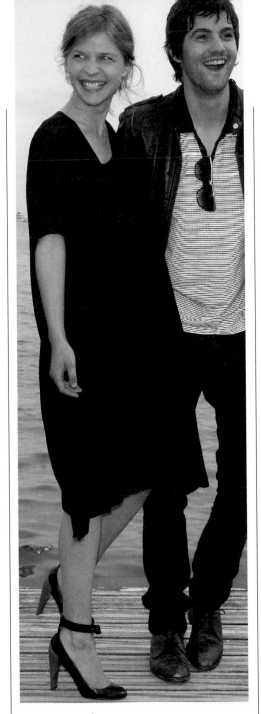

Left:
Model Kasia Smutniak at the Chanel show in Paris, 2008.

Right:
Clémence Poésy (with Jim Sturgess), 2008.

A **SIMPLE BLACK DRESS** (above) doesn't necessarily have to be stark. You can create a minimalist look from a dress that has a bow or some lace on it. There is, however, great value in a very plain black dress that fits beautifully and can be transformed into whatever style you feel like that day (think of a Diane von Furstenberg wrap dress in plain black wool jersey). Such a truly simple black dress can have one or two details— unique seams, elaborate stitching, contrasting trim—but I would leave it at that.

MINIMAL
My Favorite Things

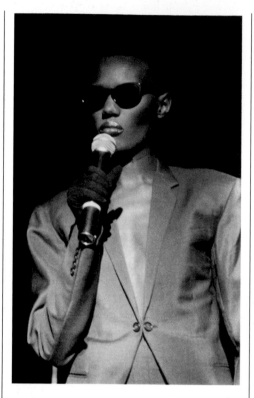

A heavy **WINTER COAT** (below) in wool or cashmere should be one of the more luxurious things you buy. It will last for years, and you can wear it every day in the colder months. Devout minimalists will instinctually avoid decoration, but if you aren't quite a purist, a simple fur collar will add warmth and detail.

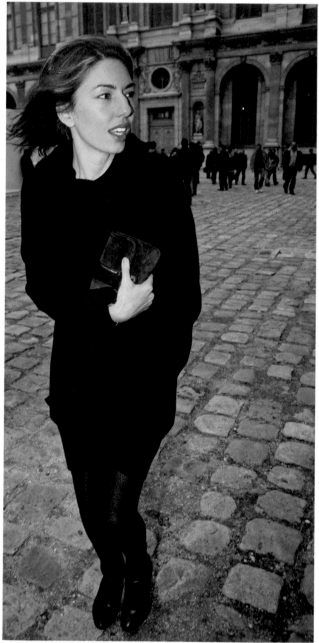

A **SIMPLE TAILORED JACKET** (above) is a must-have for minimal style. Its clean lines and strong shape are perfect, and a well-fitting, unaffected jacket will be useful for years, regardless of which style you may choose to project. My own preference is a classic blazer. Even double-breasted is great—just like a men's suit jacket but smaller.

If you choose minimal style in order to have a simpler, less cluttered life, a **SPRING/FALL COAT** that is waterproof—two coats in one—is a must-have. You can also get one with a detachable lining for warmer days—then it is three coats in one.

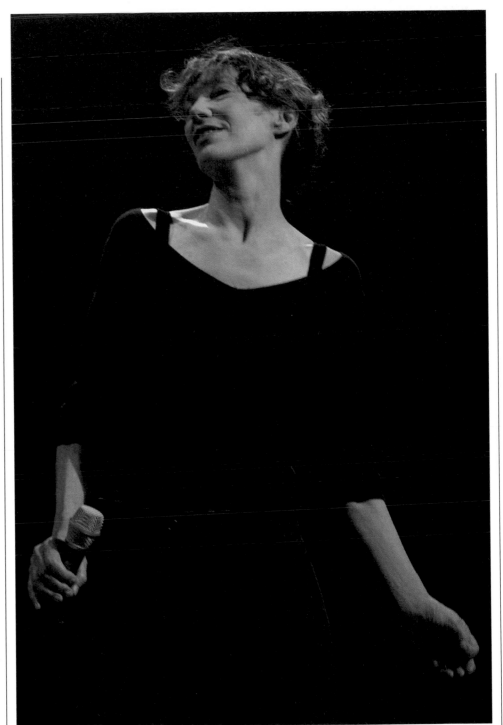

Opposite:
(Far left)
It's a stretch
to think of
Grace Jones as a
minimalist, but
she is wearing
the perfect
pared-down
jacket in this
photo, 1985.

(Left)
Sofia Coppola,
Paris, 2008.

This page:
These days
it's hard to find
a photo of
Jane Birkin
in anything
other than
a cashmere
sweater and
baggy trousers,
2008.

I find that many of my SOLID COLOR CASHMERE SWEATERS (most of them from J.Crew) have a new meaning in the context of minimalist style. The texture, the luxuriousness of the fabric, and the simple shape all work well with more streamlined, pared-down silhouettes.

MINIMAL
Accessories

SOME WOMEN WOULD RATHER DIE, BUT YOU REALLY CAN GET BY WITH ONLY ONE HANDBAG.

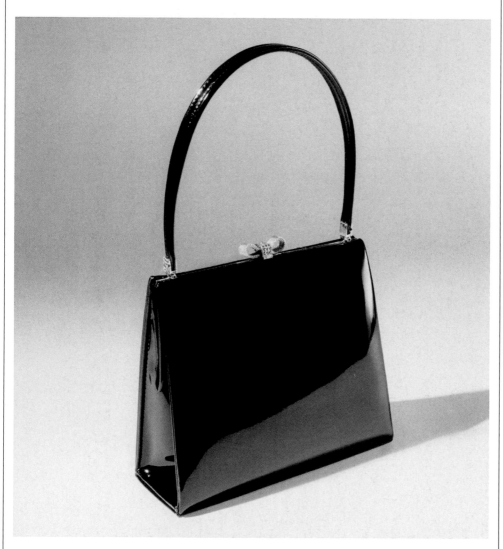

This page: A patent leather handbag from Harrods, 1965.

Opposite: (Near right) Victoria Beckham wearing classic yet minimal accessories, 2009.

(Far right) An ideal minimal watch.

Some women would rather die, but you really can get by with only one **HANDBAG**. Well, okay, maybe two would be better; black would be the obvious first choice for color, and then a neutral such as brown, tan, gray, white, or beige would be very useful as well. Some hardware might work, but sticking to the simplest rendition of a classic shape is most effective. If your budget allows, a skin bag—such as lizard, crocodile, or ostrich—would be a fantastic addition to a minimalist's closet. The texture and shine are the perfect foils for more subtle minimalist clothing fabrics such as jersey, cashmere, and matte silk.

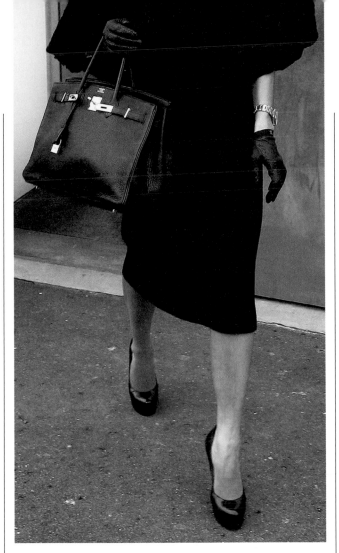

A simple WATCH is a great, chic minimalist accessory. I love the tomboy feeling of a men's watch on a woman's wrist sticking out from under a rolled-up shirt sleeve. There are some incredibly beautiful and expensive watches out there. We've all drooled over them, but I have seen Swatches and Timexes look just as chic.

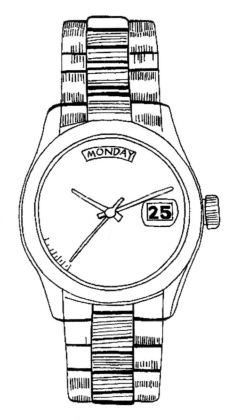

SHOES offer the minimalist a great opportunity to inject some wit into an otherwise rigorously simplified wardrobe. For example, if I were wearing all-black chic clothes I would probably wear a brown shoe and handbag just to add some contrast. And if I were wearing a 60s-inspired tailored shift dress I might wear a pump with—dare I say it?—a neat little tailored bow on the front, just to add a detail.

The 70s jewelry designer ELSA PERETTI'S SIMPLE, PERSONAL JEWELRY designs are the main reason I ever find myself inside the Tiffany store (they have the exclusive on her collection). I have been wearing her designs since I was in my early teens, starting with a silver bean necklace for my thirteenth birthday, followed by a single "diamond by the yard" chain given to me by a boyfriend when I was eighteen, then a gold heart pendant on a long chain from my mother for my thirtieth birthday, and most recently gold chain mail earrings given to me by a generous friend. I consider Elsa Peretti jewelry to be the perfect addition to a contemporary minimalist look: simple, organic, timeless.

I LOVE THE TOMBOY FEELING OF A MEN'S WATCH ON A WOMAN'S WRIST STICKING OUT FROM UNDER A ROLLED-UP SHIRT SLEEVE.

MINIMAL
Mixing It Up

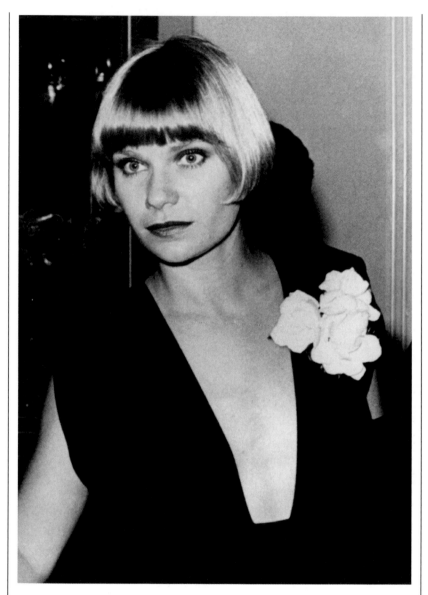

Mod dresses by Pierre Cardin, a Courrèges suit, Lanvin costume jewelry, Vionnet bias-cut dresses, and other simpler designs, especially from the 30s and 60s, all come to mind as **VINTAGE PIECES** (opposite) that could work their way suitably into a minimal wardrobe. Their clean lines, sophisticated shapes, and impeccable quality would suit the tastes of most minimalists while providing a shot of the unexpected.

> **"MY DRESSES ARE LIKE SCULPTURES. I MOLDED THEM AND THEN I PUT A WOMAN INTO IT. IT WAS MORE LIKE ARCHITECTURE OR ART."**
> —PIERRE CARDIN

Unsurprisingly, when I see a minimalist look I usually want to **DECORATE** (above) it a bit. It could be a bow on your blouse, a string of pearls around your neck, or a fresh flower in your lapel. All give a little "wink" to throw off the seriousness and rigor of minimalism.

Silk or cotton jersey is a great fabric for **SOFTER, MORE FEMININE MINIMAL PIECES.** It drapes beautifully and the fabric is not so quality-dependent (although a great quality jersey can make a stunning dress).

Even with the addition of a decorative flower, Lisa Miller's overall look still reads minimal, 1976.

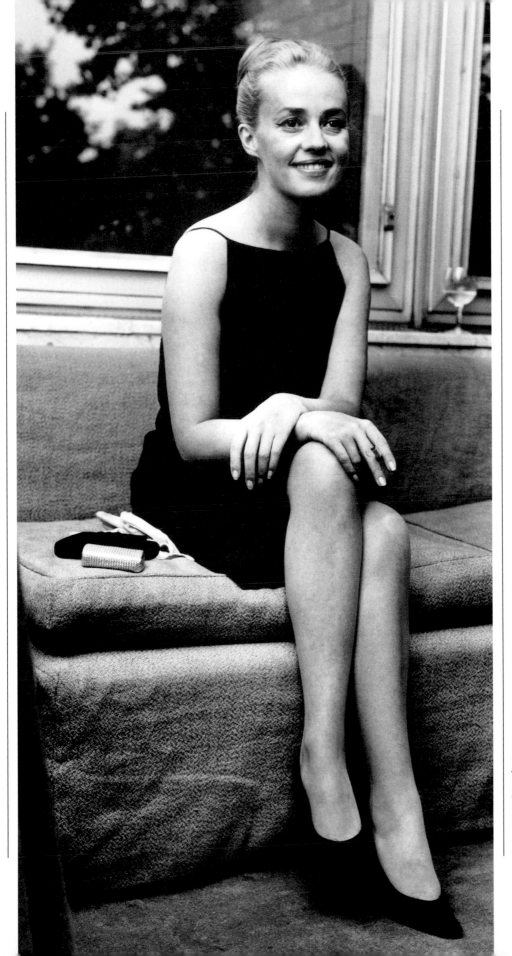

French actress Jeanne Moreau —in a simple, yet chic Pierre Cardin dress— announces her marriage to Pierre Cardin at a press conference, 1962.

MINIMAL
High Risk, High Reward

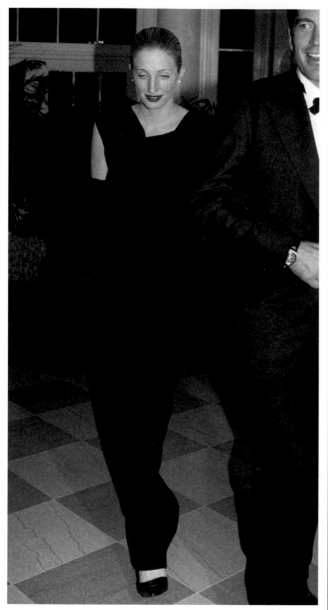

fabric, even color—so sophisticated that to some people they look outlandish rather than simple. It's hard to make them work if you don't feel completely at ease with this aesthetic.

The key to pulling off SEVERITY, by which I mean a strict, sleek, very refined look, is the structure of the face. You don't have to be a great beauty, but your face must serve the look you are going for. For example, Isabella Rossellini has always looked great with that angular Louise Brooks bob because she has such a soft, feminine face. If you have a more defined, even dramatic, bone structure, it might suit you to pull all your hair back and show your face off. Makeup is another issue. Cecilia Dean, editor of the very high-fashion *V* magazine, looks great with her hair pulled back and no makeup at all, whereas the girls dancing in the Robert Palmer videos of the 80s look stunning with very strong makeup on their very strong faces and the same pulled-back hair. As for severe clothes, there is a fine line between simply chic and willfully monastic. You don't want people to notice your clothes more than they notice you, and you certainly don't want to scare away your date. So look in the mirror and make sure that you feel completely comfortable and happy, or ask a friend to level with you about whether your severe look is working.

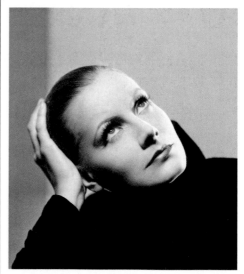

HIGH-CONCEPT DESIGN can be intriguing but tricky. Carolyn Bessette Kennedy, for example, looked amazing in her Yohji Yamamoto looks. It was her classic face, chic hair, and casual attitude that gave those high-concept looks a wearable platform. Designers such as Yamamoto and Rei Kawakubo (for Comme des Garçons) make clothes that are very sophisticated in cut, shape,

*Above:
Carolyn Bessette
Kennedy, with
John Kennedy,
at a state dinner
at the White
House in a
Comme des
Garçons dress,
1998.*

*Right:
Greta Garbo,
1931.*

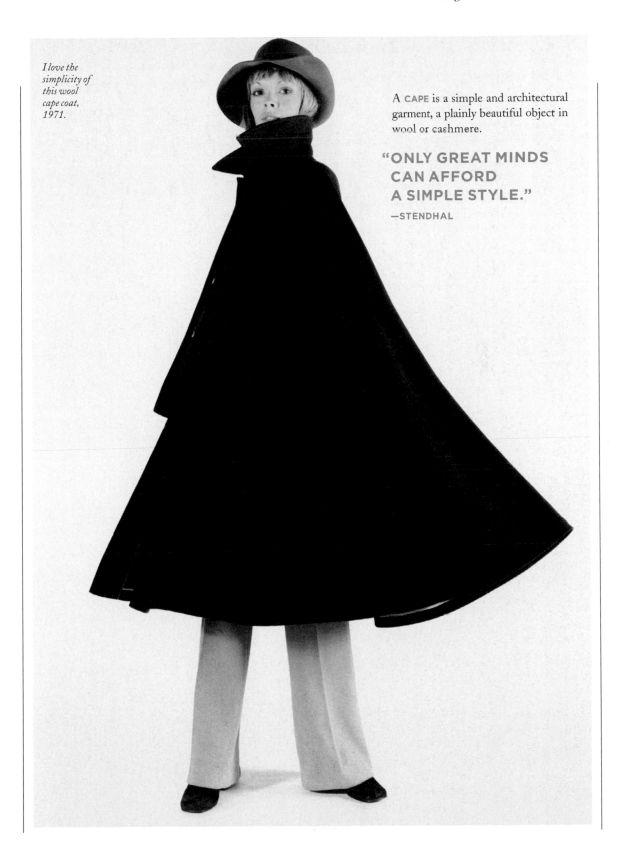

*I love the
simplicity of
this wool
cape coat,
1971.*

A CAPE is a simple and architectural garment, a plainly beautiful object in wool or cashmere.

"ONLY GREAT MINDS CAN AFFORD A SIMPLE STYLE."
—STENDHAL

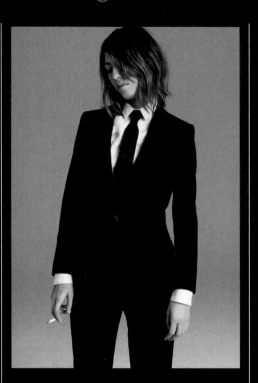

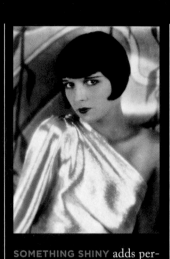

SOMETHING SHINY adds personality to an evening look. A patent leather clutch, simple gold or silver earrings, metallic shoes, even a lamé scarf worn with a tuxedo adds shimmer and flash to the most basic evening shapes.

Louise Brooks, 1929.

A MINIMAL TUXEDO is one of my all-time favorite evening looks for a woman. Style it right, and it will look minimal rather than classic: strict hair, black eye makeup, nude lips, and a tailored suit with very clean simple lines.

Sofia Coppola, 2004.

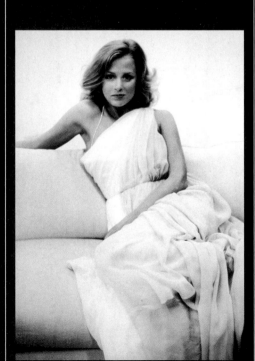

The GREEK GODDESS LOOK is a great choice for evening, soft and feminine but still utterly pared back. It avoids all ornament save beautiful layers of fabric draped over a beautiful body, a truly minimal concept, so don't overdo the accessories. A chic low bun and a simple clutch bag should do the trick.

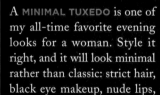

Lauren Hutton, c.1975.

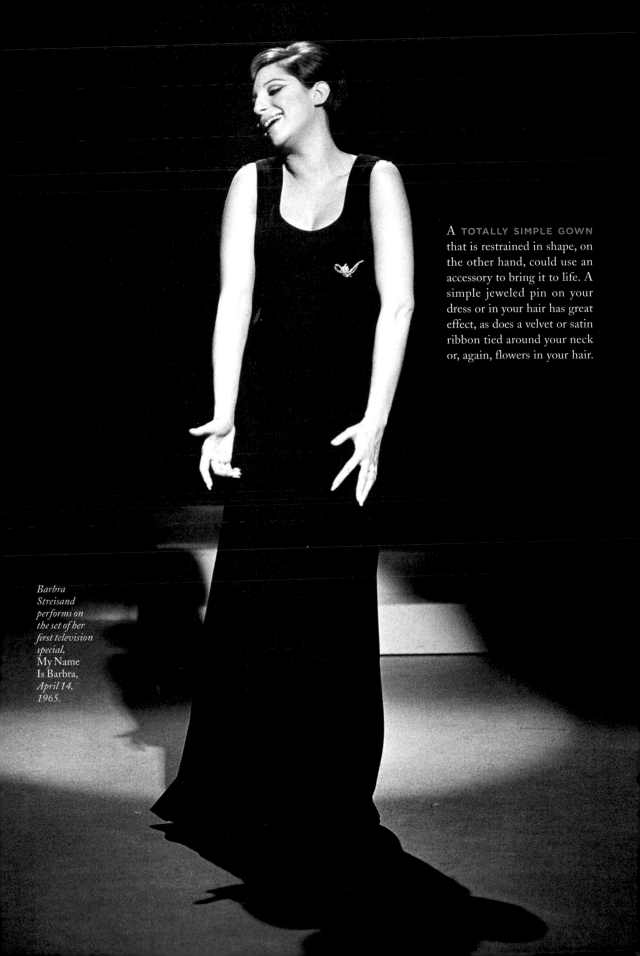

A **TOTALLY SIMPLE GOWN** that is restrained in shape, on the other hand, could use an accessory to bring it to life. A simple jeweled pin on your dress or in your hair has great effect, as does a velvet or satin ribbon tied around your neck or, again, flowers in your hair.

Barbra Streisand performs on the set of her first television special, My Name Is Barbra, *April 14, 1965.*

MINIMAL
Getting It Right

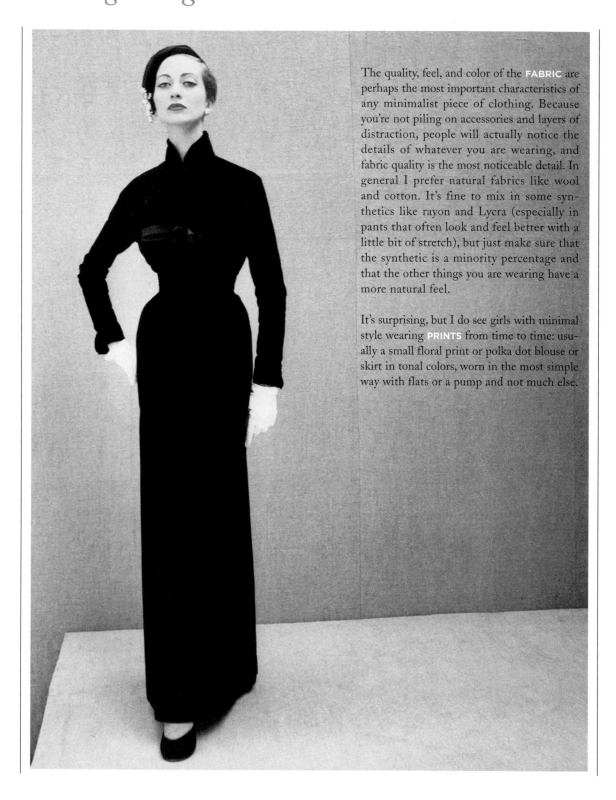

The quality, feel, and color of the **FABRIC** are perhaps the most important characteristics of any minimalist piece of clothing. Because you're not piling on accessories and layers of distraction, people will actually notice the details of whatever you are wearing, and fabric quality is the most noticeable detail. In general I prefer natural fabrics like wool and cotton. It's fine to mix in some synthetics like rayon and Lycra (especially in pants that often look and feel better with a little bit of stretch), but just make sure that the synthetic is a minority percentage and that the other things you are wearing have a more natural feel.

It's surprising, but I do see girls with minimal style wearing **PRINTS** from time to time: usually a small floral print or polka dot blouse or skirt in tonal colors, worn in the most simple way with flats or a pump and not much else.

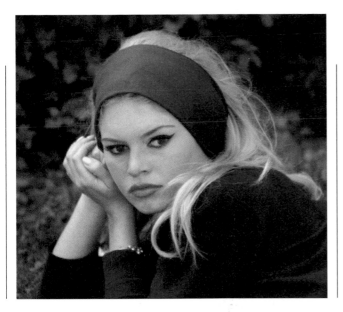

Although wearing all black is a quick shortcut to a minimalist look, it's not necessarily the most interesting path to take. You could just as easily WEAR ANY SOLID COLOR. Think of a pale pink jersey gown with simple hair, little makeup, and spare accessories—you'll look just as minimal but perhaps slightly prettier. I'm not recommending an explosion of jewel tones, but the parameters of color in minimalist dressing could perhaps relax a bit. Some people seem to think minimal has to be black, brown, gray, or white, but to me it is more about simplicity of shape, styling, and general aesthetic than it is about the color.

The most bare-bones versions of classic pieces can look minimal when worn in the context of a SIMPLE, CLEAN PROPORTION. This might be the easiest place for a virgin minimalist to start: a beautifully cut white cotton shirt, a great fitting pair of trousers, and a simple cashmere coat.

TO ME MINIMAL IS MORE ABOUT SIMPLICITY OF SHAPE, STYLING, AND GENERAL AESTHETIC THAN IT IS ABOUT THE COLOR.

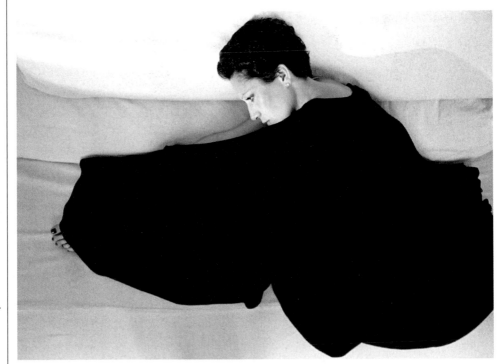

*Opposite:
A remarkably
simple and
refined Dior
gown, 1951.*

*This page:
(Above)
Brigitte
Bardot,
on the set of
Contempt,
1963.*

*(Right)
Elsa Peretti,
1975.*

MINIMAL
Icons

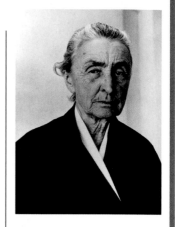

Artist **GEORGIA O'KEEFE** perfectly defines minimalism. Just look at her. She emanates discipline and a quest for simplicity. I can't say that I am a huge fan of her paintings, but her clothing style really works for me.

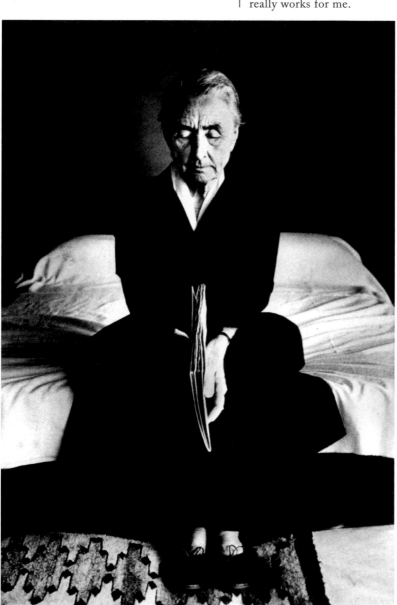

"TO CREATE ONE'S OWN WORLD IN ANY OF THE ARTS TAKES COURAGE."
—GEORGIA O'KEEFE

*Left:
Georgia
O'Keefe at her
ranch home,
1966.*

*Top:
O'Keefe, 1970.*

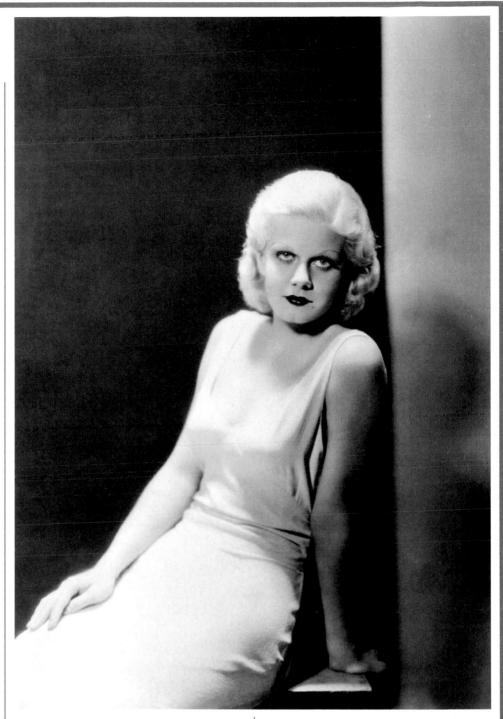

*Jean Harlow,
1932.*

Sex symbol and 30s actress **JEAN HARLOW** was *so* not an obvious choice for this chapter. But I came across pictures of her that emphasized how pared down, focused, and downright simple her approach to dressing was. It makes sense when I remember how influential fashion designer Madeleine Vionnet's work was during the 30s; Harlow certainly seems to have been paying attention. Platinum blonde curls, graphic (bordering on freakish) painted-on eyebrows, and simple slip and bias-cut dresses were her look, and it would become more and more relevant as the century progressed.

MINIMAL
The New Originals

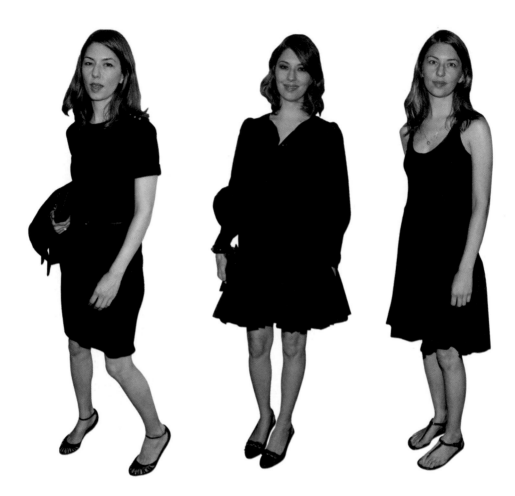

SOFIA COPPOLA screenwriter and director Sofia's style is my idea of modern minimalism. She's simple (hardly ever wears a noticeable accessory), she's disciplined (never changes her hairstyle and mostly sticks to one designer—Marc Jacobs), and she dresses in a way that is modern and focused (all of those black dresses are perfect for her). She

"MY MOTHER WAS ALWAYS VERY UNDERSTATED AND LOW-KEY TOO. IT'S NOT SOMETHING I DELIBERATELY CULTIVATE BUT I THINK THERE ARE PEOPLE WHO WANT TO BE LOOKED AT. AS A WRITER OR OBSERVER, I'M MORE INTERESTED IN LOOKING."

—SOFIA COPPOLA

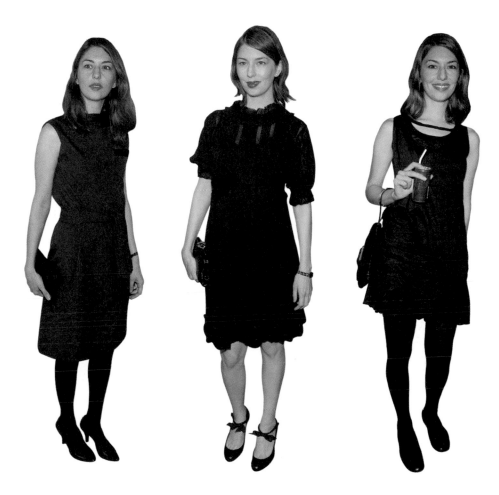

can even wear a bow on her shoulder or a ruffle on her hem and she still looks modern and elegant. She is not screaming for attention, yet everyone notices her. It's hard to believe she came out of Hollywood alongside so much manufactured beauty. She is a breath of fresh air.

The New Originals

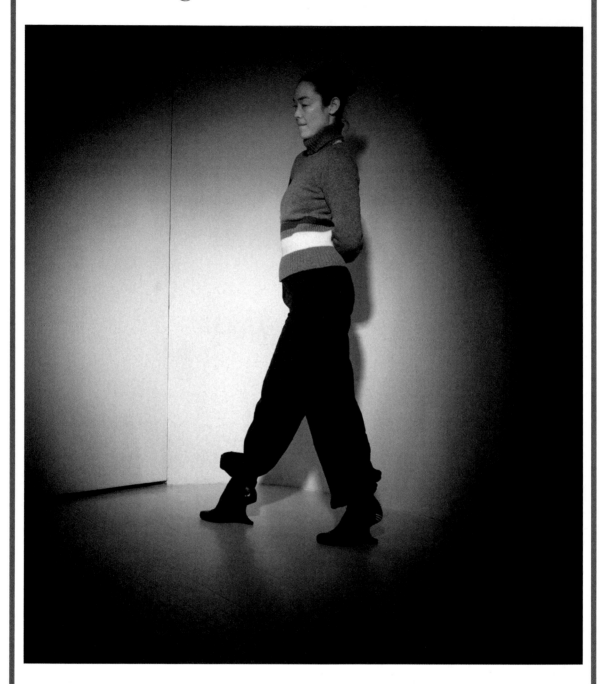

CECILIA DEAN editor and creator of *V* magazine and *Visionaire*

Ninety percent of the time Cecilia Dean is dressed in chic black and white, with a sleek (verging on severe) low bun, and a simple, modern sensibility. But every now and then she pulls out a "peacock look"—a rainbow dress, a red patent coat, a gown composed entirely of ruffles—that is highly decorative. The unpredictability is what I love about her.

Cecilia Dean, 2008.

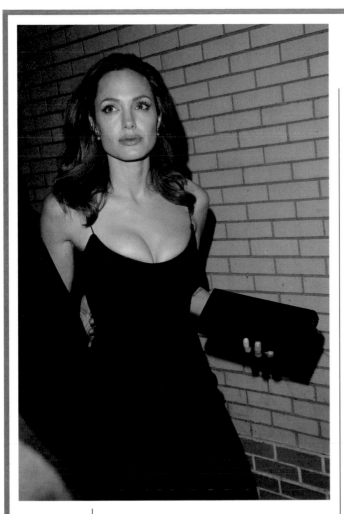

ON THE WHOLE SHE IS VERY GOOD AT WEARING JUST ENOUGH TO MAKE HER LOOK CHIC WITHOUT ADDING ANYTHING TO DISTRACT FROM HER NATURAL BEAUTY.

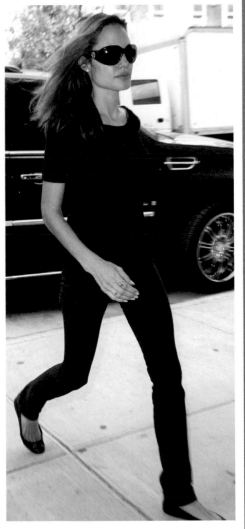

Angelina Jolie, both 2007.

ANGELINA JOLIE actress and humanitarian

It's clear to me that Angelina chooses simple clothes that make it easy for her to get dressed and look good. The message I get from her outfit choices says that she likes to look good, but that she has more important things to think about than what she wears every day. The result is a look that displays a very easy and affordable way to be a minimalist by wearing classic shapes in muted colors. For day she usually wears flat shoes, skinny jeans or loose trousers, an unfussy blouse or T-shirt, and her signature sunglasses. For evening it's classic pumps and a body-hugging cocktail dress or sexy tailored pants and a jacket. She wears very little jewelry, and she may curl her hair or wear more eyeliner to soften the effect of her more severe clothes, but on the whole she is very good at wearing just enough to make her look chic without adding anything to distract from her natural beauty.

MINIMAL
Refining Your Style

Kate Moss, 1995.

> "FASHION IS ARCHITECTURE. IT IS A MATTER OF PROPORTIONS."
> —COCO CHANEL

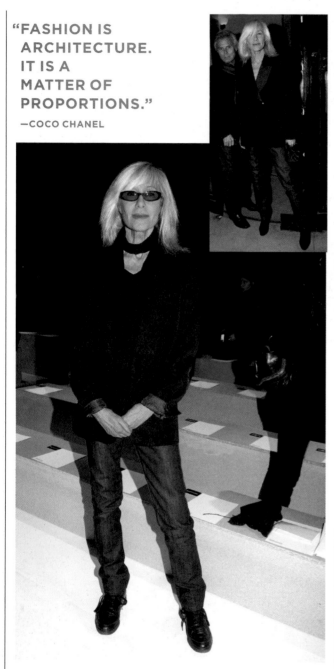

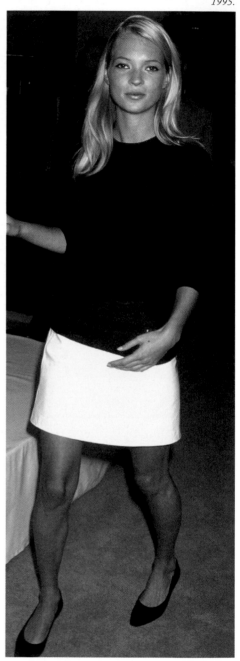

UNIFORM MINIMAL
Wearing a slight variation of the same outfit every day (Betty Catroux is a perfect example).

YSL muse Betty Catroux almost always wears tight black pants and a men's-style black blazer, 2007 (above) and 2004 (top).

CLASSIC MINIMAL
Perfectly tailored black pants, crisp white button-up shirts, sleek blazers, modest black dresses, simple watches, practical anonymous handbags.

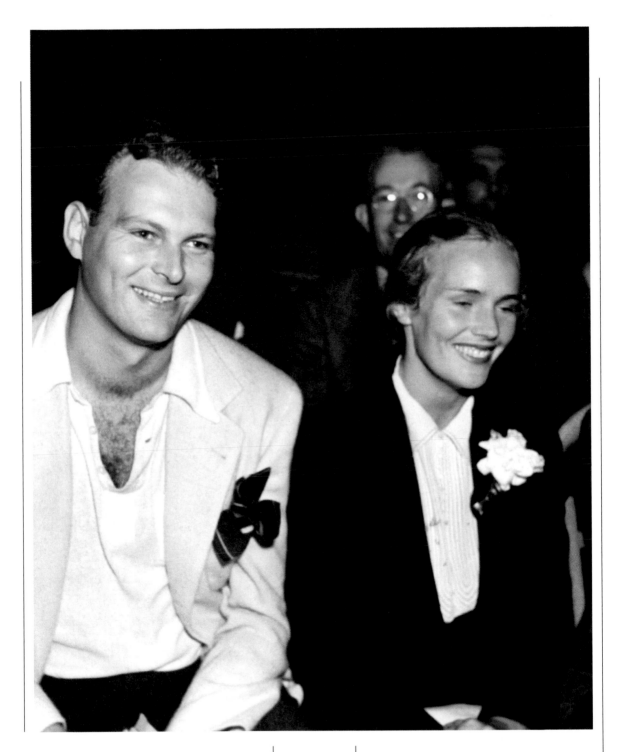

Frances Farmer and Leif Erickson in matching outfits, 1934. I love the flower on her lapel.

ANDROGYNOUS MINIMAL

Beatle boots, oxfords, slim-cut suit (ideally by Dior Homme), oversized men's shirts, vests, skinny ties, leather tote bag, no makeup, a boyish hairstyle is preferable.

MINIMAL
Inspiration

BOOKS

Madeleine Vionnet
by Betty Kirke

The founding mother of minimalism in fashion. She disliked the volatility of fashion and would be proud to know that her bias-cut gowns and Greek goddess-inspired pleats could be worn today, almost a century later, without looking a year out of place. She was a major inspiration for Calvin Klein and should be your first stop for minimalist inspiration too.

Halston
by Steven Bluttal

I love this book and over the years have referred to it countless times for inspiration. The clothes Halston designed are famously chic and glamorous, and the photos of Halston's lifestyle—his friends, his house, his studio—are amazing to look at.

Minimalism
by James Meyer

I wanted to include this book on the minimalist art of the 1960s because I don't think minimalism has been as clearly defined in fashion as it has been in other areas. Check this book out and see for yourself whether it influences the way you look at clothes.

Minimum
by John Pawson

This book heightened my alertness to color, shape, and materials. John Pawson writes in a clear and accessible way about the underlying principles and philosophy of minimalism.

French New Wave
by Jean Douchet
and Robert Bononno

I wouldn't describe the films of the French New Wave as minimal, but the actresses' clothes are beautifully so. This book features tons of gorgeous photos of stylish starlets including Anna Karina, Jeanne Moreau, Brigitte Bardot, and Jean Seberg.

FILMS

Gattaca
Uma Thurman's sleek bun, collared white shirts, and black tailored suits all have a distinctly minimalist look. These clothes are classic with minimal styling, not the wild (and totally unconvincing) fantasies you might expect from a movie that takes place in the future. The architectural sets are inspiring too.

Contempt
Brigitte Bardot's black headband and simple black-and-white basics demonstrate a feminized 60s minimalism.

Repulsion
Catherine Deneuve is the picture of minimalist chic in this Roman Polanski film. Her classic features and icy persona perfectly compliment her ladylike wardrobe of trench coats and simple shift dresses.

Darling
Julie Christie plays a charismatic fashion model in this lovely film set in 1960s London. Her simple ladylike style is timelessly cool, and there are enough costume changes to make your head spin.

Masculin Féminin
French New Wave films are full of cool-looking girls in miniskirts, but Chantal Goya's style in *Masculin Féminin* has always stood out to me. Her look is modest and understated, but she always brings a youthful edge to her cardigans, A-line skirts, and simple wool coats. Cameo appearances by Brigitte Bardot and Françoise Hardy are also a bonus.

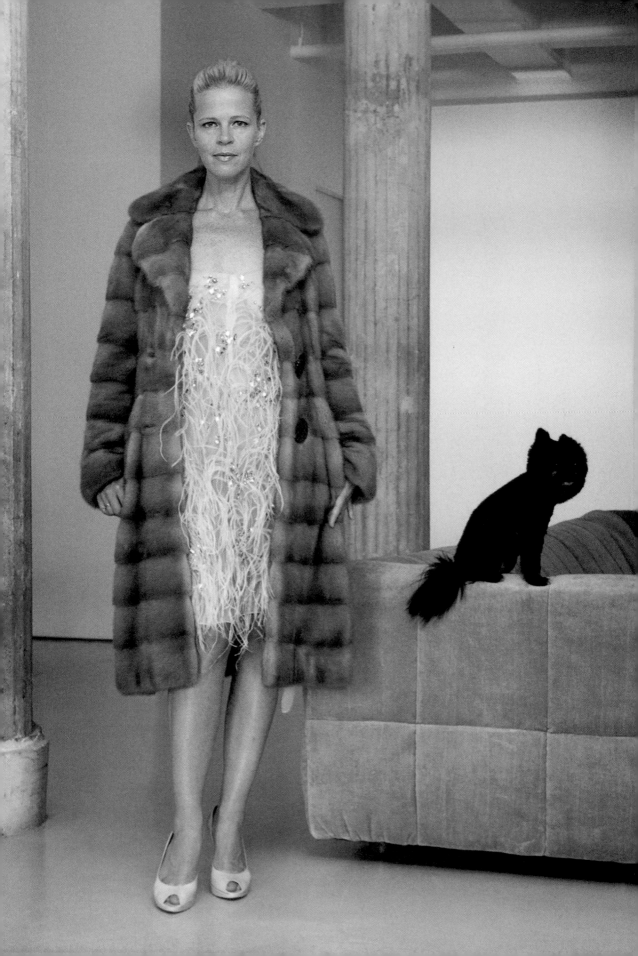

HIGH FASHION

" YOU ARE WHO YOU PRETEND TO BE."
—YVONNE FORCE

High fashion is not easy to pinpoint. Anything trendy could be considered high fashion, but high fashion needn't necessarily take part in today's trends. You can make any style you want into a high fashion look simply by taking it a bit further than the average person would likely do: Wear platform shoes with a minidress, throw a voluminous fur coat over your outfit, or simply add dramatic hair and makeup to whatever you are wearing. You can choose to make a high fashion statement at any time, just because you like the look, not because everyone else is doing it. A 60s space-age shift dress worn at a time when bohemian styles were all the rage would look high fashion but not trendy. Get it?

High fashion clothing requires self-knowledge, nerve, and a creative spirit. What is not required is a designer label or a shocking price tag (although if your budget allows, fashion designers do make some pretty amazing things). Some of the most high fashion pieces in my closet—a feather cape, a metallic brocade dress, a lace caftan with matching head scarf—have come from thrift stores, flea markets, cheap chic chain stores, even yard sales.

I want to clarify something before I begin: A fashion victim is someone who wears what someone else—a designer, a magazine, a high-minded friend—dictates. That said, I am a *major* fashion victim. The key to being a *successful* fashion victim is to embrace your affliction and dress with a great deal of confidence. I indulge in trends because I feel secure that I have enough that is personal and original in my style that I can (usually) get away with the ridiculously high wedge heel, the retro 70s sunglasses, or the leather patchwork skirt that I am wearing.

Yvonne Force (with Puff Baby) in head-to-toe Dolce and Gabbana, 2008.

My High Fashion Style

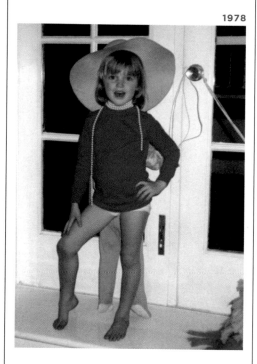

1978

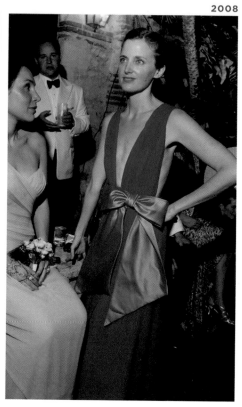

2008

The risk involved in wearing a "high fashion" look always gets my adrenaline going! Feeling nervous about a look before I wear it is usually a good thing. It means I'm really going for it. When I think about the best outfits I have worn in the last five years, I anticipated wearing each one with anxiety but felt amazing as soon as I walked out my front door. I still feel great about them. There was my mother's 1980s feather-covered evening gown that I'd waited twenty years to wear, but I wasn't sure if it would translate to today. It did. There was the Giambatista Valli giant fur coat I saw at a sample sale that I loved but thought maybe I'd feel silly in once I actually put it on to wear in reality. I don't. And then there are the countless trendy belts, scarves, and sunglasses that I buy at the flea market or from street stalls on Broadway because they're cheap and it doesn't matter if I'm bored with them in a week. Sometimes I am, sometimes not.

Yet I do, on occasion, go a little over-the-top and feel silly afterward, and sometimes I commit a full-on fashion disaster. But it's OK. I'd rather take risks and make a mistake here and there than feel bored by my look, or, even worse, "appropriate."

When I do mess up, however, I know right away. That predeparture uncertainty just doesn't go away, no matter how many compliments I get. The night I wore what I consider to be my worst outfit ever (pictured on page 24 if you need a laugh), both Serena Williams and Renée Zellweger came running up to me and told me how much they liked my dress. All I could do was look at them quizzically and say, "You do?" Not good. I can't even say I learned anything from that hideous dress. It didn't stop me from taking risks thereafter. I just thought I liked it before I left for the party, but then by the time I got home I thought it was the most awful thing I'd ever worn. The one insight I can make is that the dress came together in a big hurry. I had been

This page: (Left) Me, having early fashion fantasies at a friend's house, 1978.

(Right) Me, in a Zac Posen gown at Lauren and Andrés Santo Domingo's wedding in Cartagena, Colombia, 2009.

Opposite: A feature about my house in Vogue Living. I was scared that people would think I usually style myself that way, but I think it became clear in the photos that it's a fashion shoot, 2006.

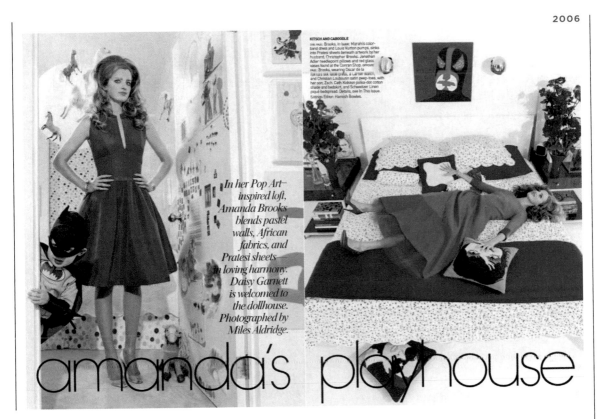

KITSCH AND CABOODLE

THIS PAGE: Brooks, in Isaac Mizrahi's color-band dress and Louis Vuitton pumps, sinks into Pratesi sheets beneath artwork by her husband, Christopher Brooks. Jonathan Adler needlepoint pillows and red glass vases found at the Conran Shop. OPPOSITE PAGE: Brooks, wearing Oscar de la Renta's silk faille sundress, a Cartier watch, and Christian Louboutin satin peep-toes, with her son, Zach. Cath Kidston polka-dot cotton shade and bedskirt, and Schweitzer Linen piqué bedspread. Details, see In This Issue.
Sittings Editor: Hamish Bowles.

In her Pop Art–inspired loft, Amanda Brooks blends pastel walls, African fabrics, and Pratesi sheets in loving harmony. Daisy Garnett is welcomed to the dollhouse. Photographed by Miles Aldridge.

amanda's playhouse

planning to wear a different, much safer dress, but I felt bored by it so Tuleh designer Bryan Bradley whipped me up something daring in a flash on his way out of town. Neither one of us put a whole lot of thought into it, and because I didn't have time to change it I just told myself it was good enough. Maybe if I'd had another day to think about it I would have gone with the safer option. But imagine if I always chose the safer option? I'd be nowhere! I hope that fashion disaster never strikes me again, but I'm sure it will. That's fashion. Designers are allowed to have good and bad reviews, and I should be too.

Regarding trends, some people might view them with skepticism, but I am a cautiously enthusiastic fan. Being ahead of the trend—anticipating it even before it goes down the runway—is ideal. But when I miss the cue, I'm usually happy riding the trend's wave with everyone else, as long as it is a trend that I feel is "me." My favorite way to be super

trendy is with vintage clothing. If the runways show a lot of plaid one season, instead of running to a department store to buy a designer piece or to the cheap chic store to buy a knockoff (that someone else will undoubtedly have), I prefer to scour eBay or thrift stores for my plaid. It saves me money and all but guarantees I'll be the only one wearing whatever treasure I found.

I also like pairing a trendy designer piece—something really expensive and of-the-moment like, say, a pair of black patent leather ankle boots, with a metallic gold platform—with something completely unrecognizable, like a no-name 70s hippie dress. That way I'm putting the trend in a new context to make it my own and to give it a different meaning. Whether I discover my take on a trend in the thrift store or buy it straight from the designer, it is especially important with trendy or high fashion clothes to make sure my look is personalized.

HIGH FASHION
My Favorite Things

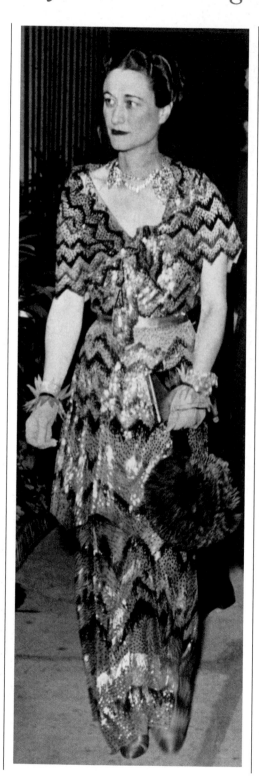

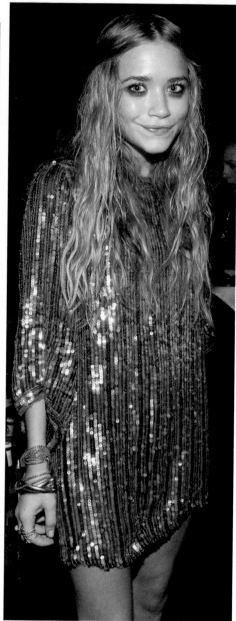

I like **SEQUINS** best when they are accompanied by a dose of good taste. Though sequins are, by definition, in stunningly bad taste, they can be carried off to great effect in the right context. When I'm wearing sequins I don't go crazy with them *and* the hair *and* the makeup. I let the sequins themselves be the main attraction and play everything else down a bit.

This page:
(Far left)
The Duchess of Windsor, 1937.
I love the sequin cape over the sequin dress.

(Left)
These days you don't need a special occasion to wear sequins. I see girls, like Mary Kate Olsen in 2006, wearing sequins out to a casual restaurant or even during the day.

Opposite:
Bianca Jagger, at the Christian Dior Haute Couture show in Paris, 1977.

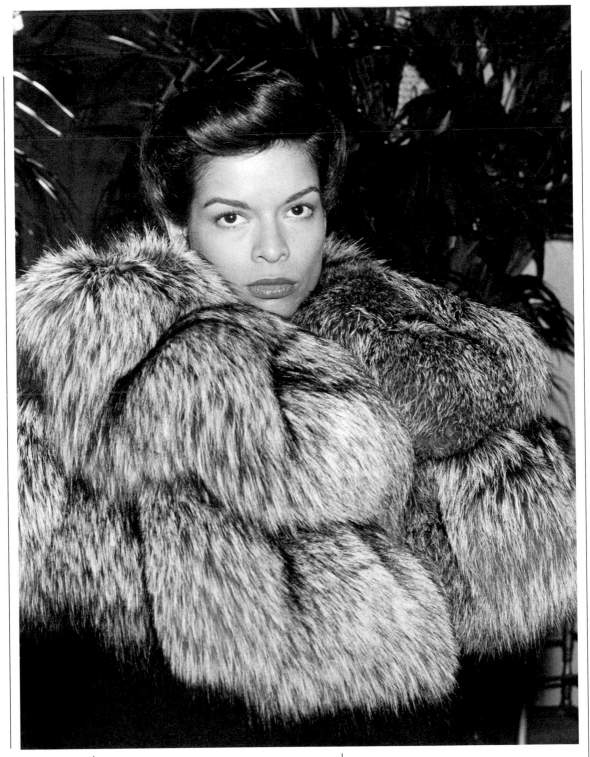

Any kind of **FUR THAT MAKES A BIG STATEMENT** will instantly give you an air of high fashion. I am, as you can probably tell, obsessed with fur. It's soft, flattering, feminine, glamorous, and warm! And it looks great with everything, from my rattiest old jeans to my shiniest, most outrageous evening gown.

Amanda Brooks

HIGH FASHION
My Favorite Things

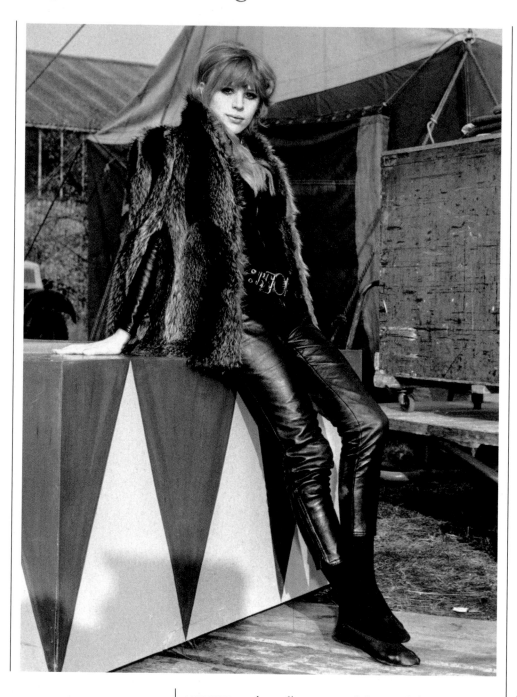

LEATHER can be really scary: reminiscent of the worst of 80s fashion. Something about it can look too harsh against soft, feminine features. But when leather looks good, it looks fantastic. I love the tough attitude of a pretty girl wearing leather in a way that adds an edge but doesn't overshadow her beauty.

Marianne Faithfull at Shepperton Studios in London, 1967. I like that she's wearing ballet flats with her leather "skins."

I can think of about three people in the world who can wear **SHORT SHORTS** (below), myself *not* included. But that doesn't mean I don't love them and wish that I could. Short shorts on the runway at a fashion show always thrill me; they create an unexpected and incredibly sexy proportion. If you're one of the lucky few who can pull them off, you have an obligation to wear them!

JUMPSUITS . . . LOOK GREAT WITH A PAIR OF SKY-HIGH HEELS AND CONFIDENCE TO MATCH.

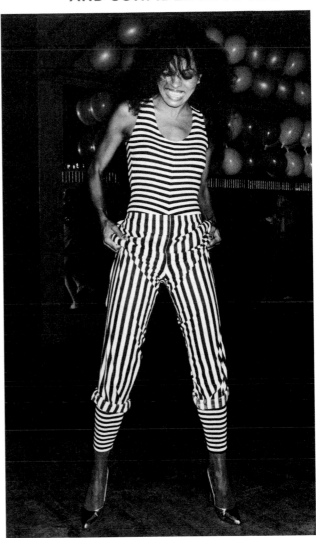

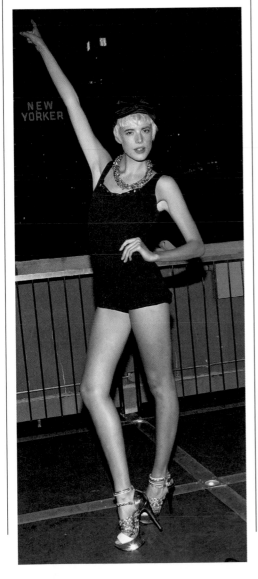

*Left:
If Agyness
Deyn's shorts
were any
shorter,
they may be
classified as
underwear.
2008.*

*Above:
Diana Ross,
1983.*

What does it take to pull off a **JUMPSUIT** (above)? A long, thin body and a lot of guts. There were a lot of wonderful, fluid jumpsuits produced in the 70s (the best ones are by Halston), and they look great with a pair of sky-high heels and confidence to match. Women who wear jumpsuits are really going for it. You gotta love them.

Amanda Brooks

HIGH FASHION
Accessories

STYLIZED BOOTS CAN TRANSFORM A SIMPLE OUTFIT SUCH AS SLIM JEANS AND A LOOSE T-SHIRT FROM SOMETHING STRAIGHTFORWARD INTO SOMETHING UNIQUELY STYLISH.

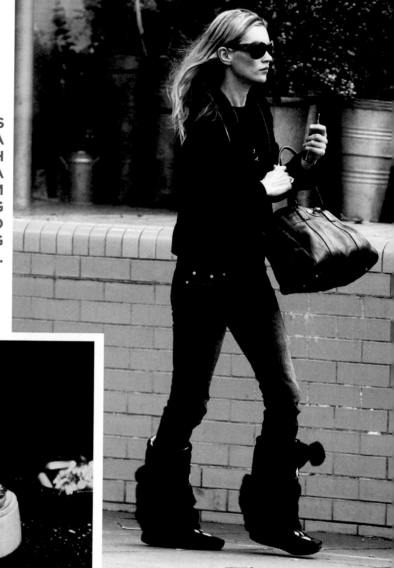

PLATFORM SHOES, in my opinion, are no longer trendy. They are a high fashion classic. They may not be in the mainstream every year, but if you are marching to the tune of your own style, platforms look good whenever you feel the desire to wear them.

Top left: Bianca Jagger's platform shoe with her Rolling Stones backstage pass attached, 1975.

Top right: Kate Moss, doing errands in London in her mukluks, traditional Eskimo moccasin boots, 2004.

STYLIZED BOOTS such as thigh highs, motorcycle boots, pirate boots, and cowboy boots have a lot of impact on an outfit. They can transform a simple outfit such as slim jeans and a loose T-shirt from something straightforward into something uniquely stylish. The trick here is to remember not to overaccessorize. The style of the boots is just about enough to cover your whole look.

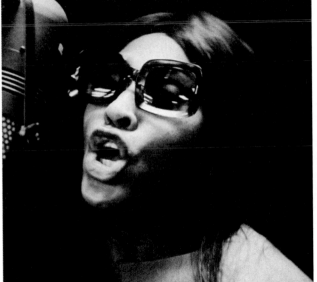

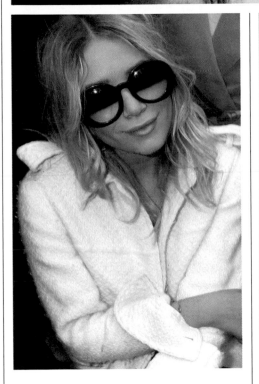

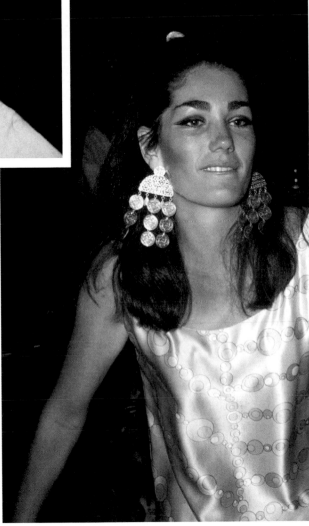

DRAMATIC SUNGLASSES have a big impact, and cheap chic ones are easy to find. Make sure they flatter you. Oversized frames, for example, can do wonders for some women but make others look like a bug. Trust your instincts: Put them on and really look at yourself—not just the glasses but what they do for your face and your overall appearance. If you feel good, go for it. If you have doubts, bring a friend back to help you evaluate or just move on to the next pair.

Clockwise from top: Tina Turner in a Los Angeles recording studio, 1961.

American society girl Minnie Cushing in Acapulco, 1966.

Mary Kate Olsen in Chanel sunglasses, 2008.

There are two ways to go with BIG STATEMENT JEWELRY. One is to wear jewelry of outrageous proportion: oversized gold hoop earrings, super long chandeliers, a huge cocktail ring, a big chunky necklace, all, perhaps, encrusted with something shiny—diamonds or rhinestones. But you can also go for quantity: ten gold chains layered on top of each other, rings on many fingers, bangles piled all the way up your forearm. Make an impact, and make it big.

HIGH FASHION
Accessories

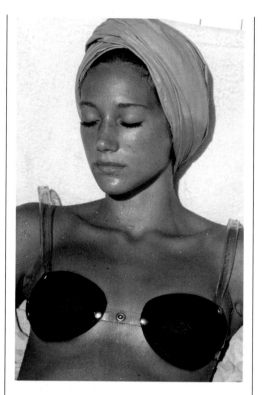

FASHION HATS (below) can attract all the attention in the room, in a good way, when they are worn convincingly.

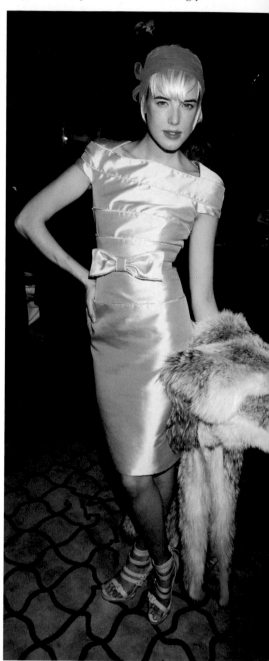

All I know about **TURBANS** (above) is that they look fabulous on some women and ridiculous on others. I once found an incredibly beautiful dark pink vintage velvet turban and tried it on with great anticipation. But when I looked in the mirror I instantly knew it wasn't me. On me it was cumbersome and overbearing, but it looked fabulous on my mom, whose facial bone structure is much more elegant than mine. I couldn't talk her into it, though.

In Palm Beach I knew an eccentric, stylish woman named Ancky Johnson who was married to my dad's best friend (her third husband, the previous two having been an Austrian count and the Revlon founder Charles Revson). I spent quite a lot of time around her; yet the only image of Ancky I can call to mind now is of her in a solid-colored caftan with a matching turban. I'm pretty sure that's all she ever wore, regardless of the occasion. She had this same outfit—turban and caftan—in many different colors and fabric variations and looked stunning in each of them.

Left: Marisa Berenson doing some high fashion sunbathing in Capri, 1968. Even her eye shadow matches her turban and bikini.

Right: Agyness Deyn, 2008.

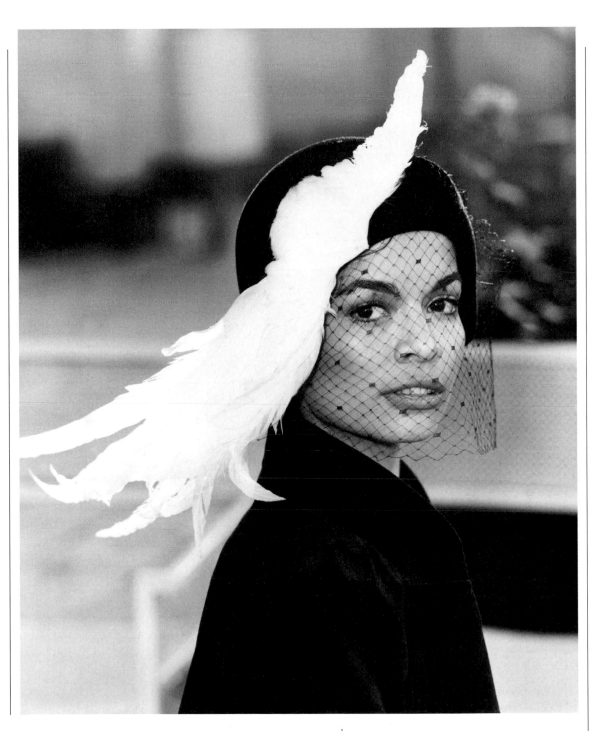

Bianca Jagger, winner of the 1972 Woman of the Year Hat Award.

You don't see too many people wearing **VEILS** today, but I think more people should. So chic, and in truth easier to wear than most hats. In order to avoid looking old-fashioned in a veil, strive for serious simplicity in the outfit. A veil like Bianca Jagger's (above) would look stunning with a simple black dress or even a silk blouse and classically tailored trousers.

Amanda Brooks

HIGH FASHION
Mixing It Up

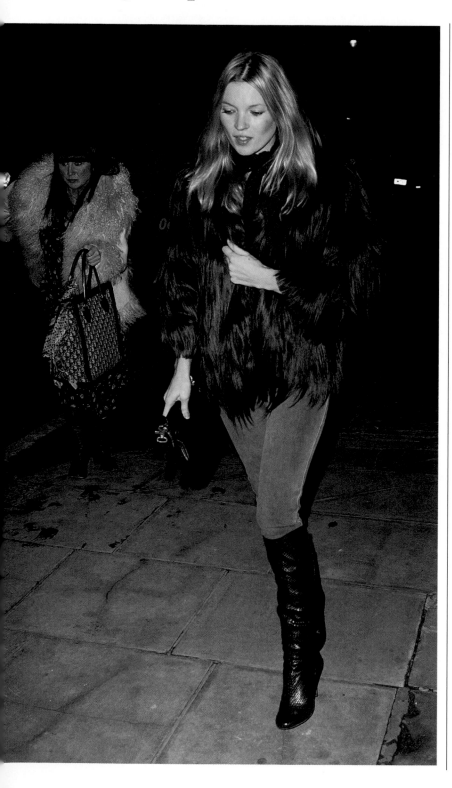

WELL-LOVED, WORN-IN DENIM (left) in any incarnation—a skirt, jeans, jacket, or vest—provides a great foil to the overt stylishness of high fashion clothes. Think of an ornate evening jacket with jeans, a sequined skirt with a worn-in jean jacket, or a classically tailored pantsuit with a denim vest under the jacket. Instant chic.

Balance trendy pieces with your favorite **CLASSIC BASICS**, like a white shirt, a trench coat, or khaki pants. It's like having an anchor for your outfit. Ninety percent of the clothes I wear today are classic basics with a little high fashion thrown in.

DENIM . . . PROVIDES A GREAT FOIL TO THE OVERT STYLISHNESS OF HIGH FASHION CLOTHES.

This page: Kate Moss dressing down her fur with jeans and boots, 2003.

Opposite: A 1966 André Courrèges outfit mixing sequins with sportswear.

HIGH FASHION
Getting It Right

Choose your **FOCAL POINT**. The "more is more" look just doesn't look right on many people. Begin with a loud piece of clothing or jewelry (a boldly printed skirt, voluminous blouse, or large necklace, for example) and construct your outfit around it, choosing more understated pieces that compliment it without competing for attention.

If you can't resist the fun of trying on a cliché, try **MIXING TWO CLICHÉS TOGETHER**. For example, when wearing something overtly glamorous, like sequins, create some irony by mixing it with sportswear, like in the photo at right. Inspired by this photo I went to an informal but festive Christmas party once in a gold sequin T-shirt with faded black jeans and worn-in leather riding boots. It felt much more interesting to me than being so straightforward.

When going for a trend, try **MIXING VINTAGE WITH NEW CLOTHES**. Vintage adds authenticity to any look and is particularly helpful in toning down trendiness.

MIXING TEXTURES is also effective. Try a leather vest over a silk dress, wear a rope bracelet next to a diamond one, or wear velvet shoes with a denim dress.

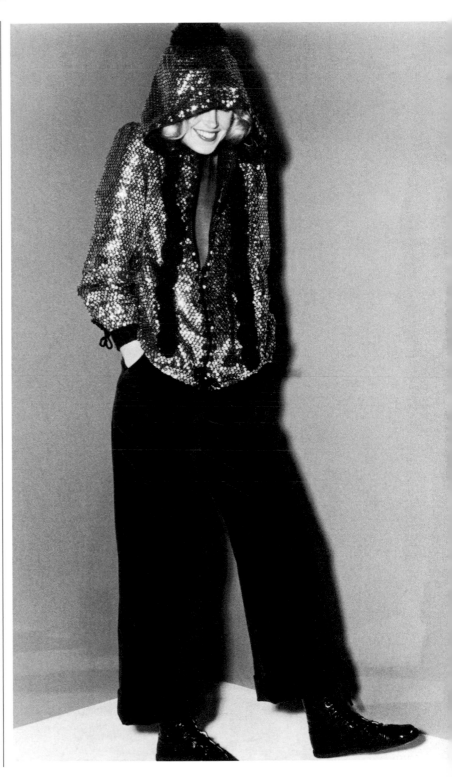

The most important part of putting together a high fashion evening look is considering every aspect and detail that make up your outfit: the clothes, the shoes, the hair, the makeup, the undergarments. And then there is the fun part, which are the inessentials, which are, of course, essential: Stockings? Shawl? Cape? Belt? Fresh flowers? Shoe clips? Hair clips? Nail color? Jewelry? Try thinking of yourself as the stylist of a fashion shoot and make yourself the subject. Every detail—whether "done" or "undone"—counts.

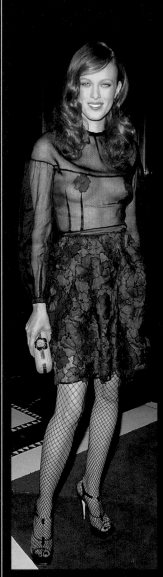

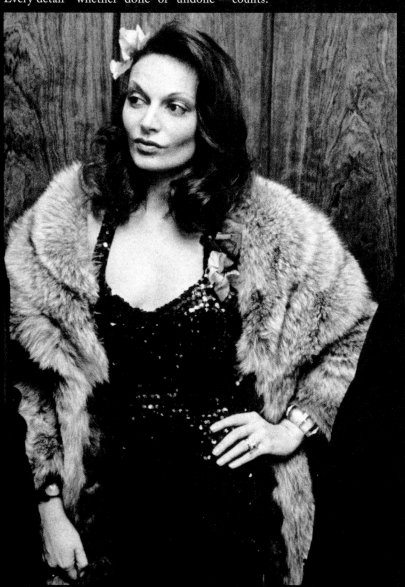

TRY THINKING OF YOURSELF AS THE STYLIST OF A FASHION SHOOT AND MAKE YOURSELF THE SUBJECT.

ORNATE MATERIALS like feathers, sequins, fur, embroidery, and beading are all easy shortcuts to a high fashion evening look. Whether new or vintage, clothes made in these materials guarantee a strong impact.

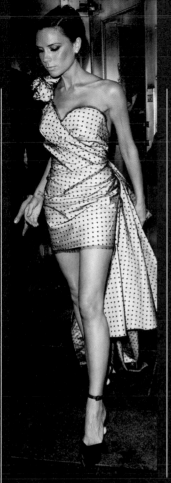

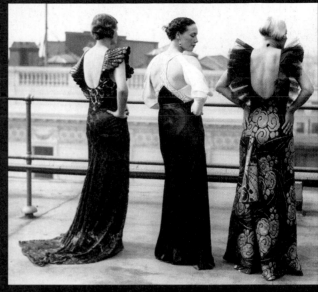

Opposite:
(Far left)
Diane von
Furstenberg at
the Rainbow
Room, 1972.

(Left)
Karen Elson in
Yves Saint
Laurent, 2006.

This page:
(Clockwise
from left)
Victoria
Beckham in
Marc Jacobs,
2009.

High fashion
evening gowns,
1933.

Cher, 1971.

VOLUME—whether in the sleeve or the skirt—also creates drama for evening.

Pay attention to BALANCE: A great way to make an overtly decorative dress look modern is to wear it simply, without major hair, much makeup, or any jewelry. Putting the focus on the dress itself can be a refreshing and novel experience. If, on the other hand, your dress is more pared down, go for it with the accessories and styling.

Don't be afraid to IMPROVISE: Belt your dress, add a bolero to a long gown, or wear plain pants with a decorative jacket. I was once at a wedding in Germany and realized that my ruffly floral chiffon dress would look that much better with a belt, but the only belt I had with me was a brown leather jeans belt—not something I'd imagine wearing in the evening, let alone to a wedding. But oddly enough I kind of liked the way it contrasted with my formal dress and the fresh flowers I'd put in my hair, so I just went for it. Whatever everyone else thought, I felt great.

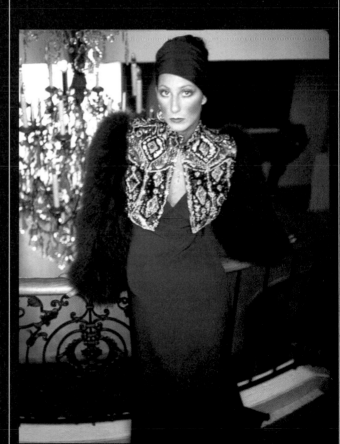

HIGH FASHION
Icons

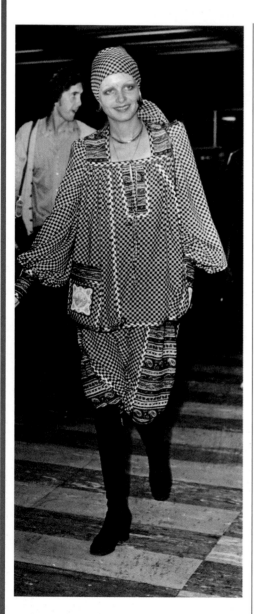

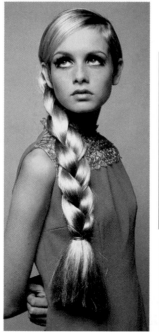

Twiggy,
1971, 1966,
and 1967.

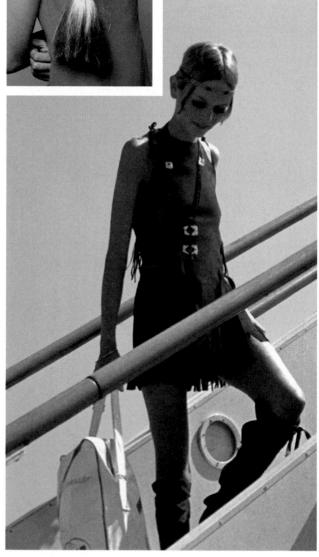

Although the 60s and 70s differed drastically in their styles, supermodel **TWIGGY** looked enviably amazing in both decades. She was often photographed in tent dresses, miniskirts, and children's-wear-inspired fashions in the 60s, and then lo and behold she seamlessly adopted a softer, more romantic hippie look in the 70s, with fringed suede boots, long ethnic dresses, and floppy hats. Cropped hair and mascara-laden doe eyes completed her signature look.

> **"THERE ARE NO CHIC AMERICAN WOMEN.**
> **THE ONE EXCEPTION IS NAN KEMPNER."**
> —DIANA VREELAND

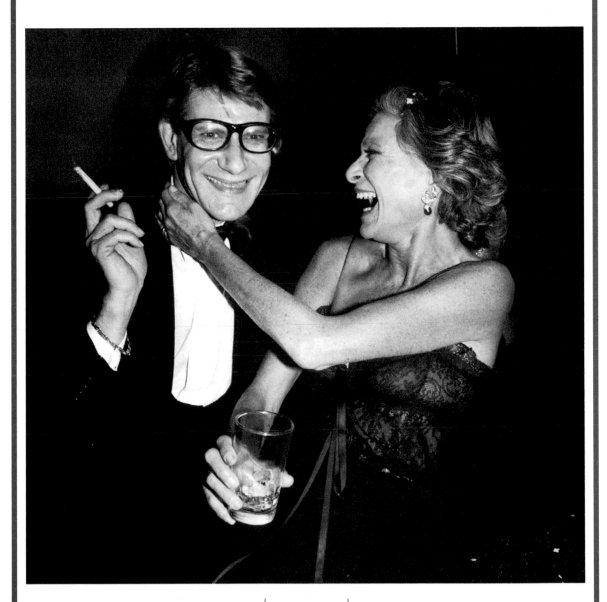

Society queen and renowned couture client **NAN KEMPNER** was such a remarkable fashion icon that an entire exhibit at the Metropolitan Museum of Art was dedicated to her clothes and her style after she died in 2005. Her lifelong passion for clothes led to the acquisition of a massive couture collection, including legendary pieces by Bill Blass, Yves Saint Laurent, and Mainbocher. Her uptown classic style did not prevent her from indulging in loud colors and bold jewelry, which let us know she didn't take it all so seriously. She was even known to show some skin, right into her seventies.

Nan Kempner with Yves Saint Laurent, 1978.

Amanda Brooks

HIGH FASHION
Icons

**"YOU CAN ALWAYS TELL WHERE
DIANA ROSS HAS BEEN
BY THE HAIR THAT'S LEFT BEHIND!"**
—DIANA ROSS

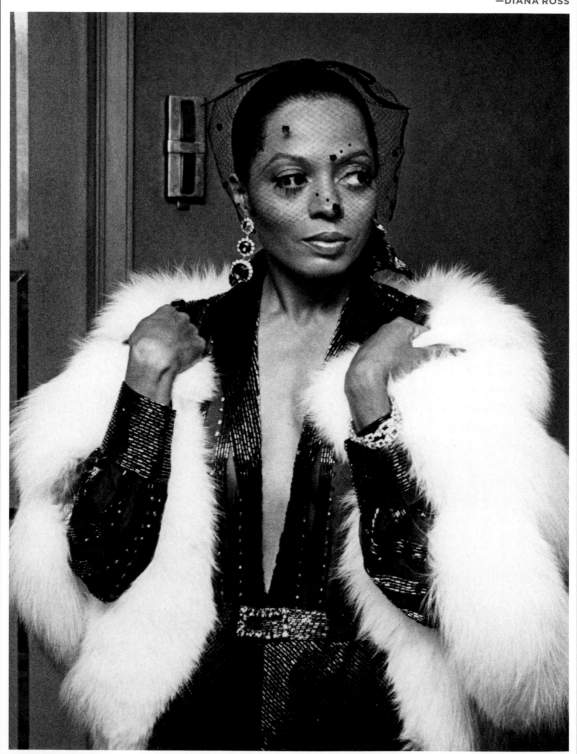

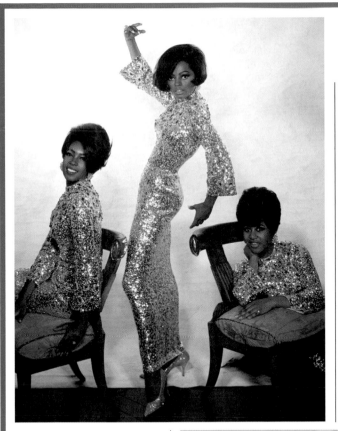

The thing I love most about DIANA ROSS's style is the fact that she has never been afraid to change it. She's been a chic 60s "lady," a groovy hipster, an onstage drama queen, an elegant champion of black style, a preppy girl, and simply a beautiful face, all while distinctly maintaining her Diana Ross aura. My personal favorite era for her is the 70s—at once groovy and chic.

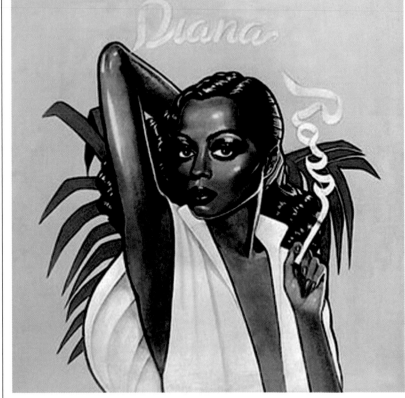

Opposite: Diana Ross, 1978

This page: (Above) With the Supremes, 1960s.

(Right) Diana Ross album cover, 1978.

HIGH FASHION
Icons

**"I WASN'T REALLY NAKED.
I SIMPLY DIDN'T
HAVE ANY CLOTHES ON."**
—JOSEPHINE BAKER

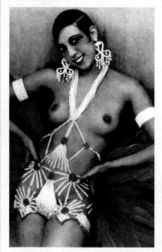

JOSEPHINE BAKER's style is an exercise in outrageousness. Originally an exotic dancer, Baker went on to be a successful singer, dancer, and actress. Ernest Hemingway called her "the most sensational woman anyone ever saw," and she played muse for Langston Hughes, F. Scott Fitzgerald, and Pablo Picasso, among others. Who could fail to be inspired by a woman who often appeared onstage dressed only in high heels and a skirt made of bananas, or elaborate headdresses, oversized feathers, turbans, cumbersome jewelry, and dramatic makeup? She walked her pet cheetah on a diamond leash. Many would follow but few would match her outrageous glamour.

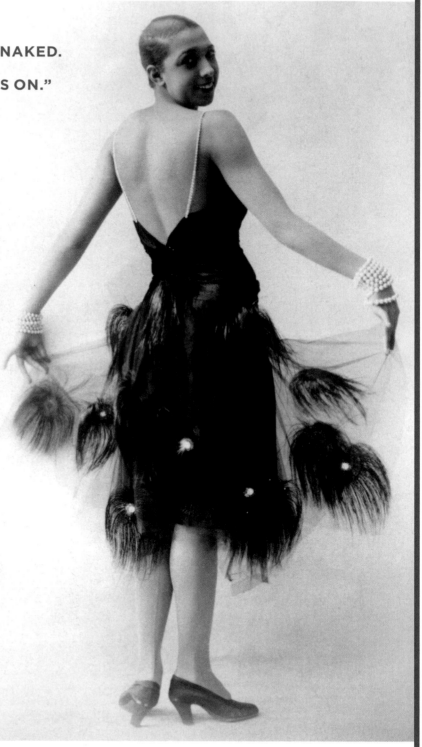

I was in Paris the first time I laid eyes on fashion muse **ISABELLA BLOW**. It was 1997, and I had recently started dating Christopher, the man who would become my husband. We were in Paris for a wedding, and he said he wanted us to have lunch with a childhood friend of his. As we walked into the eternally glamorous Brasserie Lipp, I was about to tap Christopher on the shoulder and say, "Check out that girl in the crazy hat!" when I realized that he was steering me straight toward her! She jumped up, gave us both a hug and kiss, and sat back down to continue savagely gnawing the chicken bone she'd been occupied with before we walked in. I thought I knew high fashion; I lived in New York, and in college I had friends who thought nothing of attending class in head-to-toe Chanel. But I had never in my life seen someone dressed as dramatically as Isabella. She was wearing a tight black corset with a silk taffeta coat and a black hat that looked like a black beanie topped by a large silk rose and a black veil—*to lunch!* I would later learn that Issy *always* dressed like that—even to walk her dogs in the country. She was a true fashion original. She always wore a crazy hat, an edgy dress, and outrageous shoes (with, say, a silk poppy six inches in diameter perched on the toe). She was the one who actually wore designers' most far-flung fantasies, the ones cynics say exist only to sell perfume and win licensing deals. For that reason she had a symbiotic relationship with some of the most famous designers in the world. She was credited with discovering Alexander McQueen, and her role as muse to Philip Treacy was so fruitful that there is an entire book about their relationship (*Philip Treacy: When Philip Met Isabella*, published by Assouline). Isabella died in May 2007, and I don't exaggerate when I say that the entire fashion world misses her.

Opposite: Josephine Baker, 1925 and 1930.

This page: (Right) Isabella Blow in her signature Philip Treacy hat, 2004.

(Far right) The photo I took of Issy the first day I met her, Paris, 1997.

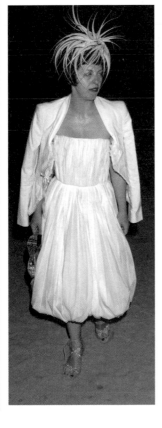

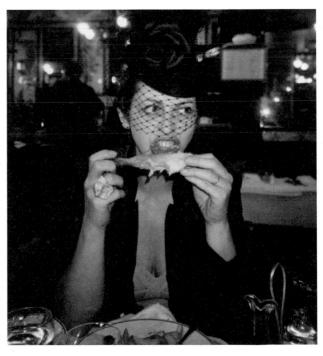

"MY STYLE ICON IS ANYONE WHO MAKES A BLOODY EFFORT."
—ISABELLA BLOW

HIGH FASHION
The New Originals

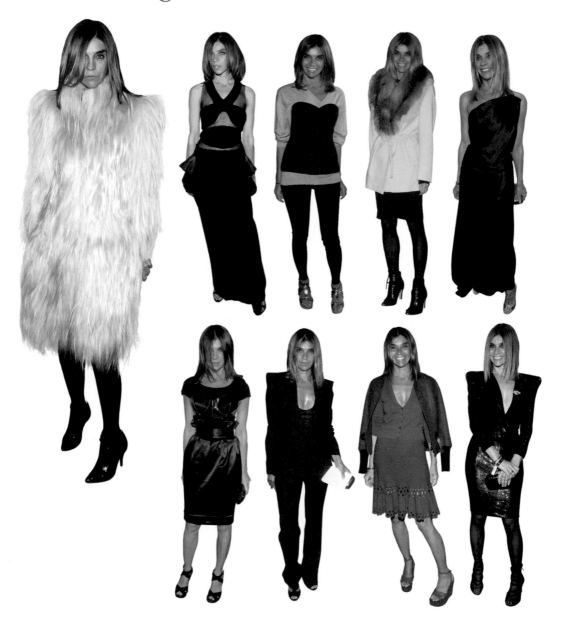

CARINE ROITFELD editor in chief, French *Vogue* Everyone in the fashion world is in awe of Carine. Her signature sexy Goth-ish look is so strong and consistent and yet somehow completely organic; it is *her* look, not something fabricated by a designer or a magazine. As the editor in chief of super cool French *Vogue* and a former muse to Tom Ford (at both Yves Saint Laurent and Gucci), she has wielded incredible influence. The flavor-of-the-week celebrity may have thousands of teenage copycats, but inspiring fashion bibles and designer labels is a whole other story. She is amazing.

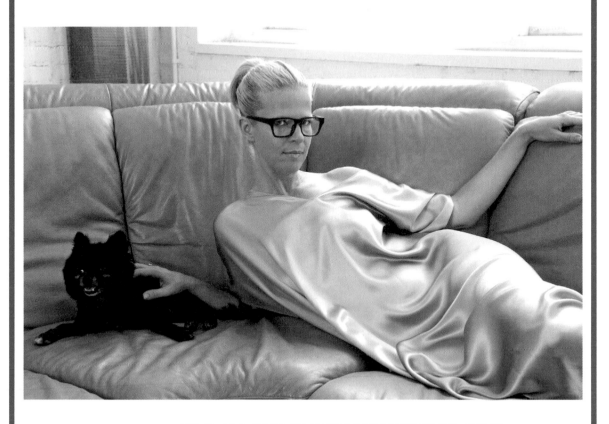

FOR ALL THE ICONS YVONNE EMULATES, THE PERSON SHE'S BEST AT CHANNELING IS ACTUALLY HERSELF.

Yvonne Force at home, with Puff Baby, 2008.

YVONNE FORCE co-founder, Art Production Fund
Yvonne is a remarkable woman. As a public art producer, mother, lead singer of her own band, and style icon, she is ambitious in all the best ways. Fashion is only a sidebar, an asterisk when I think of all the factors that go into making her fabulous. But it is exactly her fabulousity that informs her fashion. She is the only girl I know who can wear an exact look (right down to the bag, the shoes, the hair, and the makeup) from a designer's runway and not lose herself in the look. She has no fear of taking on an image or persona that she has in her mind and fully inhabiting that. "You are what you pretend to be," she says. But she also says that she is very careful in picking the personas she chooses to emulate. They have to fit in with her own personal rules of style, which revolve around big blonde hair, dark eye makeup, pale lipstick, and monochrome clothes. No prints, no bright colors. So, one day she's channeling Bianca Jagger in a white pantsuit and the next day she's strutting her stuff like a model from the Gucci runway in a pale pink silk gown, pale pink fur chubby jacket, pale pink silk sandals with fur pompoms, and a pink fur clutch. The month after that, she's a 60s drama queen with teased hair, thick eyeliner, and black mod clothes. Next, she'll add black glasses to add a little Gloria Steinem to her already established Brigitte Bardot. For all the icons Yvonne emulates, the person she's best at channeling is actually herself.

HIGH FASHION
The New Originals

"EVERY TIME I SEE A PHOTO OF MYSELF FROM THE PAST MONTH I THINK, 'WHAT WAS I THINKING?'"
—CHLOË SEVIGNY

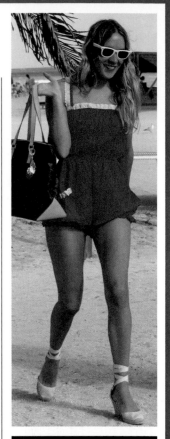

CHLOË SEVIGNY
actress, *fashion muse*

Chloë is one of the most high fashion celebrities out there. And she's *really* good at it. So good that she is a muse to many designers: Alber Elbaz at Lanvin, Dolce and Gabbana, Stefano Pilati at Yves Saint Laurent. She has good taste, she has a sophisticated understanding of inspiration, and she's excellent at adding her own style to a designer look (retro hair, secretary glasses, vintage jewelry). She's also not afraid of trying daring new looks. I ran into her at the Costume Institute benefit at the Metropolitan Museum of Art once. She had straight bangs with ringlets hanging down the side and the rest swept up into a bun. She was definitely going for some look, but I didn't quite get it. That said, it actually made me like her style more. People with personal style often make mistakes. That's how we learn what suits us. It's that fearlessness in trying a new idea. Sometimes it works and sometimes it doesn't. But on the whole, Chloë has a way of combining her classic New England looks and her traditional sense of taste (cultivated in her Darien, Connecticut, upbringing) with a bit of edge and a bit of irony. It works for me.

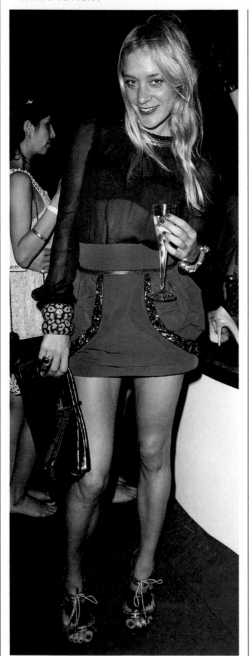

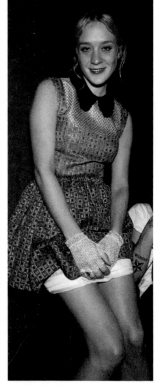

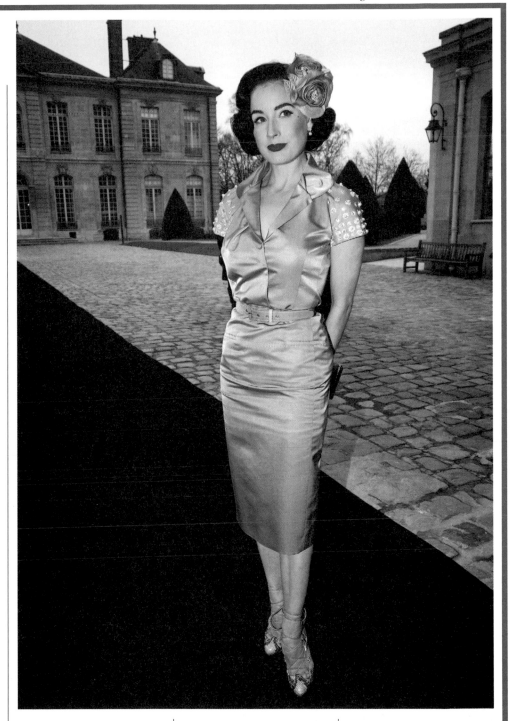

Opposite:
Chloë Sevigny
in 2008, 2005,
and 2008.

This page:
Dita von
Teese, at the
Christian Dior
Haute Couture
show in Paris,
2009.

DITA VON TEESE
burlesque dancer

I first saw Dita von Teese perform at a party Diane von Furstenberg gave for Christian Louboutin in 2005. I loved her fresh take on burlesque, but I was even more transfixed by her offstage look after the show—the combination of her sexy body, immaculate hair and makeup, and her vintage-inspired clothes. It would be so easy to look old-fashioned in the outfits she wears, but she manages to make the overall effect so clean and refined that she pulls it off. And she might just be the only one that could pull it off. Her style is truly one of a kind.

Refining Your Style

Left:
Peggy
Guggenheim in
Venice, 1968.
She was the
ultimate
eccentric.

Below:
Capucine in
Paris, 1964.

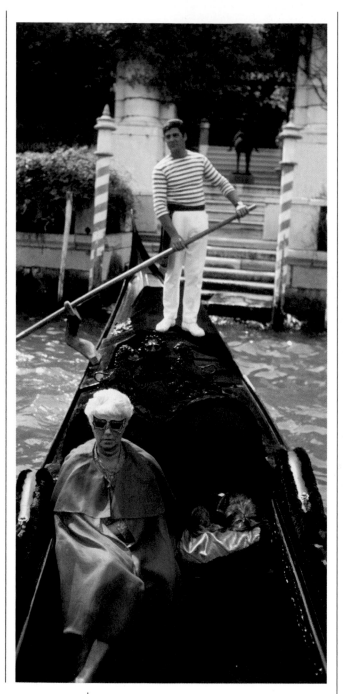

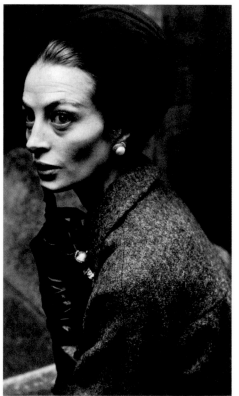

ECCENTRIC HIGH FASHION
Exotic animal skins, excessive amounts of feathers and sequins, fashion hats, sky-high heels, capes, heavily embellished evening gowns, statement jewelry.

PARISIAN HIGH FASHION
Silk trench coat, bondage shoes, tuxedos, waist belts, impeccably tailored little black dresses, silk scarves.

I Love Your Style

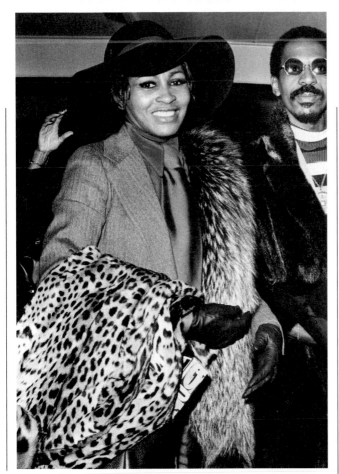

> **"I TELL PEOPLE ALL THE TIME I WANT TO BE BURIED NAKED. I KNOW THERE WILL BE A STORE WHERE I'M GOING."**
> —NAN KEMPNER

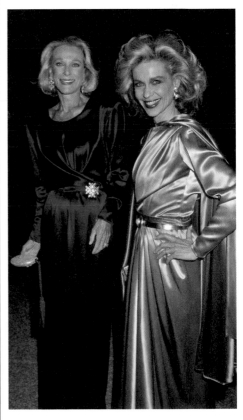

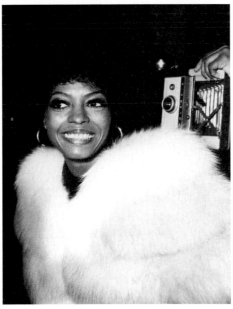

Clockwise from top: I couldn't get over this picture when I found it. Tina Turner (seen here with her husband Ike) really has it going on, 1972.

Nan Kempner and Lynn Wyatt exemplifying the excess of the 80s in 1988.

Diana Ross, 1971.

GHETTO FABULOUS
Over-the-top fur coats, gold and diamond jewelry, fedoras, bold animal prints, high-heeled boots, embellished minidresses, logos galore.

PARK AVENUE HIGH FASHION
Hermès Kelly bag, fur coats, stiletto pumps, fitted suits, designer sunglasses, lots of jewelry, coiffed hair.

HIGH FASHION
Refining Your Style / *Editorial High Fashion*

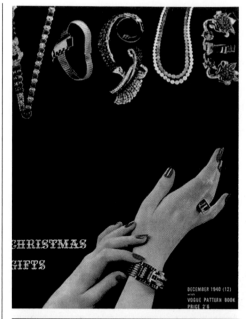
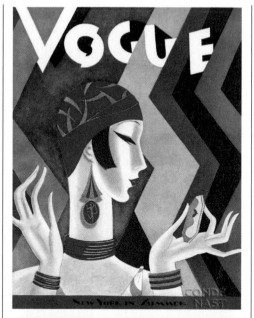
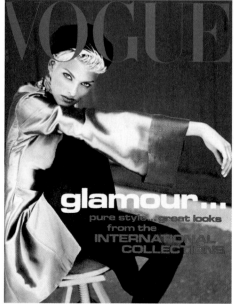
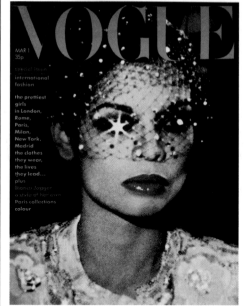

*Clockwise from
top left:
1940, 1926,
1974, 1991.*

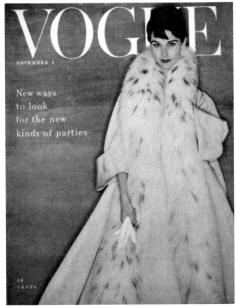

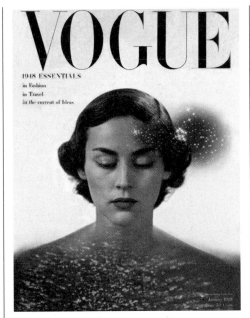

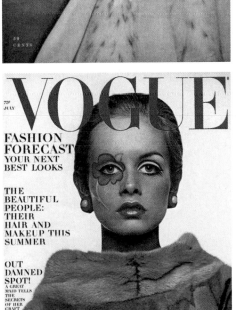

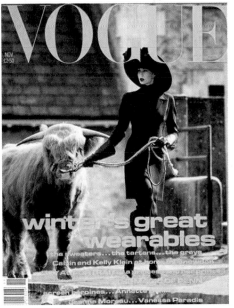

Clockwise from top left: 1954, 1948, 1991, 1967.

**"YOU'RE CONSIDERED SUPERFICIAL
AND SILLY IF YOU ARE INTERESTED IN FASHION,
BUT I THINK YOU CAN BE SUBSTANTIAL
AND STILL BE INTERESTED IN FRIVOLITY."**
—SOFIA COPPOLA

Amanda Brooks

HIGH FASHION
Inspiration

BOOKS

Louise Dahl-Wolfe
foreword by
Dorothy Twining Globus;
essays by Vicki Goldberg
and Nan Richardson
These meticulous and stylized magazine photographs taken by Louise Dahl-Wolfe in the 1940s and 50s are great inspiration for anyone who loves vintage high fashion.

**Decades of Beauty:
The Changing Images of
Women, 1890s to 1990s**
by Kate Mulvey and
Melissa Richards
A really well-organized look at each decade of fashion and style in the twentieth century: designers, stars, icons, current events, makeup, clothes. If historical dressing interests you at all, you gotta have this book.

**Yves Saint Laurent:
Images of Design 1958–1988**
by David Teboul
Since just about every current designer is inspired by Yves Saint Laurent, you might as well be too. All the books about his work are good, but this one is my favorite. It focuses on his earlier work, which I prefer. I love 1970s Yves Saint Laurent.

**In Vogue: The Illustrated
History of the World's Most
Famous Fashion Magazine**
by Alberto Oliva
and Norberto Angeletti
A bible of iconic fashion images from the twentieth century, this book is filled with inspiration, history, and fantastic photos—previously unseen.

D.V.
by Diana Vreeland
The memoir of a woman this passionately devoted to fashion and engaged with life is obviously a must-have. *D.V.* perfectly captures the delightfully witty personality of one of fashion's most treasured icons, plus it has tons of great candid photos and portraits.

Height of Fashion
by Amy Spindler, Lisa Eisner, and Roman Alonso
This hysterical record of the trials and triumphs of people's fashion lives is the result of its brilliant editors having asked their friends (including Tom Ford, Carine Roitfeld, Anh Duong, and others both famous and unknown) to send in a personal snapshot they consider their "height of fashion." One of the most amusing aspects of the book is to witness how seriously—or not—people take themselves in their choice of photo. You'll have a good time looking at this book.

Clifford Coffin
by Robin Muir
Sometimes when I'm looking for inspiration for an evening outfit I open my Clifford Coffin book. He was an amazing fashion photographer who often worked for *Vogue* in the 40s and 50s. These are pictures of rich women dressed to the nines, and the details are incredible. The picture of Lisa Fonssagrives on page 63 is one of my all-time favorite fashion images. She has a *red* french manicure (which I copied for the rehearsal dinner of my wedding). And Babe Paley on page 133 in a short fur jacket with creased trousers is as chic as anything I've ever seen.

FILMS

Grey Gardens

This brilliant documentary captures the bold fashion sensibility of Edith "Edie" Bouvier Beale, an eccentric relative of Jackie O. She refers to her outfits as "revolutionary costumes," and hordes of fans adore her topsy-turvy but oddly glamorous way with clothes: skirts worn upside down, sweaters worn as head scarves. Her fondness for house cats is also quite memorable.

3 Women

Sissy Spacek and Shelley Duvall look incredible in this surreal Robert Altman classic. They wear a mix of pastel summer dresses, ruffled blouses, and surprisingly fashionable high-waisted pants. I dream of finding clothes like these in thrift stores.

Rosemary's Baby

Aside from the whole Satan-spawn thing, what could be cuter than Mia Farrow in *Rosemary's Baby*? Her famous hairstyle looks as good today as it did then, as does her girlish mix of baby-doll dresses and Mary Janes.

The Women

Joan Crawford looks stylish as ever in this 1939 film, which features spectacular costumes by famed Hollywood costume designer Adrian. A must-rent for anyone with a love for 30s clothing and cat fights.

The Discreet Charm of the Bourgeoisie

Delphine Seyrig and Stephane Audran play ambassadors' wives as incredibly chic as this Luis Buñuel classic is surreal. Seyrig looks flawless in a dramatic pussycat bow blouse paired with a little black dress. A great resource for European high fashion.

The Bitter Tears of Petra von Kant

This gorgeous film explores the life of Petra von Kant, an eccentric, arrogant fashion designer on the verge of a nervous breakdown. She makes Joan Crawford look tame! The deeply embellished couturelike gowns that she wears are not to be missed.

Mahogany

Diana Ross plays a model turned fashion designer in this highly enjoyable rags-to-riches story with frequent costume changes. It's the ultimate black style movie.

Rear Window

Somehow seductive and impeccably prim at once, Grace Kelly brings a breath of fresh, uptown air into bohemian photographer Jimmy Stewart's sweltering Greenwich Village apartment, eventually winning him over with her full skirts, pearls, and bright red lipstick.

Shampoo

Julie Christie always looks great, but I am particularly fond of her style in *Shampoo*. Her black sequined column dress is a memorable highlight; Kate Moss loved it so much that she wore a custom-made replica to the CFDA Awards. And Goldie Hawn looks amazing in thigh-grazing dresses and punchy colors. A total treat for fans of 60s and 70s fashion.

Charade

Audrey Hepburn looks impeccable in *Charade*. The fact that she's decked out in head-to-toe Givenchy probably has something to do with it. Her big sunglasses and head scarves are the icing on the cake.

The Hunger

I am obsessed with Catherine Deneuve's style in *The Hunger*. She looks so elegant in her black Yves Saint Laurent column dresses, and her accessories—everything from studded leather gloves to quirky cat-eye sunglasses—add an edgy (and very 80s) touch to her polished look.

Blow-Up

Set in London during the 60s, *Blow-Up* revolves around the life of a fashion photographer. The mod fashions are incredible, and it features Jane Birkin *and* Veruschka.

Picnic at Hanging Rock

Set at a girls' boarding school in 1900, this film is a fashion gold mine for those with a passion for Victorian clothing. The lovely white lace dresses that the schoolgirls wear recently inspired an Alexander McQueen collection.

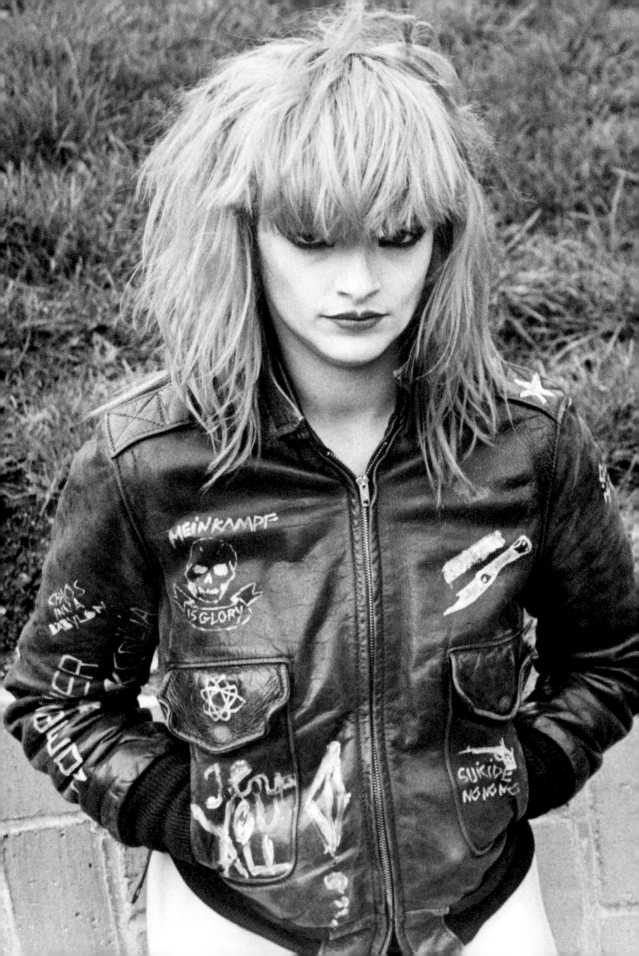

STREET

"

MY INTEREST IN FASHION STEMS FROM THE WAY PEOPLE EXPRESS THEMSELVES THROUGH THE CLOTHES THEY WEAR. IT DOESN'T MATTER WHAT KIND OF CLOTHES INDIVIDUAL DESIGNERS MAKE. WHAT IS IMPORTANT ARE ONE'S THOUGHTS AND THE ABILITY TO EXPRESS THEM, ONE'S LIFE AND ITS RELATIONSHIP TO THE ENVIRONMENT. WHEN SUCH ELEMENTS ARE COMBINED THEY CREATE A SCULPTURE. THIS SCULPTURE I CALL STREET FASHION."

—SHOICHI AOKI, PHOTOGRAPHER OF JAPANESE CULT STREET MAGAZINE *FRUITS*

The cool kids walking the streets of the world's great cities—whether it be Brooklyn, Mumbai, or Tokyo—are true fashion pioneers, inspiring us directly and through the work of the designers they influence. It used to be that fashion inspiration started at haute couture and worked its way down to the Gap, but today it seems that the opposite is true. Urban living inspires creative dressing by squeezing masses of people with totally different lives into the same streets. You can't help but absorb new ideas every time you get on the subway, go to the ATM, or stop in a deli for a bottle of water. In the past century we've seen mods, rappers, punks, black panthers, beatniks, and other urban dwellers establish trends, which are then studied and copied to the point of mainstream assimilation. Just when you begin to worry that convention and consumerism is all that's left, street kids think up something new.

German singer Nina Hagen, 1979.

Street style does not have a concrete definition and look book; therefore there are no suggested items in this chapter, as there are in the others. But there are lots of amazing and inspiring photos that have the potential to be more instructive than any summary of street style I can give you. I want you to open your eyes and be ready to discover new ideas in this chapter. If the idea appeals to you, you have two options: You can create your *own* street style based on your life, your ideas, and your cultural interests or political beliefs— whatever you feel strongly enough to associate yourself with. Or you can have fun experimenting with street styles from the past and present that will, of course, lead to the creation of your own style anyway.

STREET
My Street Style

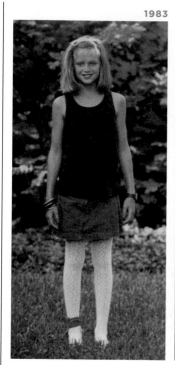

1983

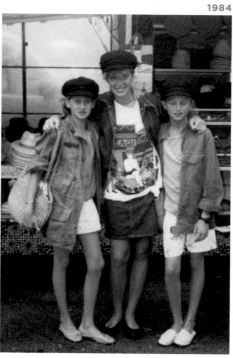

1984

MY SISTER AND I SAW LOTS OF YOUNG PARISIANS IN ARMY CLOTHES AND THOUGHT THEY WERE AMAZING.

I can thank MTV for my most profound childhood exposure to street style. Throughout fourth grade I did my best sartorial impersonation of Michael Jackson: rolled-up jeans, penny loafers (mine were brown because I wasn't allowed to wear black at that age), and T-shirts covered with Michael Jackson pins. Wow! I desperately wanted a rip-off of one of the leather jackets he wore in the "Beat It," "Thriller," or "Billie Jean" videos, but my mom (bless her!) wouldn't allow it.

When the thrill of Michael Jackson wore off, I became intrigued by the older boys who lived in my neighborhood. They were obsessed with skateboarding and BMX biking, and my best friend, Alexandra (the only other girl who lived in my neighborhood), and I talked our way into their crowd. Soon we were wearing Vans sneakers, cropped pants, and trying to make our hair more "skater" by spraying it with Sun-In (we applied in the shower so our mothers wouldn't notice).

When I was ten I spent a summer in France with my family. My sister and I saw lots of young Parisians in army clothes and thought they were amazing. We went to the flea markets and discovered piles and piles of intricately styled army coats and navy blue wool marines' hats. We bought the smallest ones we could find. They were still huge on us, but we loved them anyway.

The neighborhood I now call home, New York City's Lower East Side, exposes me to street style every day. When I moved here in 2002, I was cautious when I ventured out into the street; it seemed a world away from my parents' home on East Sixty-seventh Street. But it was already undergoing dramatic changes, for better or for worse. Young hipsters and aspiring artists mixed in with kids from nearby housing projects and struggling city schools, and inventive restaurants and vintage boutiques were opening next door to the old fabric clearance warehouses and run-down bodegas. The clash and harmony and history add up to a few square blocks with great style. It's real, it's original, and it's *young*. On my block a hip-hop store with the best sneakers and brightly colored logo T-shirts sits next

Left:
Me, dressing up as Madonna for a talent contest at summer camp in Palm Beach, 1983.

Right:
My sister, my friend Celerie, and me, wearing our army jackets purchased from a street vendor in Bordeaux, France, 1984. We felt so cool that day.

1985

2002

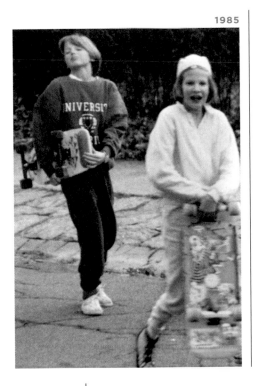

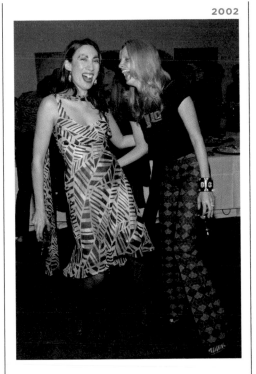

*Left:
My friend
Alexandra
(right) and
me (left),
trying the
skateboarder
look on for
size, 1985.*

*Right:
If you look
closely you'll see
I'm wearing a
rhinestone-
encrusted J.Lo
T-shirt and
African
lady-printed
jeans. Don't
know what
that was about.
Maybe that's
what my friend
Anh Duong
was laughing
at (2002).*

to an old-school barber/custom-fit tailor. The kids who walk down my street have way more personal style than you'll find in a magazine or on a runway. There are girls with matching parkas, Timberland boots, nails, and eye shadow—all in the same color. There are grungy fashion lovers wearing thrift store trends with a new sense of proportion. (Not to mention a group of guys who walk down the street looking like extras from *Star Trek*. They must make their own clothes, because I've never seen anything like them in a store!)

But I haven't forgotten myself. I always really go for it when I dress for evening, even if the overall look is more Upper East Side than Lower East Side. When I take my kids to school in the morning on my way to the gym, I'm sure I look more suburban mom than urban mom. But my neighbors have affected my style in bits and pieces. Their street style has seeped in, put ideas in my head, and changed my perspective and my expectations. My favorite thing is to see a girl walking down my street who looks completely enviable but

whose look has nothing to do with what's going on in the fashion world. She's found her own style, and that's inspiring.

There are more immediate effects of downtown living too. The hip-hop store makes me consider bright colors when I only feel like wearing neutrals. The barber shop once made me think about lumberjack plaids because I saw an old red-and-black wool Pendleton jacket sitting in the window. I wear sneakers with almost everything—even furs and designer jackets—because they feel right in my surroundings. At least once a week I see a girl who challenges my traditional sense of proportion: dresses over pants, short vests over long winter coats, long sweaters worn as dresses, cropped jackets with long skirts. I worry less about roots in my hair and chipped nail polish on my toes; uptown these lapses might be more noticed, but here they just don't stand out—in fact they make me feel more at home in my neighborhood.

I hope I always live in a place that inspires me as much as Chrystie Street.

STREET
Icons

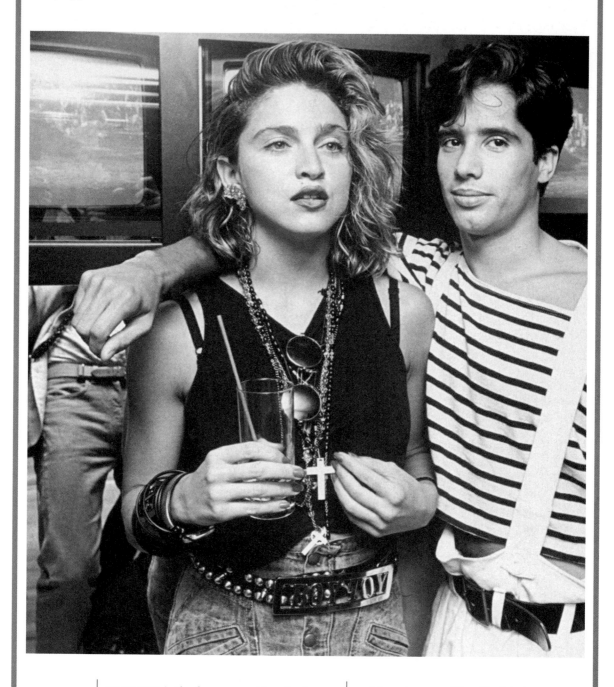

Madonna, with Jellybean Benitez, 1984.

MADONNA is the foremost emblem (and practitioner) of self-invention in our time, and she got her start as, what else, a downtown girl. That's my favorite Madonna phase: scrappy 80s East Village punk. She wore armloads of rubber bracelets, ripped T-shirts, leggings, and her signature "Boy Toy" belt, and soon thousands of other girls did too. Now we see her in Versace and Stella McCartney, but she proved her fashion chops without the designer clothes and celebrity stylist that seem always to be attached to fame today.

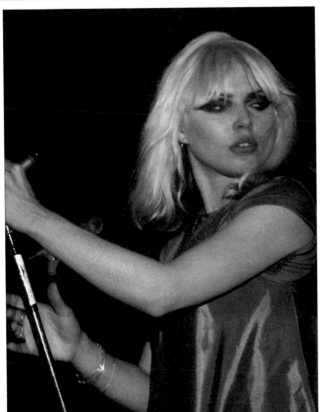

How amazing is **DEBBIE HARRY** of Blondie? The New Wave pioneer made high, high style out of the most basic clothes. Blondie created her own radical and cutting-edge look by means of dramatically different styling. T-shirts, jeans, leggings, sweatshirts, sneakers, and cut-offs were ripped, hiked up, layered, and mixed with major hair and makeup to create one of the iconic music-scene looks of the late 70s. She's one of the few women who actually pulled off spandex!

Left:
Debbie Harry,
1980.

Below:
Debbie Harry,
1977. She
reminds me of
Kate Moss in
this photo.

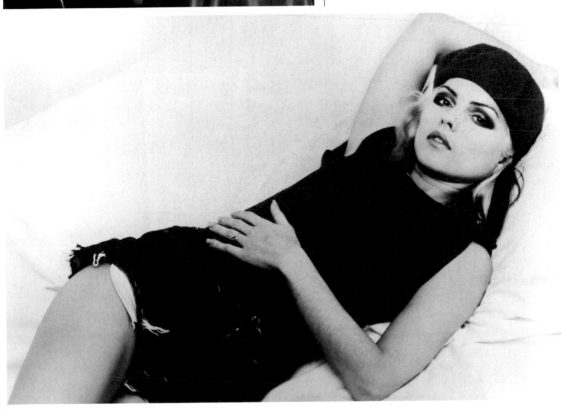

Amanda Brooks

STREET
Icons

Keith Richards, 1967 and 1974.

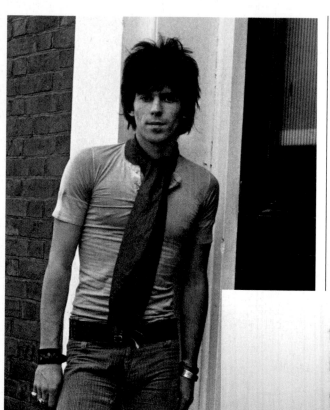

> **"WHEN I GOT OLDER
> I WORE MY OLD LADY'S
> CLOTHES. IF YOU NOTICE,
> ALL THE BUTTONS
> ARE THE OTHER SIDE."**
> —KEITH RICHARDS

I would do anything to raid KEITH RICHARDS's closet! He exemplifies rock 'n' roll style, and I cannot think of better inspiration for a cheap chic look. He brought an instant edge (and undeniable sex appeal) to the tight jeans, unbuttoned shirts, slim blazers, and scarves he wore, and he never looked the least bit contrived.

As a black feminist and political activist from the 70s, ANGELA DAVIS wasn't trying to be overtly stylish, I know, but she was undeniably beautiful and chic. Her courage and motivation inspired both John Lennon and the Rolling Stones to write songs about her, respectively "Angela" and "Sweet Black Angel." She embraced black beauty, adopting an outsized afro and mostly black clothing as her signature.

Angela Davis, sits with her head on her hand, shortly after she was fired from her job as philosophy professor at UCLA due to her membership in the Communist Party of America, November 27, 1969.

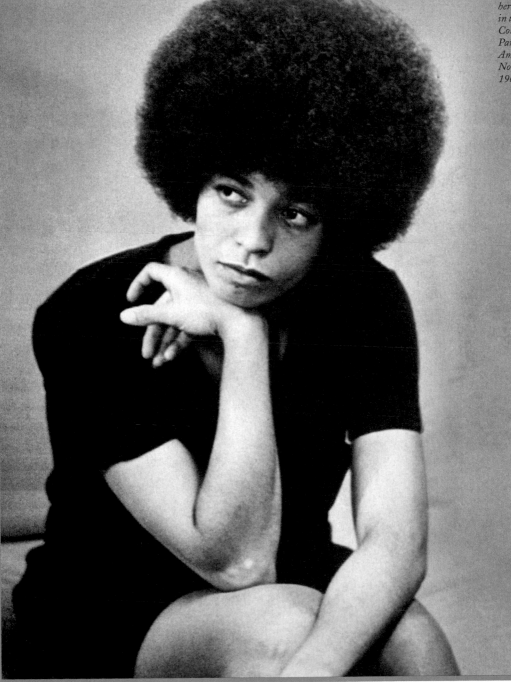

Amanda Brooks

The New Originals

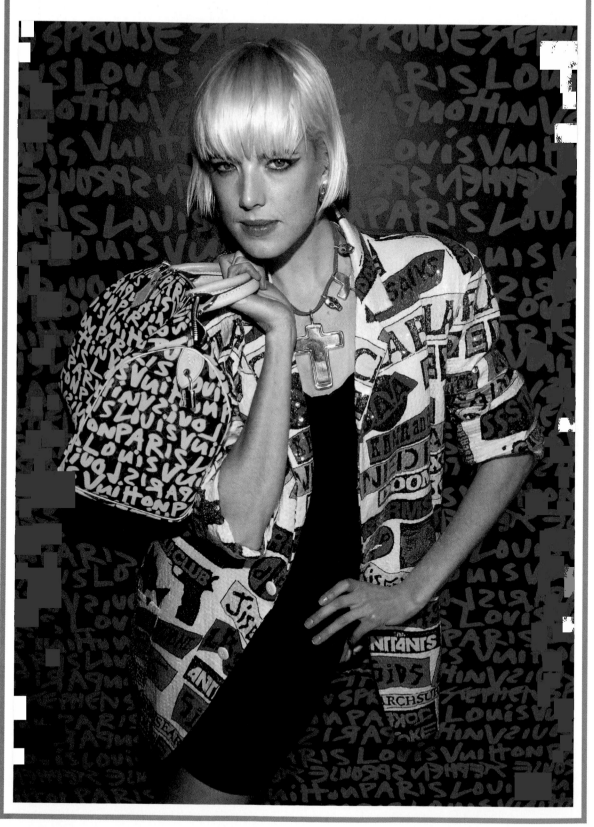

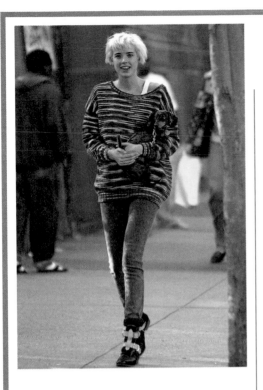

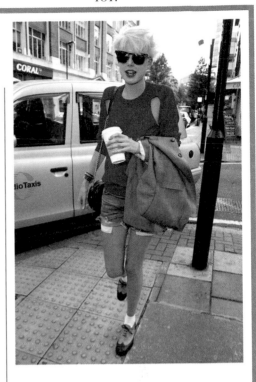

AGYNESS DEYN model

Agyness Deyn came along and took the fashion world by storm with her utterly original style. In a world that increasingly veers toward "good taste" alone, Agyness's combination of shocking color combinations, loud prints, a peroxide blonde pixie cut, and an ironic sense of proportion broke all the rules and made everyone—including me—remember how much fun it is to witness a true original.

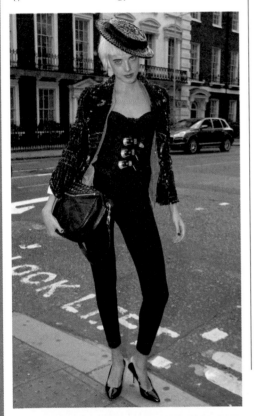

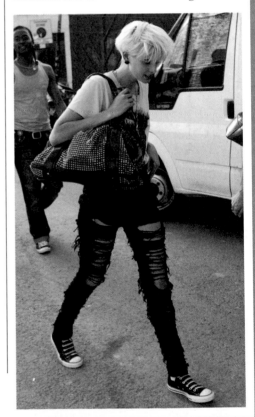

Opposite: Agyness Deyn, in a vintage Stephen Sprouse jacket with a Stephen Sprouse for Louis Vuitton bag, 2009.

This page: Agyness Deyn, all 2008.

STREET
The New Originals

SAMANTHA RONSON celebrity DJ

Despite all the flak she receives from the tabloids, I think Samantha Ronson has great style: preppy boys' clothes (she's a girl) mixed with a heavy dose of black street style (she's white). Clearly she's a contrarian, but also very certain of herself and extremely consistent. In the last ten years her style has wavered barely at all. She's the real deal when it comes to creating a personal brand of street style.

Samantha Ronson, 2004.

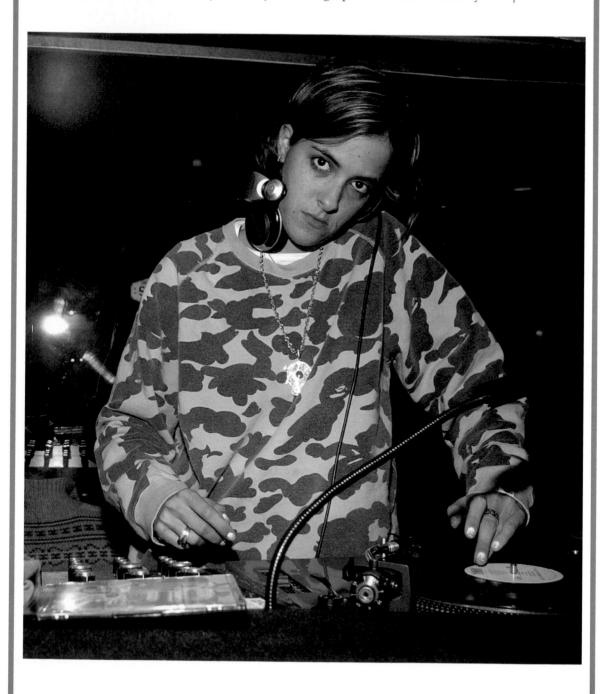

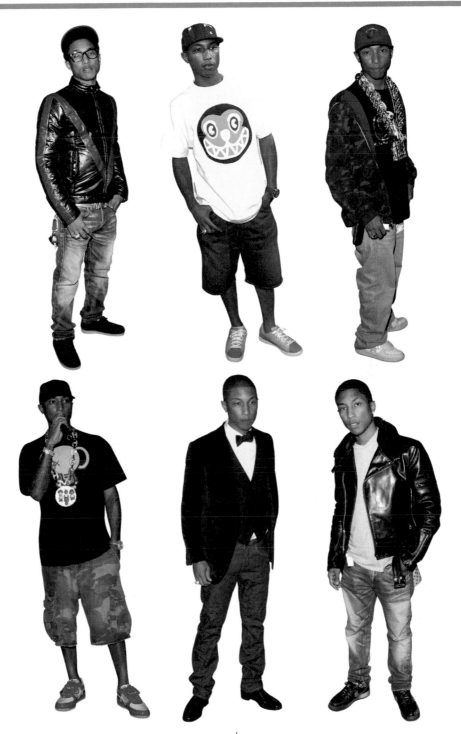

PHARRELL rapper and music producer

The first time I saw Pharrell, he was sitting across the table from me at a *Vogue* dinner. Who was this incredibly chic, preppy-meets-pop-art-meets-hip-hop guy sitting next to Anna Wintour? I asked, a friend told me all about him, and I have been keeping an eye on him ever since. He takes the best of the street, mixes it with the best of men's fashion, and then throws in his own attitude with unexpected references, proportions, and colors. He's hot.

Refining Your Style

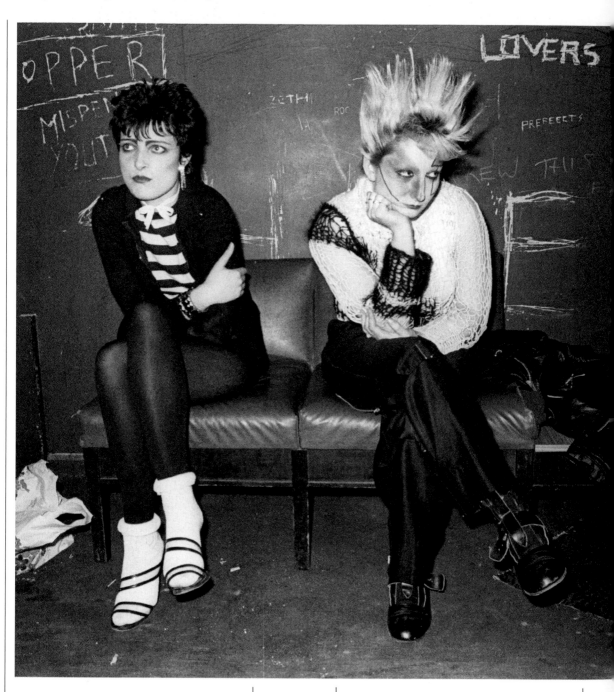

NEW WAVE
Black jeans, striped T-shirt dresses, slim belts, rubber bracelets, dramatic eye makeup, colored tights.

Siouxsie Sioux and Jordan, 1978.

PUNK
Tight tapered jeans, skinny suspenders, Doc Martens, leather jackets, decorative zippers, band T-shirts and buttons, studded belts.

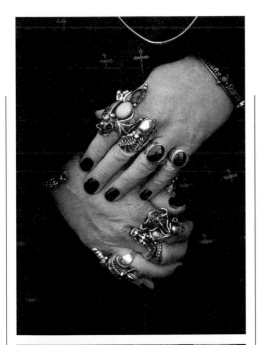

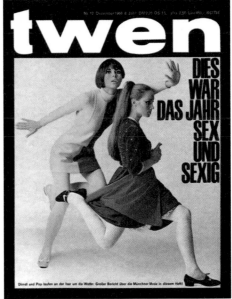

Clockwise from far left: The bejeweled hands of goth Tony Lightowler during his wedding during Whitby Gothic Weekend in England, 2007.

Twen, a German youth magazine, features mod fashions, 1966.

Courtney Love in her grunge heyday. Reading Rock Festival, Britain, 1994.

The Olsen twins doing their best high fashion goth impression during Paris fashion week, 2008.

MOD

Slim blazers and pants, baby-doll dresses, stripes, miniskirts, Mary Janes, three-quarter sleeve coats.

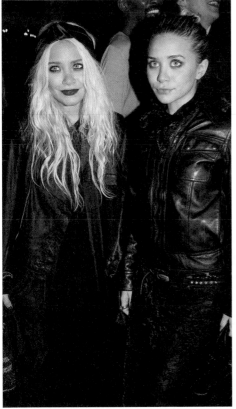

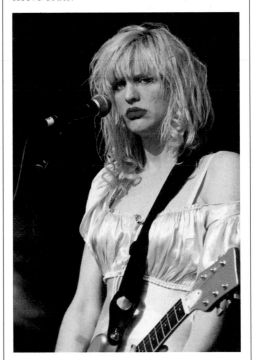

GOTH

Black clothes, makeup, and nails, dark hair, crucifixes, piercings and studs.

GRUNGE

Thermal shirts, lace-up boots, plaid flannel, slips (worn as dresses), well-worn T-shirts, ripped jeans, sweaters (preferably coming apart at the seams).

Amanda Brooks

Refining Your Style

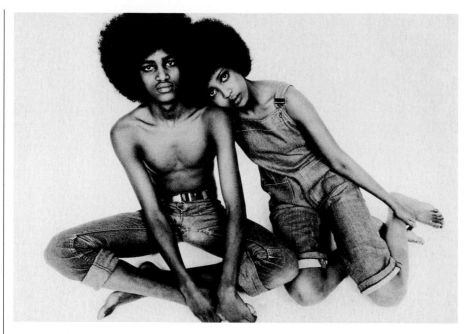

BLACK IS BEAUTIFUL
Afros, black leather, platform shoes, and plenty of saucy attitude.

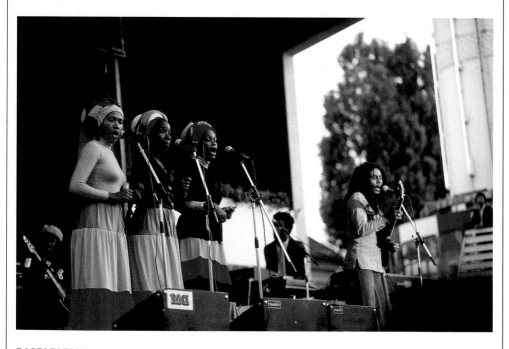

RASTAFARIAN
Crocheted hats, hemp clothes, cannabis leaf motifs, anything involving the Rasta colors: green, yellow, and red.

*This page:
(Top)
A photo from
the book*
Togetherness,
1970.

*(Bottom)
Bob Marley
and the
Wailers, 1978.*

Opposite:
The Fugees,
*2005. Lauryn
Hill is
amazing. She
has true
personal style.*

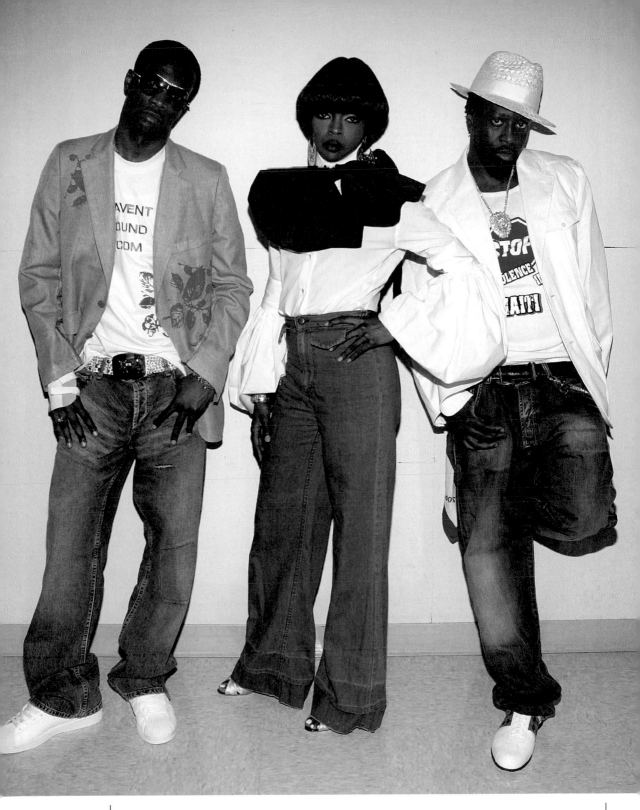

HIP-HOP
Hoodies, old-school sneakers, gold chains, track suits, logos, T-shirts with airbrushed portraits of deceased hip-hop stars.

Amanda Brooks

STREET
Inspiration

BOOKS

Nylon Street: The Nylon Book of Global Style
Nylon magazine
This extraordinarily useful book presents candid photos of people with great street style all around the world. There is some really amazing fashion in here. This book sits on my desk in my office and whenever I am waiting for a Web page to load or someone to answer the phone, I flip through it to find a new way to tie my scarf or an unusual proportion to ponder.

Roots of Street Style
by Zenshu Takamura
This book is full of fascinating fashion illustrations and photographs from different time periods, always concentrating on fashions that were popular with the general public—that is, street style. Here you'll see New Wave, mod, neo-hippie, grunge, and more. The book was published in 1996 and it covers fashion up through the 90s.

**We're Desperate:
The Punk Rock Photography of Jim Jocoy**
by Jim Jocoy
We're Desperate is a collection of photographs documenting the West Coast punk scene during the late 70s, including Iggy Pop, Lydia Lunch, and X front woman Exene Cervenka.

Maripolarama
by Maripol
The legendary scenester and stylist Maripol used a Polaroid camera to capture the faces and fashions of the 80s downtown crowd in New York City. Her book includes portraits of Grace Jones, Debbie Harry, and Madonna.

**Boutique:
A '60s Cultural Phenomenon**
by Marnie Fogg
This wonderful book documents the highly influential fashion designers and clothing boutiques that flourished in London during the 60s. Essential for fans of mod fashion.

Back in the Days and
A Time Before Crack
by Jamel Shabazz
These are two fabulous books of the photography of Jamel Shabazz, who documented the members and fashions of the early hip-hop scene in New York City. Look out for Adidas logos, oversized nerd glasses, big gold jewelry, and fat laces. Whenever I feel the urge to add some street style to my look, I turn to these books.

FILMS

Quadrophenia

Quadrophenia reminds me of the timelessness of mod fashion. The army green parkas, fitted blazers, and carefully cocked fedoras never fail to look cool. The mod look is easy to replicate on a budget and watching this film is sure to steer you the right direction.

Desperately Seeking Susan

Madonna's punky look in *Desperately Seeking Susan* is a timeless example of cheap chic style, although I do not recommend replicating her teased hair. She wore leather jackets with lacy lingerie and never hesitated to pile on the accessories.

Taxi Driver

Jodie Foster brings jailbait fashion to a whole new level in her short shorts and chunky platform shoes. She looks so quirky and carefree that it's hard to believe that anyone styled her.

Wild Style

This hip-hop classic follows the lives of teenagers living in the South Bronx during the early 80s. *Wild Style* features appearances by many prominent members of the early hip-hop scene including Fab 5 Freddy and Grandmaster Flash.

True Romance

Patricia Arquette shows us that tacky can be a good thing in this offbeat thriller about a couple on a crime spree. Her blue heart-shaped glasses and tight leopard pants seem like a bad idea on paper, but she wears them well and is a great reference point for a so-bad-it's-good street look.

Downtown 81

This cult classic (starring Jean-Michel Basquiat) presents an authentic look at the fashions of the downtown scene in 80s New York. It features cameos by several downtown luminaries from the era, including James Chance, Debbie Harry, and Vincent Gallo.

Christiane F.

This cautionary drug tale is centered on a young German girl named Christiane F., who does the street look better than anyone that I can think of. I love her grungy tomboy style and Manic Panic-d hair.

Rock 'n' Roll High School

I wish that my high school experience was more akin to the one in *Rock 'n' Roll High School*, which features an appearance by the eternally stylish Ramones. Their iconic uniform of tight jeans and leather jackets never loses its appeal.

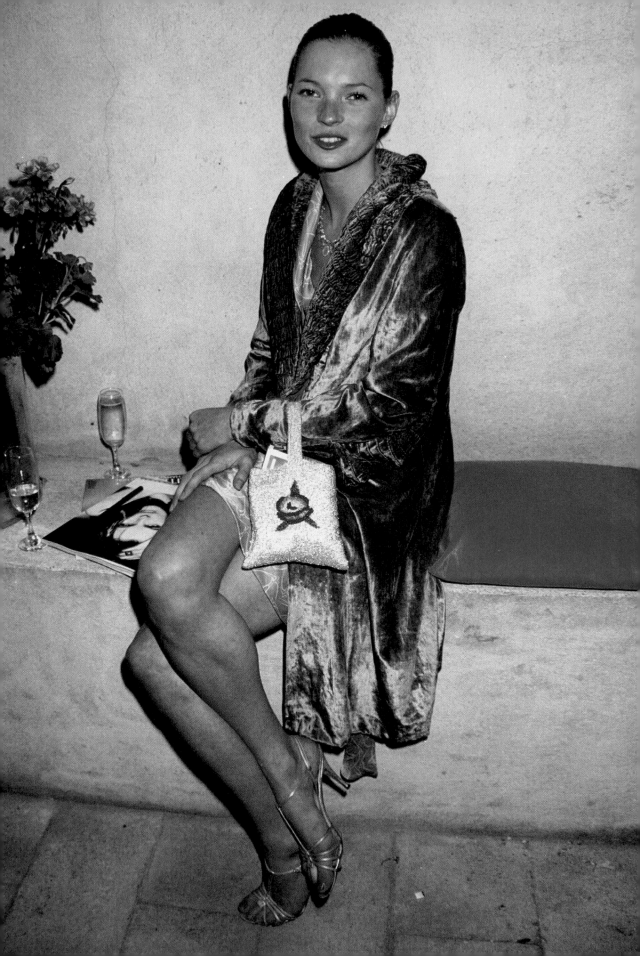

Eclectic

"

PEOPLE TODAY WANT APPROVAL FOR THE WAY THEY DRESS, WHICH IS THE KISS OF DEATH. YOU CAN'T REALLY DO YOUR OWN THING UNLESS YOU KNOW WHO YOU ARE. I THINK THERE IS A VERY DELICATE KIND OF MERGER BETWEEN YOUR CLOTHES AND YOUR PERSONALITY, A GIVE AND TAKE BETWEEN WHO YOU ARE AND WHAT YOU ARE WEARING."

—RICHARD MERKIN, 60s ARTIST

Eclectic women pick and choose their clothes from all different styles and mix them together in a way that is unique to them. There's no formula—I couldn't possibly come up with a list of favorite things; it's an invention every time. A successful eclectic look is evidence that the wearer possesses true personal style. A tried-and-true classic dresser can have her own style, too, but she relies to a certain extent on tradition; the eclectic dresser navigates the world of style with only her instincts for a compass.

Eclectic style requires a practiced editorial eye. From all the masses of merchandise out there, you must be able to cull the things that inspire you and suit you. Then you have to know how to mix them together in a way that works. It's kind of like making a salad at a salad bar: You choose all the things you like, all the while keeping in mind how they will mix together. Just because you like both raisins and onions doesn't mean you'll enjoy them in the same mouthful.

Kate Moss, 1998. This is the year I really started paying attention to Kate's amazing style.

The best thing about eclectic style is that it forces you to make your own rules because no else's apply to you.

So have fun making your own rules—and have fun breaking them too. Remember, style rules are made to be broken.

For this chapter, the only tools I have to offer you are the example and inspiration of myself and other women. Because eclectic style is indefinable and entirely unique to the person who creates it, you can't tell someone else exactly how to get there. But being excited and inspired by other people is often half the battle. I hope you are as inspired by the women in this chapter as I have been.

ECLECTIC
My Eclectic Style

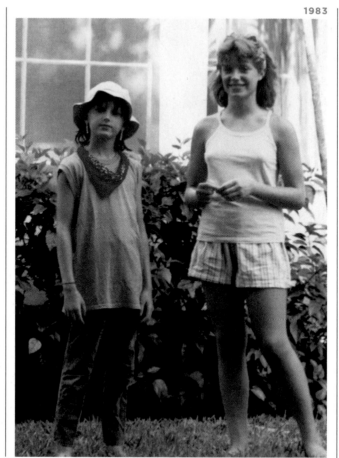

1983

1981

Left:
If you look closely you can see that I have a braid tied around my forehead in a modest attempt to subvert my obviously preppy style.

Right:
I remember this day so well. My sister Kim and I were on our way to go fishing at the Lake Worth pier in Florida. What I don't remember is what inspired me to wear yellow zigzag earrings and purple pin-striped Guess jeans.

Opposite:
My friend Jessica and me, both wearing Thakoon at the Thakoon show, 2008.

A preppy child, a bohemian teenager, a fashion-forward college coed, you know my story now, and that I've tried out many different styles over the years. And I'm not even through yet, as my foray into minimalism shows! In the beginning I adopted new looks one at a time. As I got to know myself in each style and became confident in my taste, I gradually assembled a closet full of "greatest hits," things that had become classic "Amanda" pieces, regardless of what style they conveyed to the outside world. Over the years, with a great deal of trial and probably an even greater deal of error, I learned to mix them together. I know that classic pieces—like white button-down shirts and neatly pressed trousers—are great for toning down more complicated pieces such as beaded minidresses or boho angora wool ponchos, that the oldest basic

T-shirts in my closet add contrast to the "lady" factor of tweed jackets, and that worn-in sneakers are the perfect down-to-earth foil to the trendiness of a designer bag.

I wouldn't say that I am an entirely eclectic dresser. I go through phases. When I discover a new look that I want to play with—say, androgynous dressing—I stick with it for a while, experimenting with all the men's clothes or men's-inspired clothes that I can get my hands on. Then the next inspiration strikes, and I move on. But that relationship with and understanding of men's clothes stays with me, and the best pieces from that phase remain in my closet and get mixed in with the next thing that comes along. Eclectic dressing, for me, is about keeping an open mind, trying new things, and holding on to clothes that really suit me.

FOR ME, ECLECTIC DRESSING IS ABOUT KEEPING
AN OPEN MIND, TRYING NEW THINGS, AND HOLDING
ON TO CLOTHES THAT REALLY SUIT ME.

2008

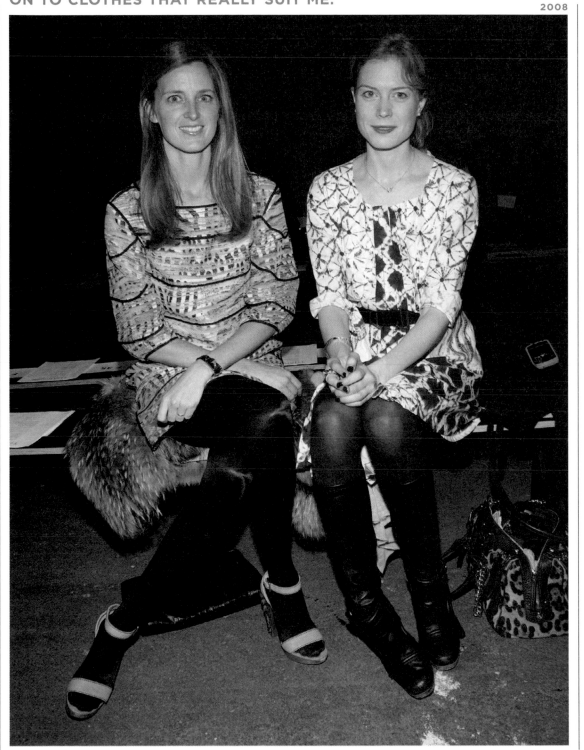

Amanda Brooks

ECLECTIC
Icons

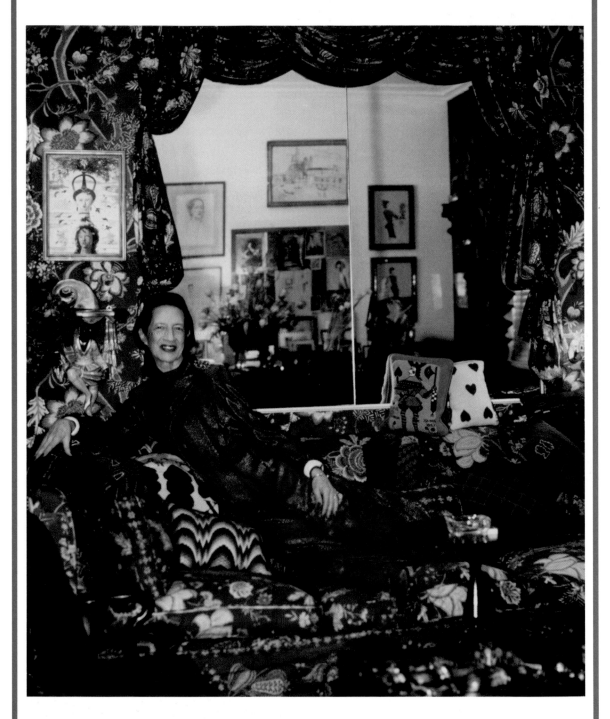

**"I WANT THIS PLACE TO LOOK LIKE A GARDEN,
BUT A GARDEN IN HELL."**
—DIANA VREELAND

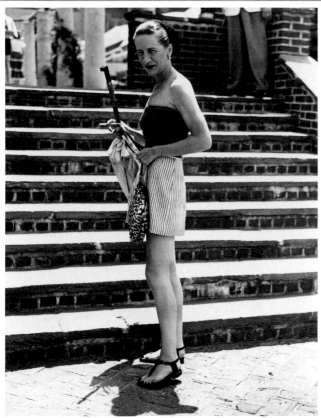

"YOU GOTTA
HAVE STYLE.
IT HELPS YOU
GET UP IN
THE MORNING."
—DIANA VREELAND

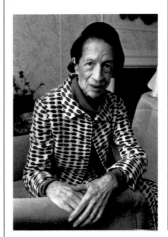

Why don't we declare DIANA VREELAND the most inherently stylish woman ever? She didn't just walk the walk, she talked the talk. She spoke about clothes, fashion, and style in a way that has never been matched, before or since. Buy the book *Why Don't You?* and you'll see what I'm talking about. Diana Vreeland was not classically beautiful, and she didn't need to be; she had enough style and personality for ten people. During her years as editor in chief of *Vogue*, and later as curator of the Costume Institute at New York's Metropolitan Museum of Art, she wore a uniform of trousers and cashmere sweaters almost every day. She accented her understated clothes with red lipstick and bold jewelry. For evening, she pulled out all the stops in brightly colored or deeply embellished couture gowns with loads of diamonds and gold jewelry.

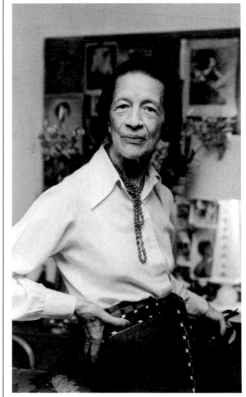

*Opposite:
Diana
Vreeland in her
living room,
1979.*

*This page:
(Clockwise
from top left)
Diana
Vreeland,
1955, 1980,
and 1980.*

Amanda Brooks

ECLECTIC
Icons

I always thought that actress ALI MACGRAW had quintessentially American style, which she did, but it was actually much more nuanced than I had realized. While wearing 70s boho for day, Hollywood glamour for evening, or casual sportswear at the airport, Ali was brilliant at indulging in trends and evolving her style, all the while maintaining her all-American grace and elegance.

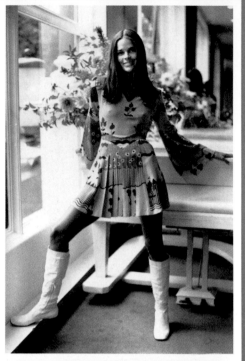

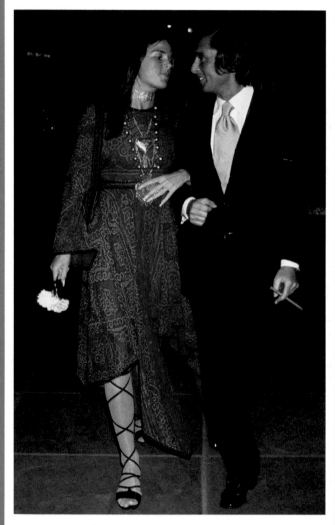

"LOOKING AT BEAUTIFUL THINGS IS WHAT MAKES ME THE HAPPIEST."
—ALI MACGRAW

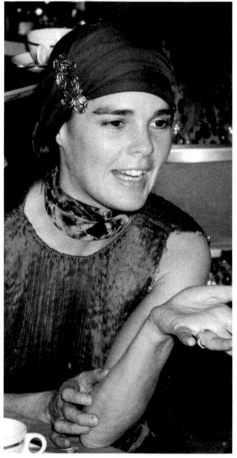

IT IS POSSIBLE TO EXPERIMENT WITH ANY STYLE AND STILL LOOK LIKE YOURSELF.

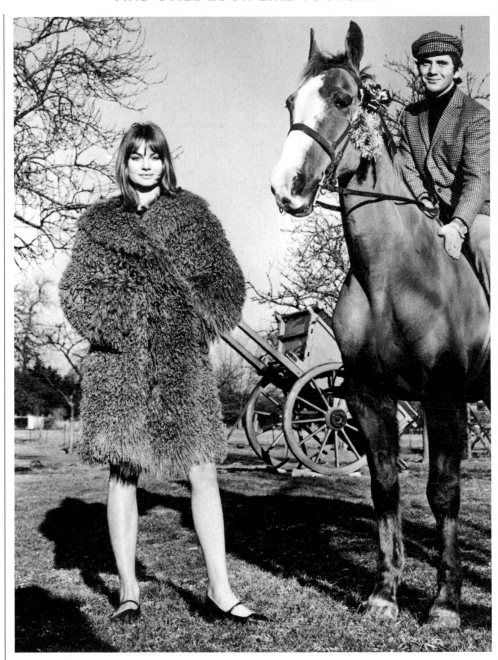

Opposite:
Ali MacGraw
and her
husband Bob
Evans, 1980.
Others are
1969.

This page:
Jean
Shrimpton and
Terence Stamp,
1965.

The secret to 60s English fashion model **JEAN SHRIMPTON**'s eclectic style is that she has great taste. Whether she wore a black pleather dress, a classic 60s shift, or a scruffy mannish pantsuit, she looked polished and put together. She knew how to tone down an over-the-top design element by wearing it simply and how to amp up a simple classic black dress with tastefully dramatic 60s hair and makeup. When you have such a strong sense of who you are and what you like, it is possible to experiment with any style and still look like yourself.

ECLECTIC
The New Originals

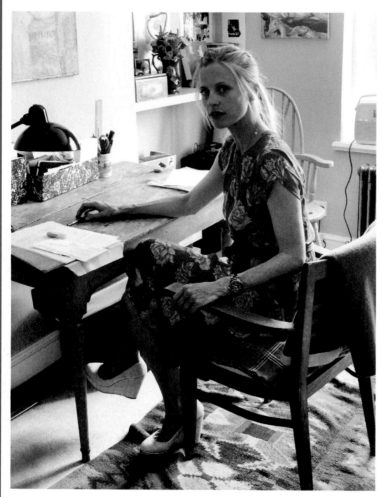

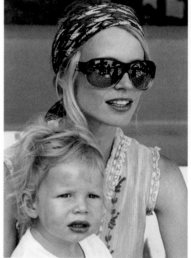

THE SCHOOLGIRL BLOUSE AND SWEATER WITH THE SEX-BOMB HAIR, MAKEUP, JEANS, AND STILETTOS— THE COMBINATION WAS SOMETHING TO BEHOLD.

LAURA BAILEY writer, model The first time I saw Laura she was having dinner at an Italian restaurant with Richard Gere. They were hidden away in a dark corner, and everyone in the place wanted to know who the gorgeous girl was, the one having dinner on the sly with such a major movie star. She was wearing a frilly 70s blouse with a vintage Fair Isle cardigan, skintight jeans, pink lizard Gucci high heels. Her hair was bleached blonde and messy, very Brigitte Bardot, and she had on loads of mascara and black eyeliner. The schoolgirl blouse and sweater with the sex-bomb hair, makeup, jeans, and stilettos— the combination was something to behold. I couldn't take my eyes off of her. Months later Laura started dating an old friend of my husband's, and she and I became close friends. She still has the same mostly cheap chic style she has always had, mixed in with a few sensible splurges (a Prada peacoat, Missoni plat- form shoes) and an enviable matching Chanel diamond ring and necklace set that was a gift from her boyfriend. She has the bombshell hair, the killer legs, and sexy schoolgirl clothes—but something is always a little off. Maybe her nails are red but chipped, or her eye makeup is smudgy, or her designer dress is wrinkled. You can almost guarantee she has a run in her stockings, and it takes lot to pull that off without looking sloppy. But she always looks fantastic.

Left: Laura Bailey in her home office in London. I was sure her dress was Prada, but it was actually vintage, 2008.

Right: Laura, with her son Luc, 2008.

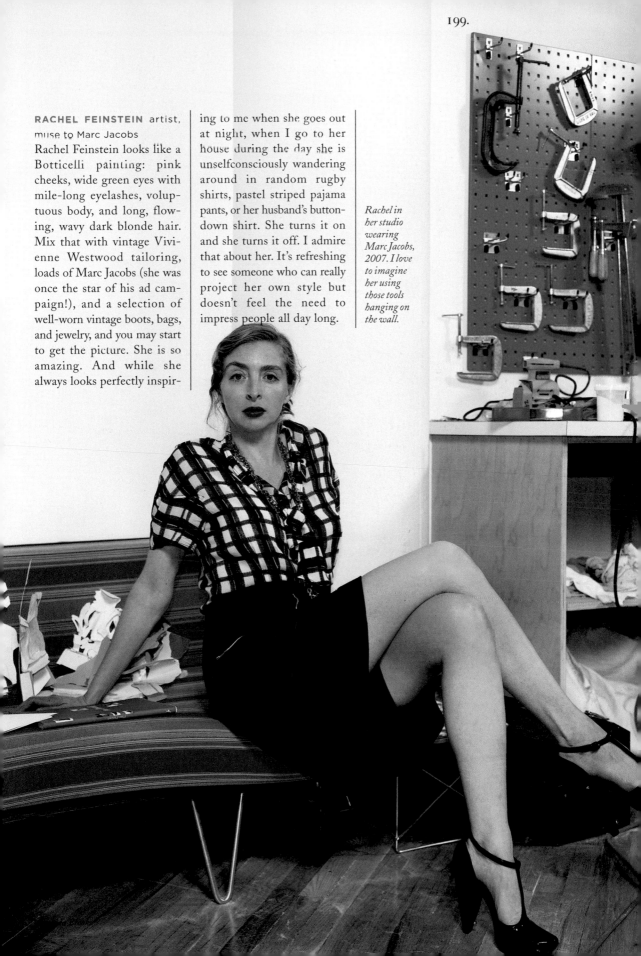

RACHEL FEINSTEIN artist, muse to Marc Jacobs

Rachel Feinstein looks like a Botticelli painting: pink cheeks, wide green eyes with mile-long eyelashes, voluptuous body, and long, flowing, wavy dark blonde hair. Mix that with vintage Vivienne Westwood tailoring, loads of Marc Jacobs (she was once the star of his ad campaign!), and a selection of well-worn vintage boots, bags, and jewelry, and you may start to get the picture. She is so amazing. And while she always looks perfectly inspiring to me when she goes out at night, when I go to her house during the day she is unselfconsciously wandering around in random rugby shirts, pastel striped pajama pants, or her husband's button-down shirt. She turns it on and she turns it off. I admire that about her. It's refreshing to see someone who can really project her own style but doesn't feel the need to impress people all day long.

Rachel in her studio wearing Marc Jacobs, 2007. I love to imagine her using those tools hanging on the wall.

ECLECTIC
The New Originals

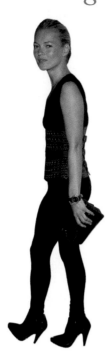

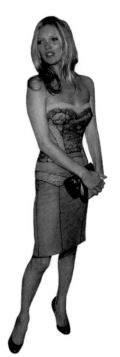

"I HAVE A DRESS-UP
CHEST AT HOME.
I LOVE TO CREATE
THIS FANTASY
KIND OF THING."
—KATE MOSS

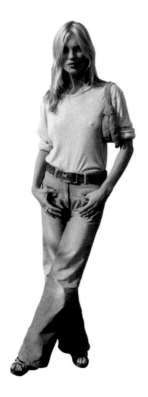

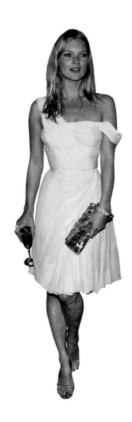

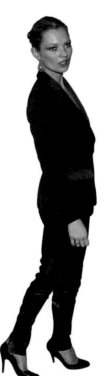

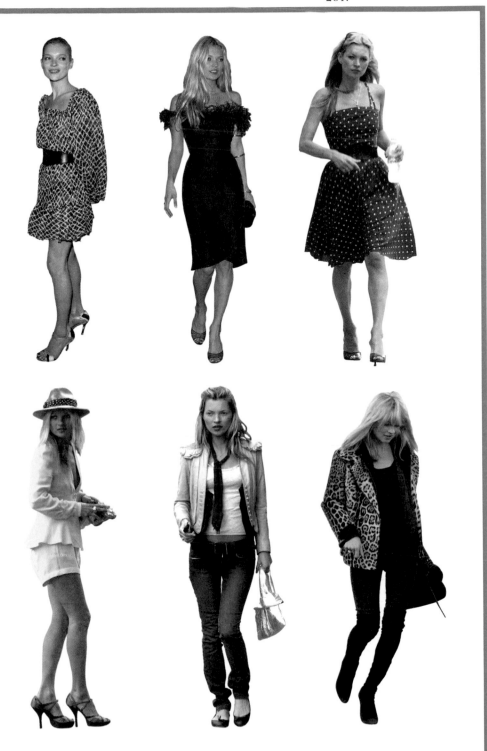

KATE MOSS supermodel

I am always excited to see what Kate Moss is going to wear next. Aren't you? No one is more unpredictable, harder to define. That's why everyone is obsessed with her. She's always reinventing herself—trendy, boho, classic, vintage, rock 'n' roll, cheap chic—yet she always looks like Kate Moss. She clearly dresses to please herself while the rest of us hang on every detail.

Amanda Brooks

ECLECTIC
The New Originals

LIZ GOLDWYN filmmaker, author, vintage clothing collector

Liz Goldwyn has been wearing and collecting vintage since way before it became the thing to do, and her relationship with these clothes is highly evolved. She doesn't just mix in something old to make her outfit look cooler. Using her upbringing in the film world (her grandfather was Samuel Goldwyn, the G in MGM), she constructs entire cinematic identities to inspire her outfits. When she went on a book tour to promote *Pretty Things*, her book about the history and costumes of burlesque dancers, she was going for a "sexy deconstructionist academic" look, meaning vintage Martin Margiela and Yohji Yamamoto worn with stiletto heels and librarian glasses. A year before that I saw her doing "sexy lumberjack" in a vintage plaid wool jacket and a pencil skirt. For her, fashion is role-play, but she doesn't leave the part about dreaming up the role to the designer. "My favorite dress for business meetings is a vintage Courrèges black wool dress with black patent leather details. I love it because it's half dominatrix, half little girl," she says. Her style is like no one else's.

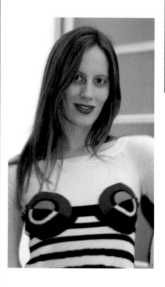

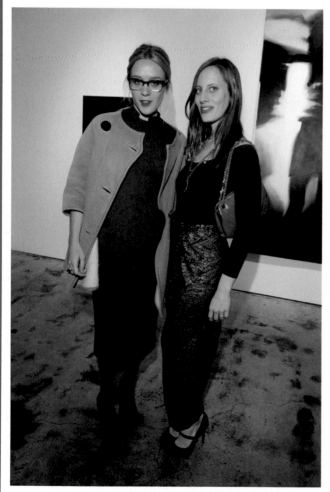

Far left: Chloë Sevigny and Liz Goldwyn at Hope Atherton's art opening in Los Angeles, 2007.

Left: Liz, in a hilarious vintage sweater (my guess is that it's vintage Sonia Rykiel), 2006.

Opposite: Margherita Missoni, at the Missoni show in Milan, 2009.

"MY FAVORITE DRESS FOR BUSINESS MEETINGS IS A VINTAGE COURRÈGES BLACK WOOL DRESS WITH BLACK PATENT LEATHER DETAILS. I LOVE IT BECAUSE IT'S HALF DOMINATRIX, HALF LITTLE GIRL."
—LIZ GOLDWYN

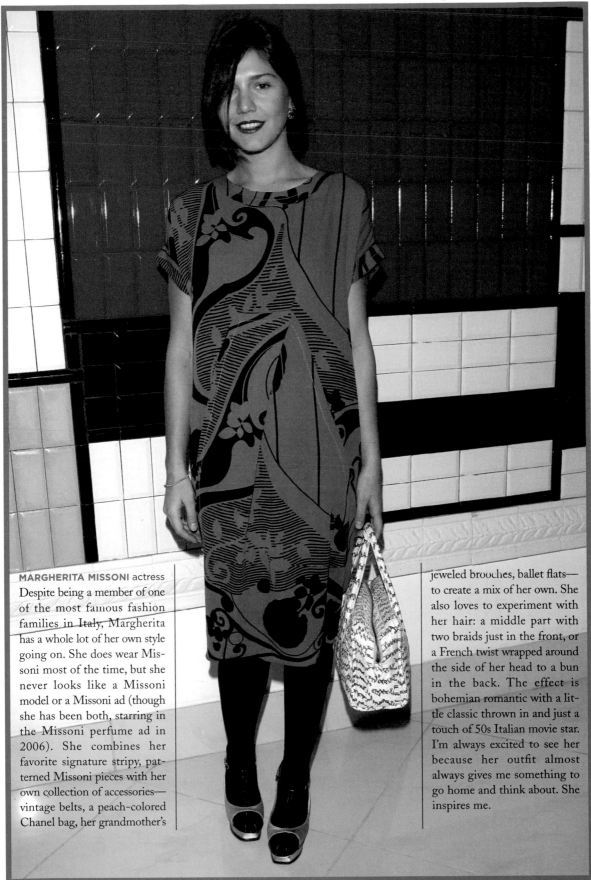

MARGHERITA MISSONI actress
Despite being a member of one of the most famous fashion families in Italy, Margherita has a whole lot of her own style going on. She does wear Missoni most of the time, but she never looks like a Missoni model or a Missoni ad (though she has been both, starring in the Missoni perfume ad in 2006). She combines her favorite signature stripy, patterned Missoni pieces with her own collection of accessories— vintage belts, a peach-colored Chanel bag, her grandmother's jeweled brooches, ballet flats— to create a mix of her own. She also loves to experiment with her hair: a middle part with two braids just in the front, or a French twist wrapped around the side of her head to a bun in the back. The effect is bohemian romantic with a little classic thrown in and just a touch of 50s Italian movie star. I'm always excited to see her because her outfit almost always gives me something to go home and think about. She inspires me.

Amanda Brooks

ECLECTIC
Mixing Styles

A great inspiration for eclectic style is mixing references. It's almost like a game—it should be fun and you don't need to think about it too much. Just choose a reference in the left column that speaks to you and then find another reference from the right column that adds the right dose of irony. I have made some suggestions below, but it's up to you to find the right mix for your style.

STEVIE NICKS

CHANEL

PUNK

GRACE KELLY

1920s

PARIS

FREDDIE MERCURY

VERSACE

NAUTICAL

KLUTE

HITCHCOCK

BETTY BOOP

1970s

AXL ROSE

DOLLY PARTON

TOKYO

PROM QUEEN

CLUELESS

SAFARI

FEMME FATALE

GOTH

KATE MOSS

BLADE RUNNER

GRACE JONES

VICTORIAN

FASSBINDER

MINIMAL

L.A.

MOSCOW

KEITH RICHARDS

1980s

EDIE BEALE

LOVE STORY

JACKIE O

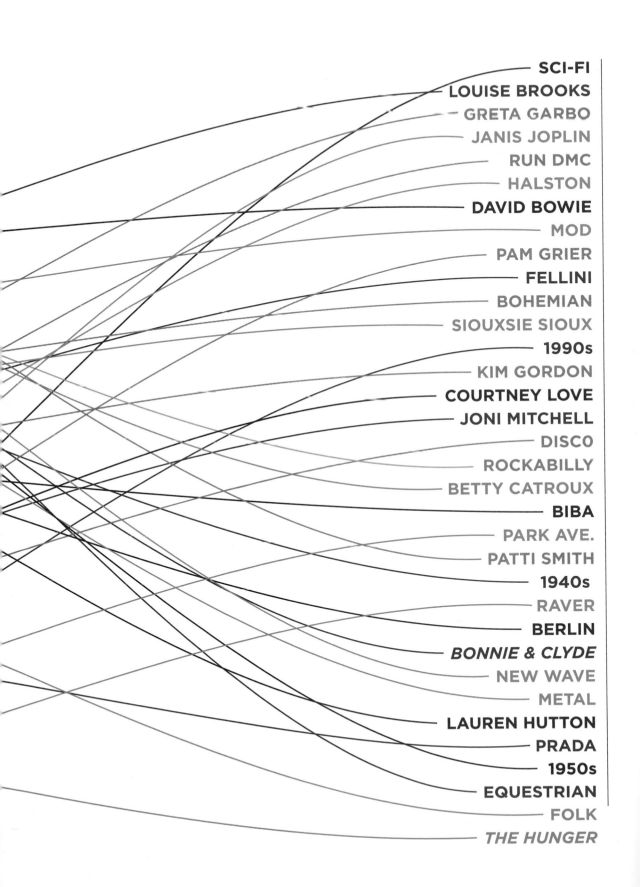

SCI-FI
LOUISE BROOKS
GRETA GARBO
JANIS JOPLIN
RUN DMC
HALSTON
DAVID BOWIE
MOD
PAM GRIER
FELLINI
BOHEMIAN
SIOUXSIE SIOUX
1990s
KIM GORDON
COURTNEY LOVE
JONI MITCHELL
DISCO
ROCKABILLY
BETTY CATROUX
BIBA
PARK AVE.
PATTI SMITH
1940s
RAVER
BERLIN
BONNIE & CLYDE
NEW WAVE
METAL
LAUREN HUTTON
PRADA
1950s
EQUESTRIAN
FOLK
THE HUNGER

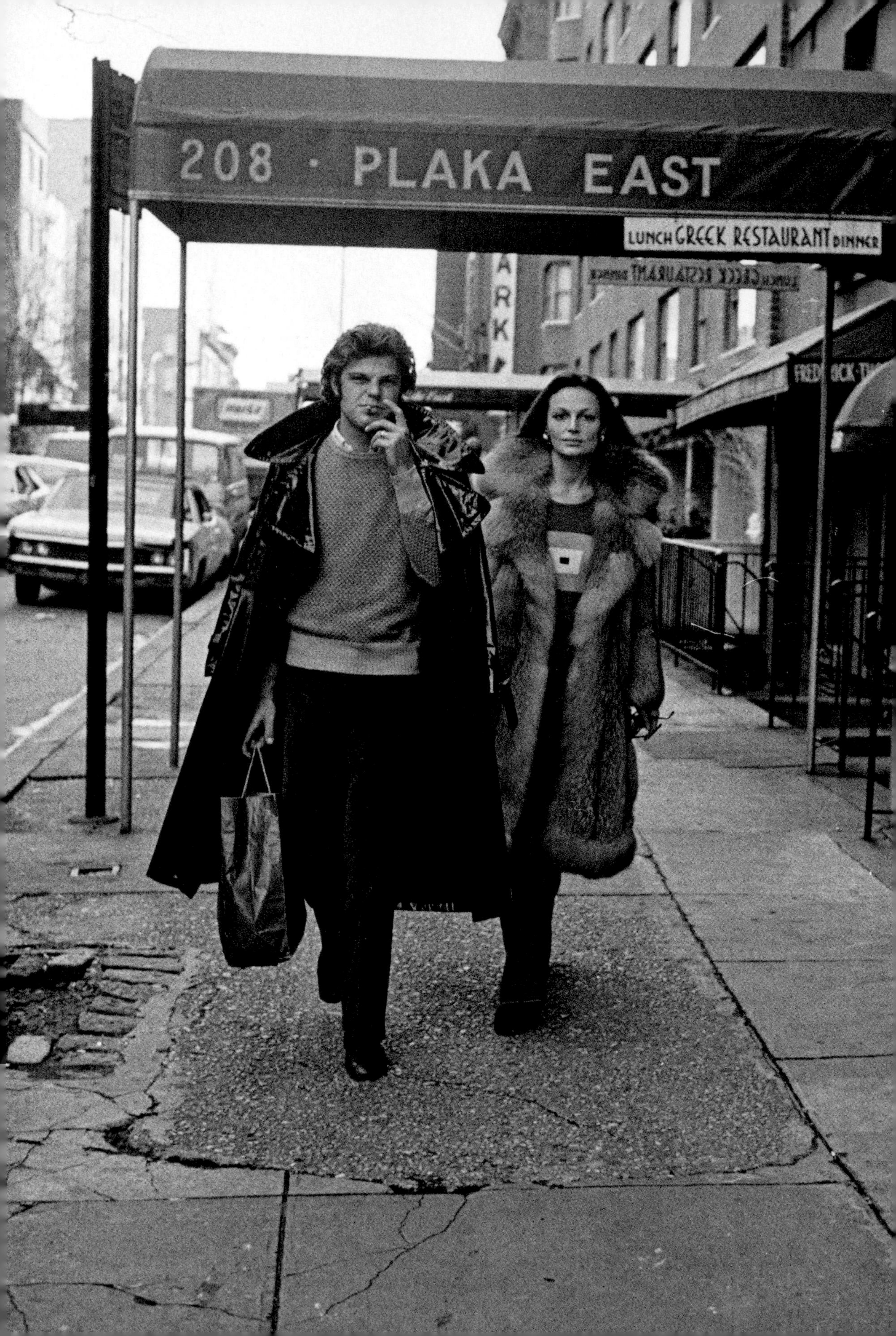
208 · PLAKA EAST
LUNCH GREEK RESTAURANT DINNER

INTRODUCTION

Shopping

**"SHOPPING IS BETTER THAN SEX.
IF YOU'RE NOT SATISFIED AFTER SHOPPING
YOU CAN MAKE AN EXCHANGE
FOR SOMETHING YOU REALLY LIKE."**
—ADRIENNE GUSOFF

Diane and Egon von Furstenberg doing errands in New York City, 1975. I wish I could look that glamorous when I go shopping.

I almost never "set out" to go shopping for clothes. Living in New York, I don't have to, and I like it that way. Just the natural movement in my day—taking the kids to school, walking to the gym, getting to and from meetings around the city—takes me past enough stores to apply some stress to my back account. When I'm feeling cash poor, I actually have to focus on breaking the habit of wandering into the Miu Miu store across from the gym or my favorite vintage store, Zachary's Smile, on my way home from the morning school drop-off. It's not easy. Putting on my iPod to tune out the temptation sometimes helps. But fresh off a paycheck, I love breezing in and out of local shops to add some new excitement to my shoe closet or stock up on my favorite T-shirts (J.Crew tissue boyfriend crewneck tee).

What I don't enjoy so much is setting out to find something specific. Looking for shoes to go with a dress for a specific party, trying to find a the perfect cream button-down silk blouse (it's perfectly designed in my head, it just doesn't seem to exist in reality), or even just shopping for winter tights because last year's have holes—can all be a big waste of time if I don't know exactly what I am looking for and where to find it. Online stores have taken away some of the pain of "must-find" shopping—I found the perfect pair of YSL patent leather platforms to go with a dress for a party on Neiman Marcus.com—but on the whole it's my least favorite part of the fashion experience.

Perhaps my favorite shopping scenario is going along to help my mom or a girlfriend. I can spend hours and hours sitting patiently in a waiting room giving the yea or nay to everything on the rack, or I can scope the floor for new things to try. Part of the joy is having the pleasure of someone who wants to hear my opinion (don't we all love that?), and the other is the satisfaction of shopping vicariously through someone else. It's their wallet that's in trouble, not mine. Some of my happiest shopping memories have been helping my mom find the perfect suit to wear to my wedding (she choose a purple tweed Chanel) or taking my friend Trinny, who visits from London a few times a year (she wrote the enormously successful fashion book *What Not to Wear*), around to show her all the cool new shops in New York.

What is most important about shopping is that it should be fun. So if, like me, there is a part of shopping that you like less than others, that means you should work extra hard to make it exciting. Take a friend, stop along the way for sustenance (a brownie and a cappuccino works for me), and keep your mind open at all times to the possibilities that are out there. You never know when the find of a decade will be staring you in the face!

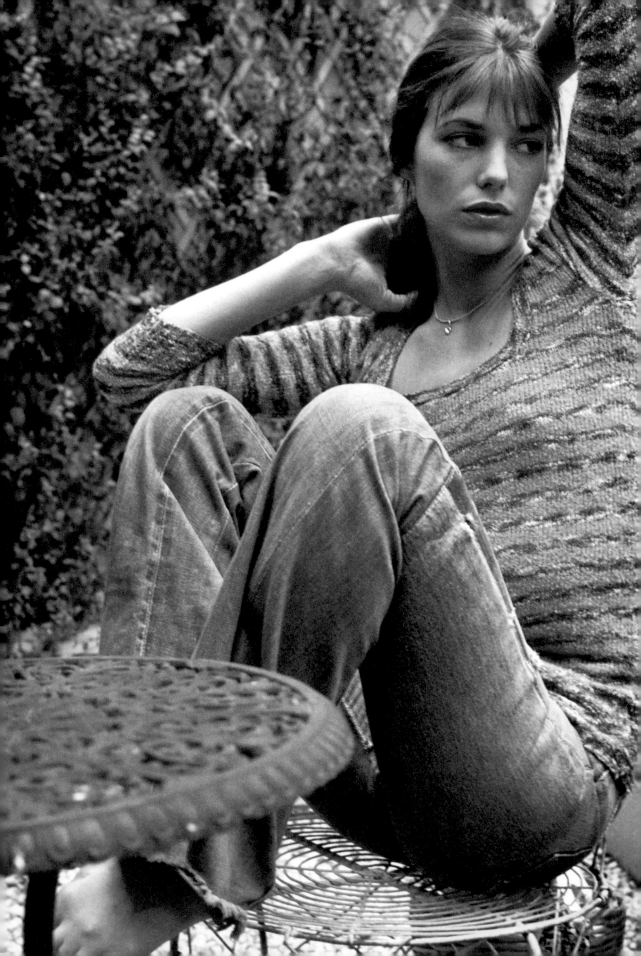

BASICS

"

I HAVE OFTEN SAID THAT I WISH I HAD INVENTED BLUE JEANS: THE MOST SPECTACULAR, THE MOST PRACTICAL, THE MOST RELAXED AND NONCHALANT. THEY HAVE EXPRESSION, MODESTY, SEX APPEAL, SIMPLICITY—ALL I HOPE FOR IN MY CLOTHES."
—YVES SAINT LAURENT

This chapter is for absolutely everyone. It is about assembling a core wardrobe of everyday pieces that make life in your closet a little easier. Basics are the jeans, T-shirts, simple sweaters, throw-on shoes—the foundations of getting dressed. Whether your shirts are skintight or baggy, your jeans tapered or boot cut, or your necklines V shaped or scooped, every single thing you put on contributes to your overall look and so deserves consideration.

Some women use basics as a starting point for a more stylized look. Imagine a stylish young woman getting dressed on the weekend: She'll wear a T-shirt, jeans, and classic Puma sneakers, and then add something with more personality, like a knit jersey blazer and a Marc by Marc Jacobs plastic necklace. Or in the summer she'll wear J.Crew khaki shorts and rubber flip-flops with an embroidered peasant blouse and a crocodile belt.

Other women create their entire look out of layered basics worn in a stylish way. This works well for women with relaxed, casual style, and a good relationship with accessories. There's a girl I often see walking on my block who has this look down. She's always wearing jeans and a layering of T-shirts, often topped off with a longish cardigan or a little vest. I always notice how at home she looks in her

Jane Birkin, 1974. I could do a whole chapter on her love of basics.

reliable basics, and with the addition of an old cowboy belt buckle, a pair of well-worn boots, or the thick band of chains, strings, and charms she has hanging off her wrist, she looks slightly different each time I see her. She also has a really good haircut—long with hippie waves and shaggy bangs. I have no idea who she is, but she is my ideal basic-basics woman. Others might look boring in similar outfits, but she looks amazing because she has found just the right basics for her body and her personality, and she wears them with style.

This is important: Basics don't have to be classic. If you don't have a classic sensibility, why would you build your outfit on a classic foundation? Your basics might be a slashed T-shirt with puff sleeves, or a tank dress to wear with jeans instead of a tank top. If they suit your style, your basics will work as long as they are simple enough to work with other things in your closet and remain relevant over time.

Figuring out the foundation of your wardrobe is arguably the most important part of knowing your fashion identity, and half the battle is finding the right shape in the right color at the right price. While it may take a few tries to find these things, whether in stores or online, it's essential that you don't stop looking until you've found the things that work for your body, your life, and your style.

BASICS
My Basics Shopping

1977–78

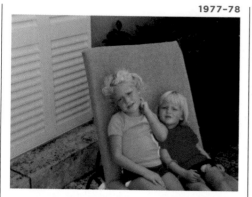

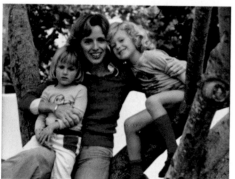

1987

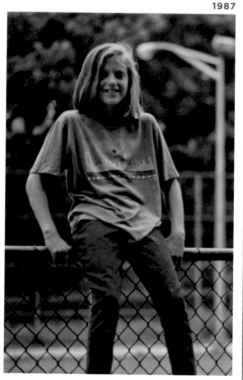

Finding the right basics is a never-ending quest for most women. I think I am just beginning to get the hang of it. Because my clothing budget has a beginning, a middle, and an end, I used to spend money where it was most noticeable, on big-ticket items. I tried wherever I could to skimp on the basics. In some areas I got away with this (I don't think I've ever spent more than $20 on solid T-shirts, and I have really great ones), and in others I haven't (inexpensive leggings often get baggy in the knees after a few hours' wear, so I now buy more costly ones that stay fitted all day and even make my butt look more firm!).

On principle, I agreed that it's wise to buy multiples of basics you love, but I had never been one to do it. I almost always regretted later that I didn't have, say, five perfect white T-shirts, but at the cash register it just seemed overindulgent (and, to tell the truth, like a boring expenditure). But I began to realize that it's actually just inefficient not to stock up. What use is a perfectly cut Phillip Lim blazer if I don't have the right shirt to wear underneath it? And then when I find the shirt that works under all my blazers, it's incredibly annoying to realize it's in the wash when I need it most. So I started to correct the problem. The first step was to buy ten pairs of my favorite underpants: low-rise lace things from Hanky Panky. At $20 a pop it wasn't too painful, and now whenever I open my underwear drawer I'm delighted to find just what I want instead of a ratty assortment of not-quite-right choices. I also went to J.Crew and bought three more T-shirts like one that I had almost beaten to death by wearing and washing many times a week.

As the demands of life continue to pull me and my wallet away from shopping, the wisdom of investing in basics seems clearer than ever. I might not know at the moment of purchase whether it will become a favorite, but if a reasonable basic enters heavy rotation right away I try to hurry back and buy more before they're gone.

*Top left:
My sister Kim and me at our grandmother's house, 1977.*

*Bottom left:
My mom, sister Kim, and me in Palm Beach, 1978.*

*Right:
Me, hanging out at the baseball field in Bronxville, 1987. Those were my first pair of Guess jeans, and they had stirrups on the bottom!*

*Opposite:
My friend Anh Duong and me, 2006. I almost never wear basics alone anymore, but they make my more fashionable things (like fur coats) that much more wearable.*

I Love Your Style

AS THE DEMANDS OF MY LIFE CONTINUE TO
PULL ME AND MY WALLET AWAY FROM SHOPPING,
THE WISDOM OF INVESTING
IN BASICS SEEMS CLEARER THAN EVER.

2006

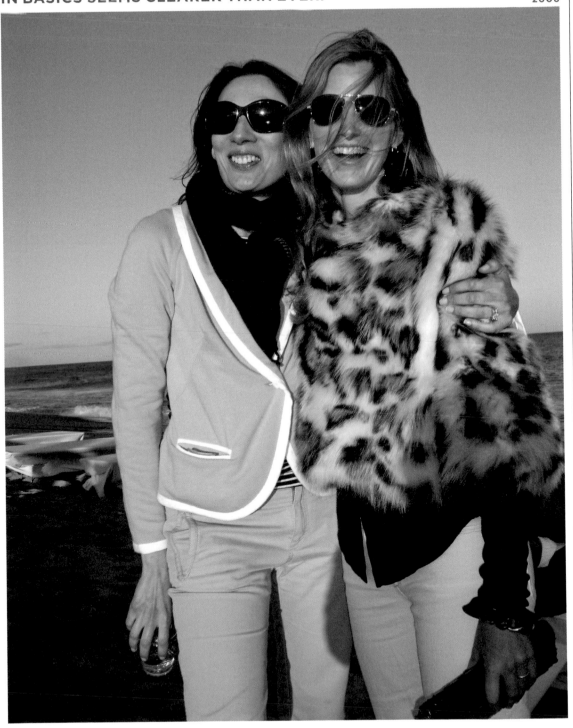

Amanda Brooks

BASICS
What to Look For

We all keep one eye out for the perfect jeans, tank tops, or easy cute dresses all the time, but only you truly know what you *must* look for right this minute. Do your blue jeans party like it's 1999 despite the fact that the rest of your clothes have moved on? Or maybe you splurge on the latest jeans every year but have trouble getting excited about buying T-shirts, so yours are all stretched out and faded. Make a list of basics you need to replace (or lack entirely) and spend an afternoon shopping for them and them only. Afterward, I promise you'll feel better about getting dressed every day, even if you don't look dramatically different.

"I'VE ALWAYS THOUGHT OF THE T-SHIRT AS THE ALPHA AND OMEGA OF THE FASHION ALPHABET."
—GIORGIO ARMANI

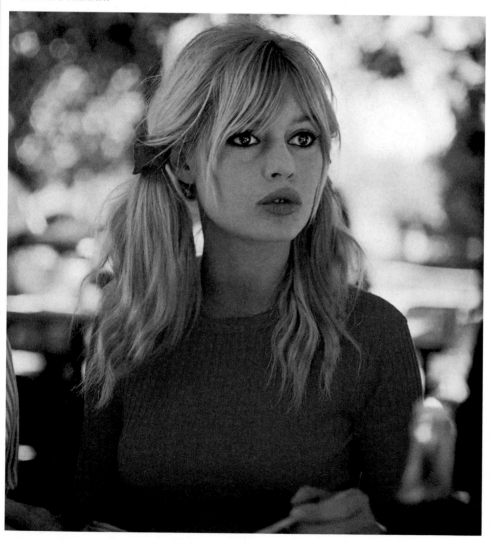

I love that Brigitte Bardot's pigtail bows match her T-shirt, and her messy hair adds some sexy irony to the cuteness of the styling, 1965.

Shopping Tip:
If something really works for you, I suggest you **BUY MULTIPLES**. *And not only different colors, but different sizes too. I often buy casual pants in two sizes: small and medium. I wear the small pair during the week because the slimmer fit looks better with flats and a tailored jacket, but on the weekend, when I want to feel flexible and relaxed, I wear the medium, which actually looks better with my baggier sweaters and sneakers.*

T-SHIRT

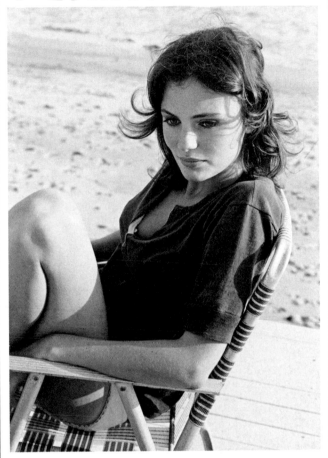

OVERSIZED ITEMS, like your boyfriend's button-down shirt or sweater, can look great if worn in a sloppy, casual way with something fitted and slim on the bottom. This look has never worked for me (except when I was pregnant), but I see other people looking good in slim jeans and an oversized sweatshirt from time to time and it always makes me want to try again. I have tried again. I just haven't left the house like that.

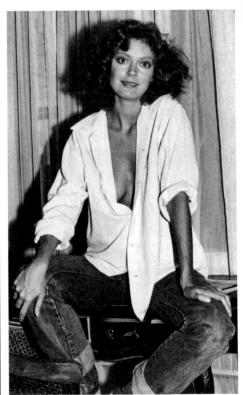

Although a **T-SHIRT** seems pretty straightforward, there are many choices and things to consider when looking for one that will serve its purpose. I am always looking for T-shirts that are *soft* and *long*. I *never* want to show my midriff, and I like the layered effect of having the T-shirt peek out from the bottom of whatever I am wearing on top: a chiffon blouse, a tailored jacket, or even a sequined tank top in the evening. The first-layer T-shirt also has to be thin, so I don't feel padded or constricted, especially in the shoulder and underarm. When finding the right T-shirt style for you, think about the use you have for T-shirts in your life and how the shape of them contributes to your look.

Top: Jacqueline Bissett, 1965.

Right: Susan Sarandon, 1978.

OVERSIZED
ITEMS

Amanda Brooks

What to Look For

JEANS

Unless you are one of those people who refuses to wear them, **JEANS** are one of the most important and personal pieces of clothing you buy. I don't believe in owning endless pairs of jeans. I buy two pairs of jeans per year—one for day, hemmed to wear with flats and sneakers, and another pair for night, long enough to wear with heels. It's usually the wash that motivates me to buy a new pair. I'll be really into a light wash for a year before suddenly feeling like stiff dark denim is all I want to wear. And although I try not to fall victim too often to trends in jeans shapes, if I feel that a trend really speaks to my own personal style (70s high-waisted wide leg jeans) I'll often go for it and keep them around long after the trend is gone. This is one place I don't skimp. After three bad pairs of jeans from cheap chic stores, I now know that the expensive ones are really worth it.

I may be unpopular for saying this, but I'm not fond of the elaborate pocket stitching that appears on many jeans today. It's basically the designers' way of slapping a logo on your butt. Frankly I'd rather sport the actual logo, like Calvin Klein and Gloria Vanderbilt made their customers do in the 80s, than have to deal with some overly decorative stitching that is often at odds with the rest of my look. Jeans are supposed to be basic and simple.

In regard to choosing the style that's right for you, I suggest you first try on a lot of pairs. Jeans should always be a *little* bit too tight because they inevitably stretch after wearing them for as little as a car ride. Think about how you will wear the jeans. Are they for every day? For weekends? For dates? Do they need to be long enough to wear with heels? Are these the only pair you are buying, or one of many? Do you want them to last for years, or just for this season? And then, after you make your decision, don't be scared to return them if after the first wearing (not after the third!) they stretch too much, don't look good with your clothes, or just don't look the same in your home mirror.

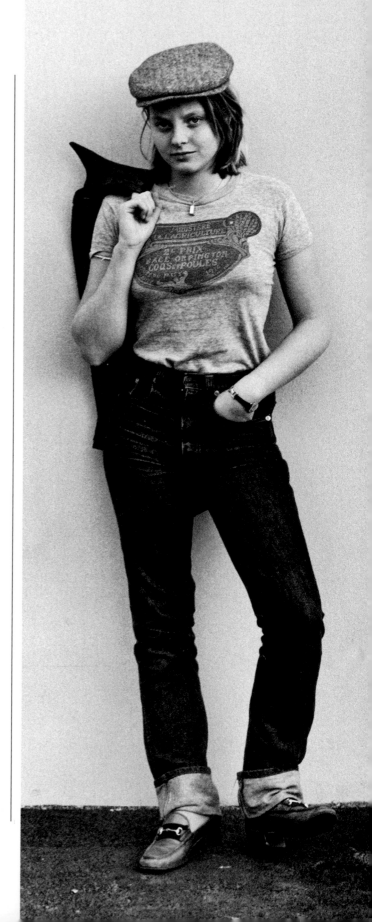

PRACTICAL
PANTS

My closet has a good selection of **PRACTICAL PANTS**: comfortable, loose-fitting pants that are not jeans. They can be cargo pants, men's tailored flat-front cotton pants, corduroys of any variety, or even just classic twill trousers. My rule is that they have to work for pretty much any situation: I wear my vintage Levi's cords with sneakers to the post office, my black wool tailored pants with ballet flats for a meeting, or plain-front khakis with flip-flops on the weekend. They're a little less casual than jeans but easy to wear all the same.

Shopping Tip:
Basics should be useful and appealing for many years. For that reason I tend to stick to **NEUTRAL COLORS**: *gray, beige, khaki, black, white, cream, and navy are all great colors for the first layer of an outfit. That said, if you are a basic dresser full stop then you will probably want to add* **MORE COLORS**. *Red is my favorite bright basic color. Red socks, or even a red sweater, are classic as well as basic. And pale pastels can also work in diverse and flattering ways.*

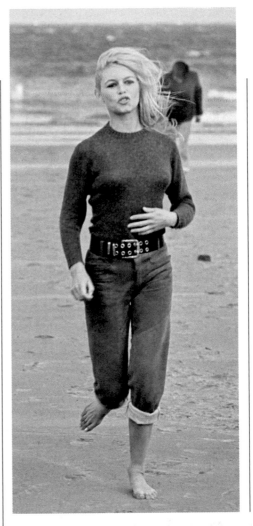

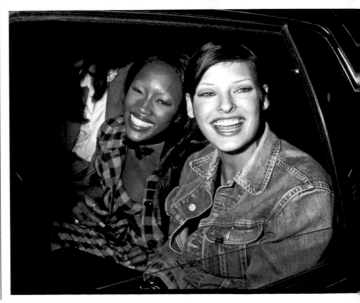

Opposite: I love this picture of Jodie Foster. It was taken in 1976, but her outfit would be every bit as relevant today.

Left: Brigitte Bardot, 1966.

Below: Linda Evangelista, with Naomi Campbell, 1992.

JEAN
JACKET

A **JEAN JACKET** is a high-risk item. If you don't agree with me then you haven't seen all the hideous ones lurking out there. There is only one kind of jean jacket that truly works: It has to be classic cut and it has to fit perfectly through the shoulder and body. Boxy jean jackets are awful. I found mine in an anonymous vintage store in New York's West Village. It's Wrangler and it is a very soft, very faded light blue denim. It must have been a child's size, because the arms are too short on me, but I like them that way. I wear it all year, whether under a fox fur vest or over a bathing suit, and I've never gotten sick of it.

What to Look For

TANK **TOP**

TANK TOPS are incredibly useful. I have many different variations of cut, fabric, and color, and I wear them with everything from sweatpants to long evening skirts. Although I do on occasion wear tank tops alone in the summer, I mostly use them as a foundation for layering. If I want to wear, say, a romantic blouse but don't want to feel too fancy, a tank top underneath is perfect for dressing down the whole outfit. Tanks also look great worn one on top of the other in different colors. I sometimes use tank tops to cover up when I feel a dress is too revealing. Once I put on a borrowed Calvin Klein silk dress that was very low cut both in the front and on the sides; I loved the dress but it wasn't flattering me. So I put a silk ribbed tank underneath it. It covered up the parts I didn't want to show and added some personality to an otherwise straightforward dress.

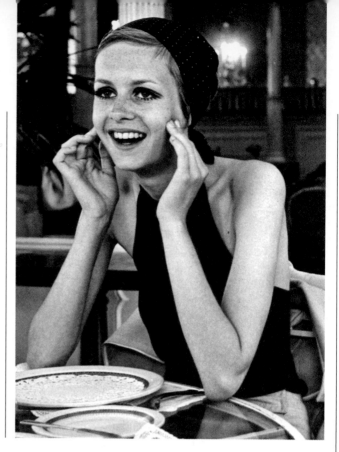

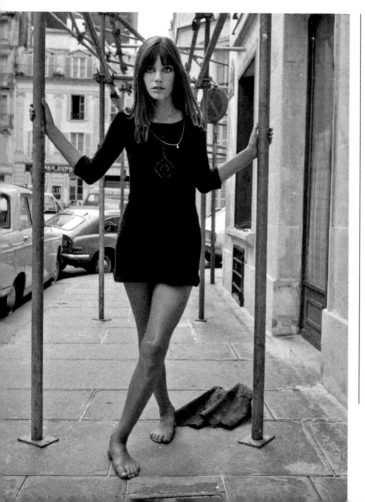

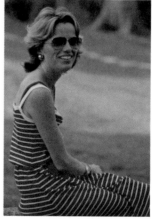

Clockwise from top: Twiggy, 1967. I always think a woman can get away with very basic clothes if she makes an effort with her hair and makeup.

My mom, 1979.

Jane Birkin, 1968.

T-SHIRT OR SWEATER **DRESS**

A **T-SHIRT DRESS** or **SWEATER DRESS** looks basic and is easy to wear with a pair of flats, maybe with a thin scarf thrown around your neck.

*Elizabeth Jagger,
Georgia Jagger and
Theodora Richards
at the Rolling
Stones after-concert
party, showing that
basics are a great
foundation for far
more elaborate
outfits, 2006.*

ANYTHING
FITTED
AND
STRETCHY

ANYTHING FITTED AND STRETCHY like leotards and leggings can be scary to attempt (and even more scary to witness), but they are worth the trouble if you get them right. I went so far as to buy a unitard from American Apparel last year and have not regretted it. In fact it has proved more useful than I imagined. I wear it most often at the gym (it makes me feel more ballerina, less jock), but it has also come in handy a few times in my everyday wardrobe—topped with a denim mini skirt or a sheer vintage summer dress. Leotards and leggings can prove equally useful under skirts or dresses, or simply worn as body-skimming basics.

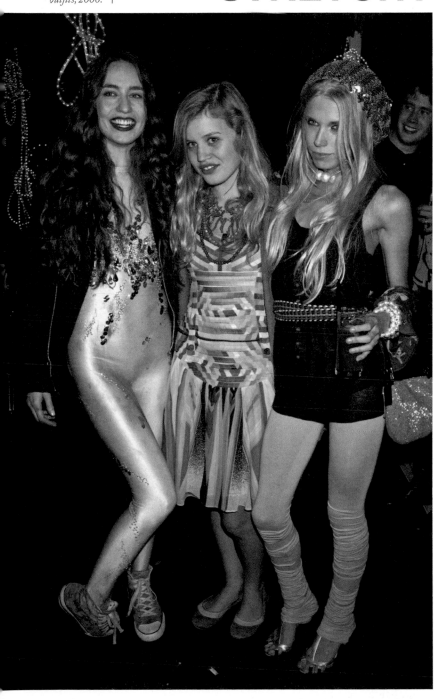

Shopping Tip:
COMFORT *is also crucial here. If you're not comfortable in your clothes it's hard to feel like yourself. There is nothing worse than trying to eat lunch with a waistline that is digging into your belly or wearing an itchy wool sweater next to your skin. Whenever I leave my house in something uncomfortable, all I want to do is go home and take it off. If you feel the slightest discomfort when trying something on, don't even think about buying it. That tightness or itchiness or pulling will almost certainly only get worse outside of the dressing room.*

BASICS
Where to Find It

KEEP AN OPEN MIND about where you buy your basics. **LOOK EVERYWHERE**: department stores, chain stores, discount stores, catalogs, etc. A six-pack of men's (or boys') undershirts from Target or K-Mart may be just what you need as a base layer, and who knows what else you'll find while you're there.

That said, while it is possible to find great basics at great prices, it can also be worth it to invest in better quality for basic items you think will become staples in your wardrobe. Many **DESIGNER BOUTIQUES**—Prada, Marc Jacobs, Phillip Lim come to mind—have a constant supply of well-fitting, beautifully made pants, shirts, and sweaters in their collections season after season. One of my biggest indulgences is silk "tissue tees" from Proenza Schouler. They are the cut of a T-shirt made in more of a blouse fabric, they fit me perfectly, and I wear them nonstop under blazers, sweaters, dresses. They do cost a bloody fortune ($315—for a glorified T-shirt!) but I wear them so often and they work so well in my wardrobe that I know they are worth it.

If basics are going to be a big feature in your wardrobe, try having a few things **CUSTOM-MADE**—shirts, pants, and even jeans can all be made to order. On the high end, traditional custom tailors are expensive but well worth the investment. My friend Alexandra has a vintage Adolfo blouse that she just lives in, so every few years she has a few more exact copies of her beloved blouse made at a custom-tailoring shop so that she will never be without it. But the tailor at your dry cleaner should be able to copy things for you, too, at a lower price. My friend Zandy has a great eye for fabric, so she buys one pair of expensive, perfectly fitting trousers and takes them to her tailor who duplicates them for her at a fraction of the cost of the original. I can't say it often enough: Building your outfit around well-made, well-fitting basics is the best way I know to look great in your clothes.

Shopping Tip:

The single most important aspect of basics is **FIT**. *If you need to spend a little more to get it right, then do. If you feel crappy in your jeans and T-shirts because they don't fit, you'll never wear them and will end up buying new ones anyway.*

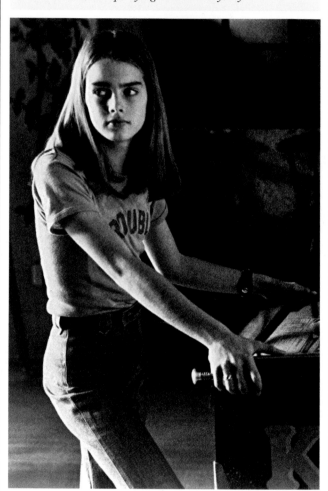

BUILDING YOUR OUTFIT AROUND WELL-MADE, WELL-FITTING BASICS IS THE BEST WAY I KNOW TO LOOK GREAT IN YOUR CLOTHES.

Brooke Shields, from the movie Tilt, *1978.*

BASIC
BITS & PIECES

"SPANX" can be a lifesaver under clingy dresses and skirts or fitted trousers. Once I was dying to wear a white jersey dress with crochet trim to a party. When I finally got my hands on the dress and tried it on before the mirror, I was humbled to say the least. I may be skinny, but I'm still a mother of two and in my thirties, and my butt did not look cute. A friend told me about Spanx, and they transformed my butt from small and saggy (and even a bit lumpy . . . when did that happen!) to still small but less saggy (and lump-free). I wouldn't want to wear them every single day, but they definitely come in handy from time to time.

I don't know how anyone today can wear jeans or trousers with anything other than a **THONG**. No matter how well they fit or how seamless they are, bikini underwear make a line on your butt that just does not look okay. Do not be intimidated by a thong; there is one out there for everyone, and I promise after the first few wears you will get used to the feeling. I've been wearing thongs since college and I feel far more comfortable than I ever did in bikini cut panties. All the women in my family wear Hanky Panky thongs—my sister and I like the low rise and my mother likes the high rise. If you are looking for the right thong, try these.

Everyone should have a couple of pairs of opaque **BLACK TIGHTS**. I also have a few pairs of charcoal gray and brown tights for adding contrast to all-black outfits or toning down a bright color. Some girls today prefer to wear leggings instead of tights, and that's cool too.

In the past decade, so much has been written and aired about the importance of well-fitting **BRAS** that you must know the drill: The only way to ensure that you are buying the right size, fit, and shape is to go to a good lingerie shop or department store to get fitted by a professional. It could dramatically change your appearance. As for me, I don't wear a bra unless I need it to hold the **SILICONE INSERTS** that help me fill out the bodice of a blouse or dress. My friends and I call them "chicken cutlets" because that's what they look like, and they are a lifesaver for me. Being a woman with AAA breasts has some advantages, such as constant comfort and never having to wear a bra. But there are some unfortunate limitations too. I wish I could wear a bikini, but I can't fill out a cup of any kind. That problem would extend to clothes were it not for chicken cutlets. When I encounter a top with any sort of cup structure in the boob area, I fill it out with the cutlets tucked into a bra. Now they even make them with adhesive to stick directly to your skin, no bra required. If you require a little filling, or even just a lift, cutlets will do the trick. As much of a naturalist as I am, I'm convinced I would have been researching a boob job by now if I hadn't discovered them.

A lot of people think **SOCKS** don't matter, but I disagree. Details are the most important thing when it comes to personal style. I'm not saying that you have to express yourself through your socks. In fact, please don't. I think "fun" socks (with cartoon kittens, martini glasses, your nation's flag) are the worst. But you also don't want your socks to distract or take away from your outfit. I like to buy socks that are good enough quality to last at least a year without pilling or developing holes, in colors that will blend in with the pants and shoes I am wearing. My basic sock colors are gray (light and dark), beige, cream, black, and brown. There's nothing worse than starting your morning with holey socks, so please, spare yourself.

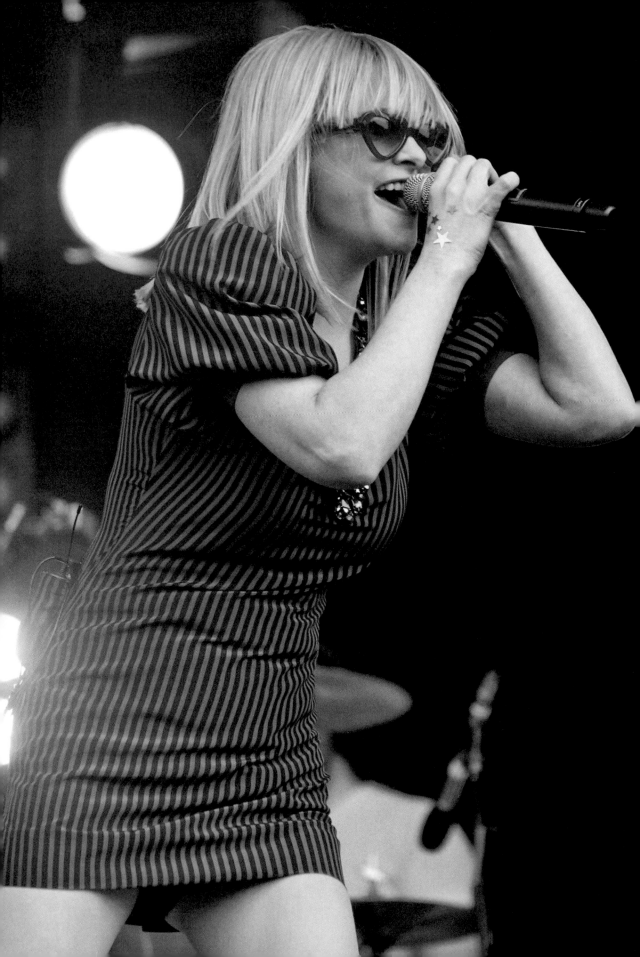

CHEAP CHIC

**I HAVE ALWAYS BELIEVED THAT
YOU DON'T HAVE TO BE RICH TO HAVE STYLE."**
—DIANE VON FURSTENBERG

True style doesn't have a price tag. Most stylish women I know pride themselves on finding inexpensive things that look great. Whether it's a jacket from the army/navy store, an embroidered dress bought on vacation in Mexico, or a ruffled cotton blouse from Zara, the thrill of the outfit you purchased for a song is anything but cheap.

There are two kinds of successful cheap chic shoppers. The **TRUE CHEAP CHIC WOMAN** has a limited budget, or just a limited interest in spending lots of money on clothes. Her closet is full of inexpensive clothes collected from a combination of thrift stores, flea markets, trendy chain stores, and purveyors of reasonably priced basics. She'll wear, say, an H&M floral dress with ballet flats and a straw tote bag; a vintage concert T-shirt with Zara tailored pants and old-school Adidas sneakers; or a J.Crew shift dress with a chunky costume jewelry necklace and platform espadrilles.

Then there is the **HIGH/LOW WOMAN**, who mixes pricy clothes with their less dear cousins. There's more than one way to go with this: One woman might base her wardrobe on expensive classics and liven it up with cheap chic trends, while another splurges on the designer pieces of the moment but wears them with cheap chic basics. High and low can mingle in a totally haphazard way in the outfits of a woman who has money to spend but who also has style and therefore buys what she loves, no matter what it costs.

Cheap chic does not suggest any one style. Any "look" can be pulled off on a cheap chic budget. All you need is a passion for shopping, a sure idea of what suits you, an eye for editing, and an open mind. You can find cool things in the unlikeliest of places, but only if you're on the lookout.

*Alison Goldfrapp
onstage in
London, 2006.*

CHEAP CHIC
My Cheap Chic Shopping

I DISCOVERED CONTEMPO CASUALS AND A WHOLE NEW WORLD OPENED UP FOR ME.

1984

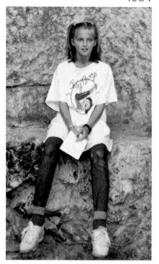

1984

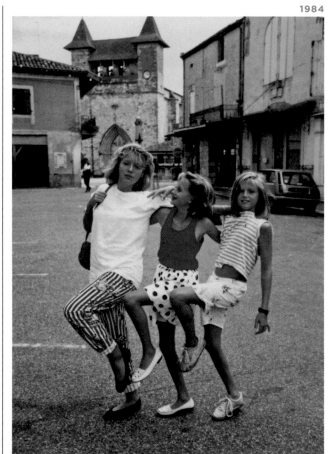

This page:
(Left)
I really loved this outfit. My Guess stirrup jeans, my pink leather Reeboks, the layered socks, and if you look closely you can also see that I have wispy bangs, 1984.

(Right)
My sister Kim, my friend Celerie, and me, all doing our best to look stylish while on vacation in France, 1984.

Opposite:
(Left)
My cheap chic nod to Chanel at the Met Ball, 2005.

(Right)
Me, with Lauren duPont, at a party, 2009. I'm wearing my favorite H&M dress. André Leon Talley told me that night he thought my dress was vintage Chanel couture!

The Woolworth's in Bronxville was my first introduction to the joys of cheap chic. When I turned ten and was finally allowed to walk from my house into town by myself, it was the only store where a few weeks' worth of allowance would buy me something I actually wanted. I bought all kinds of things there, including a hamster named Fozzy purchased without my mother's permission. (He lived in my closet for a month before he was discovered and returned, but that's another story.) On the fashion end, I brought home a rainbow of classic sweatshirts and sweatpants, flip-flops, "jelly" sandals, Hanes T-shirts, and endless cheap and colorful makeup (blue metallic wet n wild nail polish and Revlon Silver City Pink lipstick were favorites).

In college, I discovered Contempo Casu-als and a whole new world opened up for me. Contempo gave this prepster from the suburbs an affordable opportunity to *play* with fashion. I had always looked at *Vogue* with my mom and watched her buy designer clothes here and there. Real fashion, as seen in magazines, was something grown-up and out of my reach financially. But then it turned out that experimenting with trends was as easy as driving to the mall near my college and plunking down a twenty for a runway knockoff frock. Madonna was on the cover of *Vogue* dressed as a hippie and Marc Jacobs had just launched his infamous "grunge" collection. At Contempo I bought bell-bottom pants, crocheted vests, ruffled blouses, velvet chokers, and skull caps that I mixed in with my own clothes to give myself a whole new look.

2005

2009

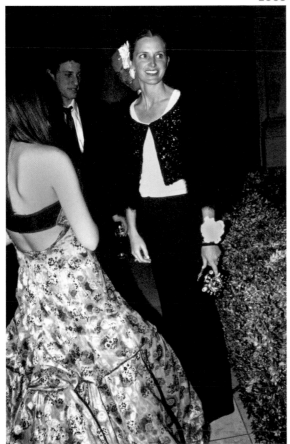

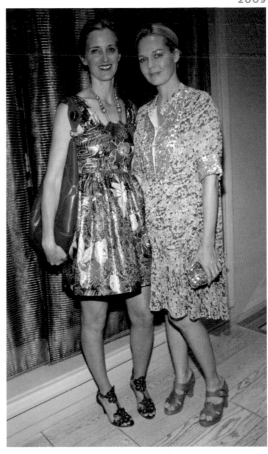

MY GREATEST COUP IS SHOWING UP AT A VERY FORMAL EVENT IN A FANTASTIC CHEAP CHIC OUTFIT.

Today, my greatest coup is showing up at a very formal event in a fantastic cheap chic outfit. One year, the Costume Institute Benefit at the Metropolitan Museum of Art, the fashion world's most important and dressiest social event of the year, was showing a retrospective of Chanel. I thought it would be fun and clever to wear something vintage Chanel that looked relevant today. A call to the public relations office at Chanel revealed that this same idea had already occurred to the likes of Nicole Kidman, Vanessa Paradis, and Selma Blair, and all the best dresses were already claimed. I next called some vintage dealers I know, but their Chanel pieces either had already been snapped up by other partygoers or were way out of my price range. Before giving in to despair, I remembered a 70s Yves Saint Laurent jacket that I'd gotten in a trade with a vintage collector friend. It was a black sequined bolero with feathered sleeves, and I'd been saving it for some time to wear to something special. When I thought about it, it was very Chanel. As a nod to Coco Chanel herself, who was one of the first women of the century to wear pants, I wore the jacket with my favorite black viscose evening pants and a $30 white silk ribbed tank top. Topped off with a fresh gardenia corsage (the official flower of Chanel), it was my favorite outfit I've ever worn.

CHEAP CHIC
What to Look For

While the variety of styles you can pull off with cheap chic clothes is endless, the success of inexpensive fabrics and shapes cut for the masses is not. Of course there are exceptions, but on the whole I find that certain categories and general items work better than others.

MILITARY-INSPIRED PIECES

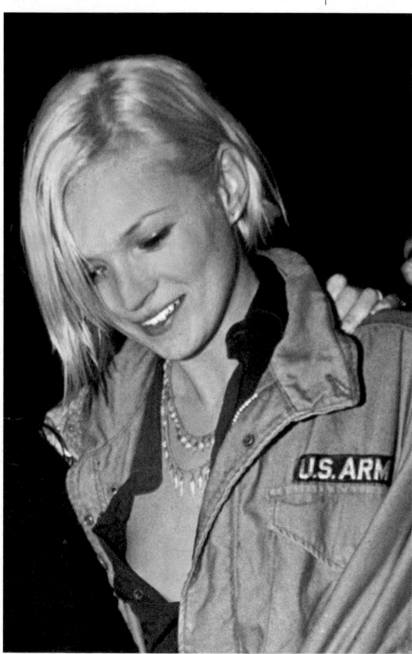

At almost any cheap chic store, whether an army/navy or an inexpensive fashion chain, you will find **MILITARY-INSPIRED PIECES:** cargo pants, army jackets, wool military coats, multipocketed vests. The army/navy store is the obvious choice if you are into authenticity, and the clothes are usually surprisingly well made—but you have to be careful about fit since most of the clothes are made for men. Chain stores offer lots of choice and a more predictable fit, but the clothes usually seem trendier and less sturdily constructed. The great thing about military clothes is that they shouldn't have a perfect, polished look, so you have flexibility in both fit and quality. My mother, who is in her early sixties and is very specific about quality, lives in a brown military-style blazer I coerced her to buy years ago. She still can't get over the low price! You can't really go wrong in this category.

*This page:
Kate Moss,
2000.*

*Opposite:
(Bottom)
Brigitte Bardot
in an authentic
military jacket,
1967.*

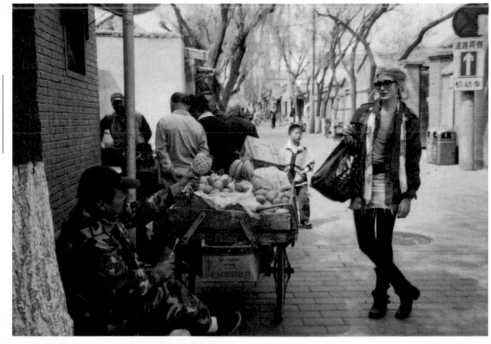

Right: My friend Amelie Torling in China, wearing an army jacket among other layers.

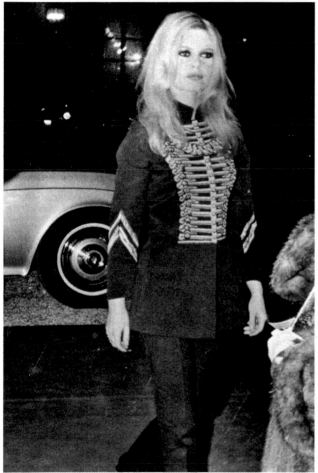

ALSO TO LOOK FOR AT ARMY/NAVY STORES:

THERMAL SHIRTS
So Marc Jacobs.

OLD-SCHOOL RAINCOATS
I like them best in bright yellow or army green.

NAVY WOOL SAILOR SWEATERS
They often have elbow patches, buttons on the shoulder, maybe even some star patches. Very chic.

ACCESSORIES
You can find belts with grommets, canvas backpacks, oversized duffels, and desert boots.

Shopping Tip:
Buy PIECES, not OUTFITS.
Shopping at cheap chic stores is about picking and choosing a few great things from a sea of potential mistakes. If you go for an "outfit" that has been merchandised by the store, it's pretty likely something in there won't actually work for you, but you won't realize it because you are too busy buying the "outfit."

CHEAP CHIC
What to Look For
STRIPES or POLKA DOTS

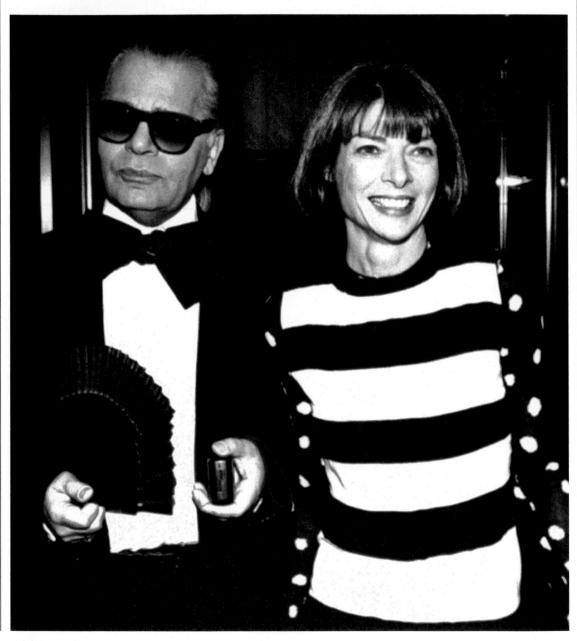

Anna Wintour (with Karl Lagerfeld) in a striped and polka dotted sweater, 1993.

Anything with STRIPES OR POLKA DOTS will add a youthful feeling to your look. T-shirts, scarves, dresses, skirts, pants, even socks that have a simple graphic pattern are easy to mix with solid colors and even can be fun to mix with one another.

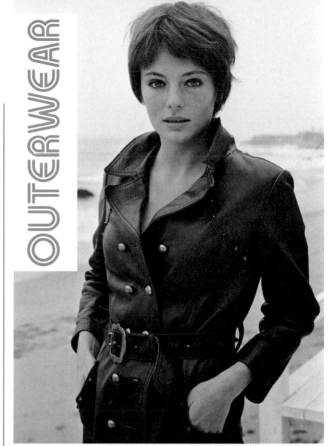

I wish I could find Jacqueline Bisset's double-breasted leather trench coat today, 1975.

OUTERWEAR is another great cheap chic purchase. Bomber jackets, rain coats, trench coats, parkas, and wind breakers are all classic pieces that look good regardless of borderline quality. Don't be scared to go for contrast: a utility vest over a feminine jersey blouse and tailored pants, a trench coat over a ball gown, or a belted military jacket over a chiffon dress.

You can't have enough plain T-shirts, but COLLECTIBLE T-SHIRTS, such as concert T-shirts, old logo shirts, or school emblem shirts, have a more specifically personal feel. I love, love, love printed T-shirts. They are a super cheap way to announce something about yourself: your favorite band, your favorite fashion brand, your political views, your home state, your favorite TV show. It's personal branding basically. My own favorite printed T-shirts are:

A classic red T-shirt with an abstract drawing of Stevie Wonder's braids and glasses. Stevie Wonder is my all-time favorite musician. I never get sick of listening to him. When I saw this T-shirt in the window of a store on my block I ran in and bought it immediately. I came home that night and found the same T-shirt waiting for me on my pillow. My husband hadn't been able to pass it by either! I wear it with gray jeans, a black-and-white striped leather belt, white leather ballet flats, and a long black sheared mink coat. I get a lot of attention on the streets of my neighborhood in this outfit.

A gray fitted cap sleeve T-shirt that says "I love you" in 70s retro metallic orange script. It's Chloe. I bought it in Paris when I was in my midtwenties and it was a big splurge at the time (although it was by far the least expensive thing in the store). I was just so excited to be buying something from Chloe. It was pretty trendy at the time so I wore it for a while and then put it away. It's been long enough now that I'm interested in it again and have been wearing it all the time. It looks great with my Tuleh black viscose capri pants and leopard print ballet flats from Marc Jacobs (talk about splurging).

Chrissie Hynde of the Pretenders in a Pretenders T-shirt, 1981.

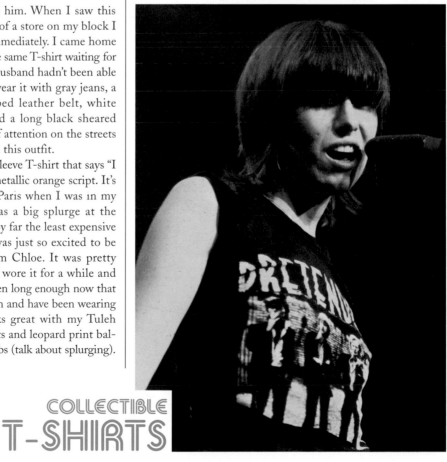

OUTERWEAR

COLLECTIBLE T-SHIRTS

Amanda Brooks

CHEAP CHIC
What to Look For

FEMININE DRESS OR BLOUSE

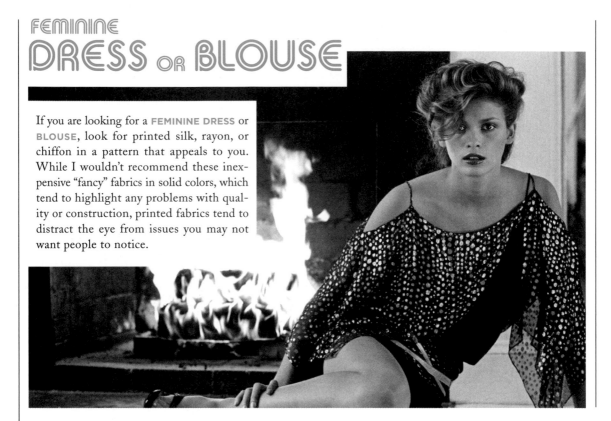

If you are looking for a FEMININE DRESS or BLOUSE, look for printed silk, rayon, or chiffon in a pattern that appeals to you. While I wouldn't recommend these inexpensive "fancy" fabrics in solid colors, which tend to highlight any problems with quality or construction, printed fabrics tend to distract the eye from issues you may not want people to notice.

Shopping Tip:
One of the best things to happen to cheap chic shoppers in years is the DEMOCRATIZATION OF DESIGNER CLOTHES. *Target sells clothes designed by Proenza Schouler, Thakoon, and Libertine; H&M sells Karl Lagerfeld, Viktor and Rolf, and Stella McCartney; and Topshop sells a line designed by Kate Moss. I went to the opening day of these collections with great anticipation and have been met by mixed results. Karl Lagerfeld for H&M was a big disappointment for me because most of the clothes were made in black chiffon and cheap black chiffon just looks cheap to me, no matter the shape or the design. So I returned to H&M with adjusted expectations for the Viktor and Rolf opening and was happily surprised to return home with bags full of clothes: a classic trench, a well-cut tuxedo jacket, some great-fitting lingerie, and a black wool peacoat among them. They were better at choosing which fabrics worked in which*

shapes and there was a larger variety of choice. While Kate Moss's clothes for Topshop looked stunning in the ads, the quality just looked really too poor for my taste to actually buy much more than an evening clutch as a gift for my assistant.

But perhaps the best designer/cheap chic collaborations I've witnessed was Proenza Schouler and Thakoon for Target: great prints, great colors, great cuts. The clothes didn't look like they were trying to be expensive so it didn't matter that they weren't. I bought bright red jeans, a white button-down shirt with black piping, a navy nylon "motorcycle jacket," some printed cotton beach dresses, and two fantastic floral bikinis. So the moral is, proceed with caution. Just because the name on the label is good doesn't mean you should buy it. Look at the clothes and judge them with the same eye as you would with more expensive clothes. If they hold up to those standards, they're probably worth a try.

Supermodel Gia Carangi in the kind of blouse I would look to buy in Topshop, 1982.

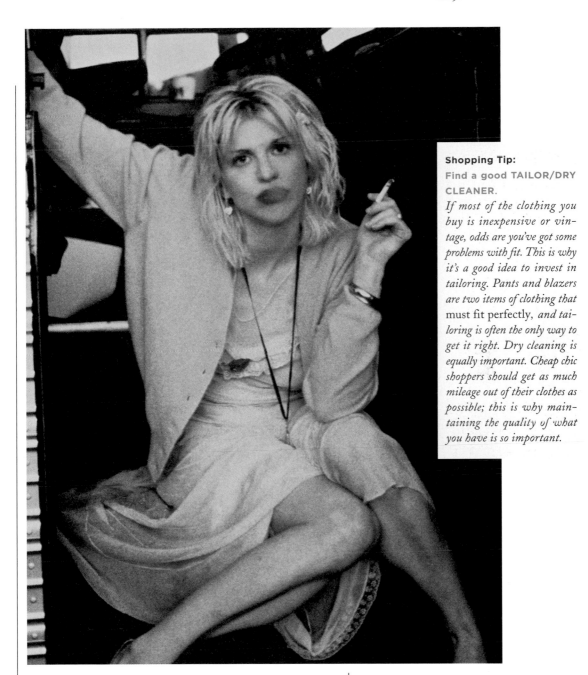

Shopping Tip:

Find a good TAILOR/DRY CLEANER.

If most of the clothing you buy is inexpensive or vintage, odds are you've got some problems with fit. This is why it's a good idea to invest in tailoring. Pants and blazers are two items of clothing that must fit perfectly, *and tailoring is often the only way to get it right. Dry cleaning is equally important. Cheap chic shoppers should get as much mileage out of their clothes as possible; this is why maintaining the quality of what you have is so important.*

If you have a tight budget for shopping, quality fabric is probably a rare luxury. That is why it can be a great joy to experience the variety of choice and relatively low price of **PRIVATE-LABEL CASHMERE** from stores such as Uniqlo, J.Crew, or almost any department store. A good cashmere sweater, scarf, hat, or gloves can last for decades if treated well (hand wash and lay flat to dry) and will always make you feel cozy and luxurious. Keep an eye out for the inevitable big sale at the end of the season!

PRIVATE-LABEL CASHMERE

Only Courtney Love could make a pink cashmere cardigan look grunge, 1993.

Amanda Brooks

CHEAP CHIC
What to Look For

Left top:
Rhinestone bracelets,
1984.

Left bottom:
Agyness Deyn, 2008.

Opposite:
Although Shakira
Caine's jewelry looks
glamorous, you can find
things like this at most
Indian or Tibetan
stores for a great price,
1989.

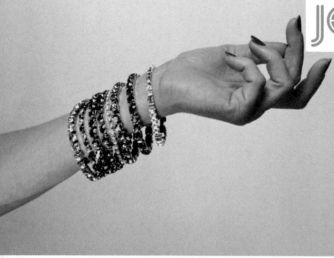

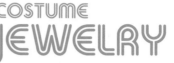

COSTUME
JEWELRY

There is such a huge variety of COSTUME JEWELRY. There's new, there's old, there are things that are supposed to look real and things that are supposed to look fake, there's designer and there's anonymous, there's precisely manufactured and there's homemade, and there's cheap and there's expensive.

HERE'S MY RUNDOWN:

DESIGNER COSTUME JEWELRY
Plastic Chanel logo earrings, a resin and rhinestone cuff from YSL, a gold snake necklace from Roberto Cavalli, a Marc by Marc Jacobs black-and-white plastic disc necklace. I own all of these pieces and they all cost under $200.

ETHNIC JEWELRY
Indian fake-jeweled chandelier earrings, African bead necklaces, Mexican fake-gold chandelier earrings.

DEPARTMENT STORE KNOCKOFFS
Fake diamond studs, fake pearls, fake gold. The key to wearing fake jewelry (that is supposed to look real) is to take good care of it and replenish it often. I feel no shame wearing fake diamonds as long as they are shiny and new.

COSTUME JEWELRY BOUTIQUES
There are costume jewelry boutiques in most upscale shopping neighborhoods (Mariko in NYC and Palm Beach is my personal favorite) that make real-looking, excellent replicas of fabulous jewelry. Most of what they sell is copies of designer jewelry from all decades of the twentieth century. The prices are definitely on the high end of the costume jewelry range but worth it if you want something that looks real, will hold up for a reasonable amount of time, and looks more sophisticated than most of the fake jewelry we see everywhere.

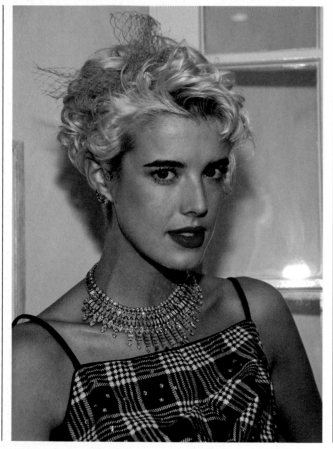

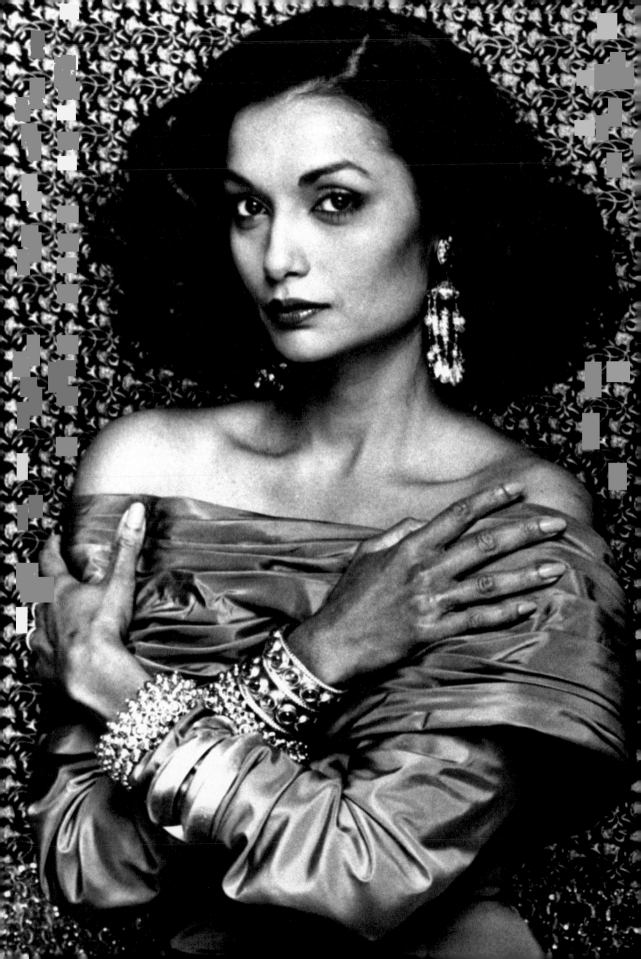

CHEAP CHIC
What to Look For

BELTS are one of the easiest things to find on a budget. Almost every variety of cheap chic store sells great belts; just look for one that speaks to you. I have a brown suede belt from the Gap that fits perfectly into the belt holes of jeans, is a really pretty color of caramel brown, and has a very simple brass d-ring buckle that seems to go with everything. Its simplicity and lack of busy decoration compelled me to buy it. It cost $19 and is more useful than all the other belts hanging in my closet.

Shopping Tip:

Be realistic about YOUR AGE. *Cheap chic chain stores encourage experimentation, but unfortunately they can also encourage us to believe that we are ten years older or younger than we actually are. The best way to avoid age deception is to shop with a girlfriend. You won't get jealous if she finds something before you (there's enough to go around for everyone), and you need someone to tell you honestly whether you can get away with such trendy looks as puff sleeves, low-slung belts, anything with sequins, fringed scarves, or shorts.*

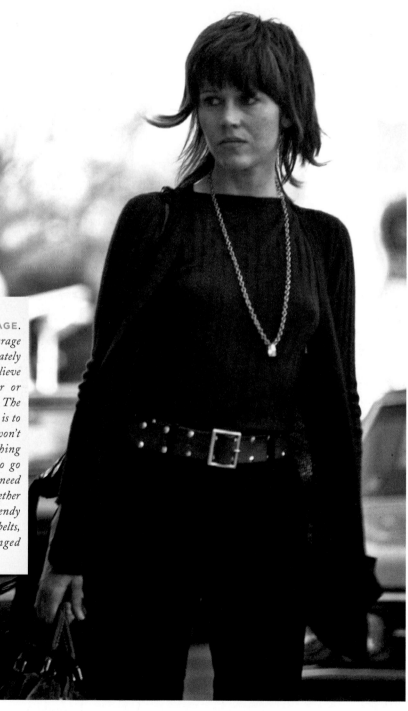

Of all the amazing outfits Jane Fonda has worn, this one (with her groovy studded belt) is my favorite, 1971.

Shopping Tip:

AVOID BUYING THINGS ONLY BECAUSE THEY ARE
"A GOOD DEAL."

We've all fallen into the trap of buying things because they are inexpensive or on sale, or because they just seem like a good deal—and then we never wear them. You spend a lot of time thinking about whether you should buy an expensive coat; lavish some thought on your cheap chic purchases, too, and you'll save money in the long run. Ask yourself the following questions:

- *What will I wear it with?*
- *Where will I where it?*
- *Does it work with the other things in my closet?*
- *Will I still like it next week?*
- *Is it me?*

REAL GOLD JEWELRY

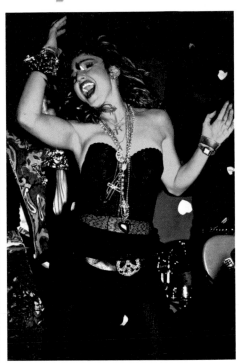

CASUAL HATS

CASUAL HATS such as baseball hats, straw sun hats, newsboy caps, and even ski hats are very inexpensive and can add a lot of style to a basic look.

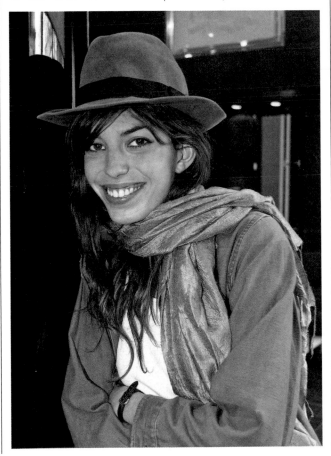

A good approach to buying REAL GOLD JEWELRY on a budget is to buy simple classic pieces—hoops, chains, charm bracelets, signet rings, rosary necklaces—from the least expensive jewelry store you can find. I particularly like jewelry stands in Chinatown, the airport, or in the mall—seriously.

*Above:
Madonna,
1985.*

*Left:
Lou Doillon,
who is a
fantastic hat
wearer, 2003.*

Amanda Brooks

What to Look For

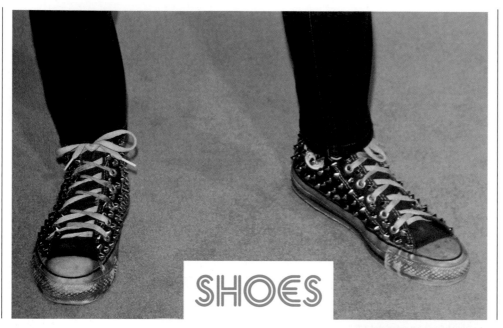

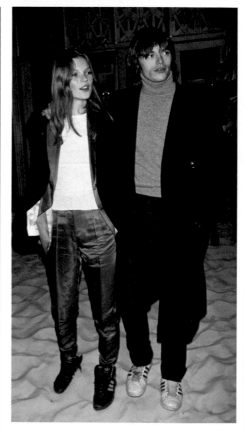

Left:
Agyness Deyn's
studded
Converse All
Stars, 2009.

Opposite:
Matching
bikinis and
espadrilles,
Monte Carlo,
1975.

SHOES

Finding a good pair of **SHOES** that don't break the bank can be tough. If you are looking for leather shoes, I beg you to buy the most expensive pair you can afford. It might hurt a little bit to spend that much money, but they will last much longer and make any outfit look better. Cheap leather shoes almost always look just that—*cheap*!

There are, however, a variety of shoes that are inexpensive but have great original style.

CONSIDER THE FOLLOWING:

One of the most practical and timeless cheap chic purchases is **OLD-SCHOOL SNEAKERS**. Puma, Adidas, Converse All-Stars, and Vans, to name just a few of the classic sneakers out there, can range in effect from traditional to edgy, from sporty to high fashion, and they mostly cost under $100. I love wearing a classically tailored suit with a men's tailored shirt and old-school sneakers. It is chic in a rock 'n' roll kind of way, and yet it's comfortable and timeless.

Right:
Kate Moss and
then-boyfriend
Mario Sorrenti,
both in matching
Adidas, 1993.
The tomboy look
really suits her.

NOVELTY SHOES such as Chinese fabric Mary Janes, rubber rain boots, and flip-flops all look great because they are authentic, hard-working shoes.

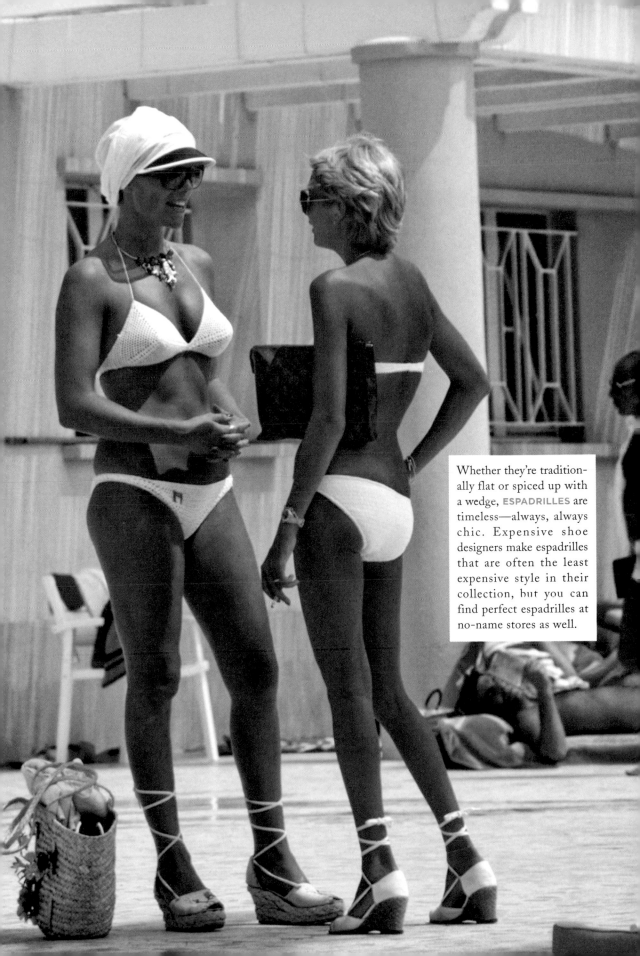

Whether they're traditionally flat or spiced up with a wedge, **ESPADRILLES** are timeless—always, always chic. Expensive shoe designers make espadrilles that are often the least expensive style in their collection, but you can find perfect espadrilles at no-name stores as well.

CHEAP CHIC

What to Look For

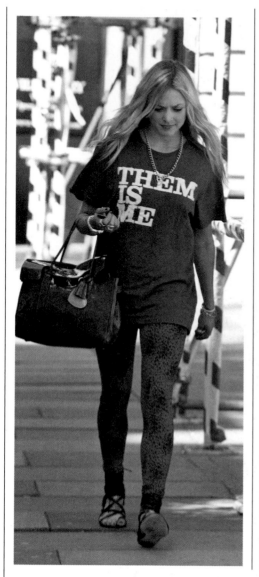

An assortment of **LEGWEAR** is easy to afford and can do a lot to create personality in your look. Besides classic opaque tights in a variety of colors, there are fishnets, knee socks, over the knee socks, leggings, and plain old socks that can portray great character. If it seems like too young an idea to you, limit yourself to playing with black tights in a variety of textures and patterns. A black dress with black lace tights can be a very classic, yet personal look.

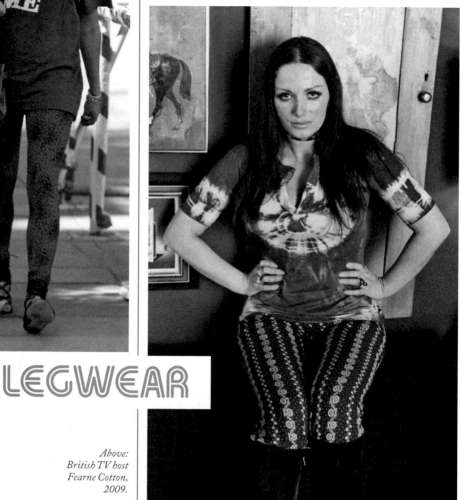

LEGWEAR

*Above:
British TV host
Fearne Cotton,
2009.*

*Right:
Isn't it hard
to believe this is
Jackie Collins?
1971.*

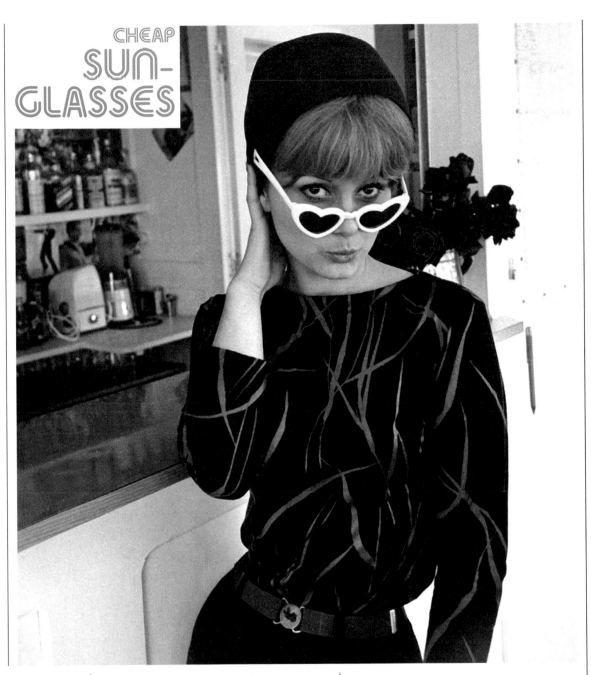

CHEAP SUN-GLASSES

French actress France Anglade at the Cannes Film Festival, 1960.

You know how when you buy a pair of **CHEAP SUNGLASSES** on the street you hold on to them forever, but when you buy a designer pair you lose them the next day. As a veteran of this phenomenon I try my best to buy sunglasses on the cheap. The key to buying cheap sunglasses is that they should be somewhat elaborate (unusual shape, signature metal detail, two-tone color) in order to distract from the fact that they are made of cheap plastic. For people who like the classic Ray-Ban Wayfarer, the drug store brand Foster Grant makes an awfully believable version.

Amanda Brooks

CHEAP CHIC
Evening

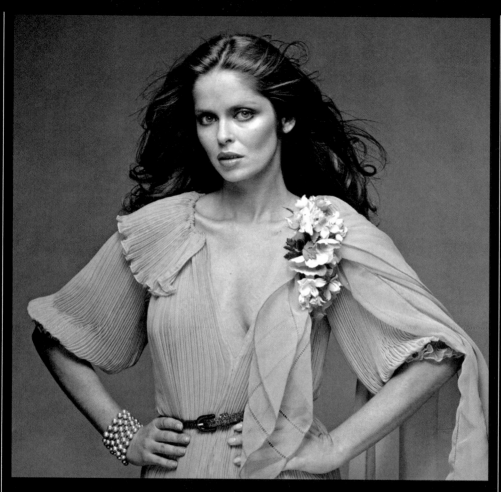

I HAVE A WHOLE COLLECTION OF BITS AND PIECES I HAVE GATHERED OVER THE YEARS THAT ADD A BIT OF DRAMA AND DECORATION.

Dressing for evening on a budget can be tough, but it is a worthy challenge. The most satisfying feeling is getting compliments on an outfit you put together on a dime, especially when you're standing in a room full of people who paid much more. You don't need a closet full of cocktail dresses and stilettos, just a small selection of clothing and accessories that you can use to dress up the clothes you already have.

ONE EXPENSIVE PIECE OF CLOTHING can be the foundation of half a dozen successful evening looks. It could be an amazing formal blouse, a long skirt, a dress, or even an evening jacket that is simple enough to mix but striking enough to make an impact. I inherited a black silk floor-length Vicky Tiel evening skirt from my mother that I have worn to countless formal occasions: with a sequined blouse, a tailored jacket, a velvet fringed shawl, a satin cape, even a tank top. The fit is beautiful and the shape works with many different proportions. If you find something similarly wonderful you might make a well-calculated investment.

This page: I love the combination of accessories in Barbara Bach's evening look, 1977.

Opposite: (Top) Agyness Deyn, with Henry Holland, brings the 80s back at the Elle Style Awards in London, 2008.

(Bottom) Catherine Deneuve and her sister Françoise Dorléac, with fresh flowers in their hair, 1967.

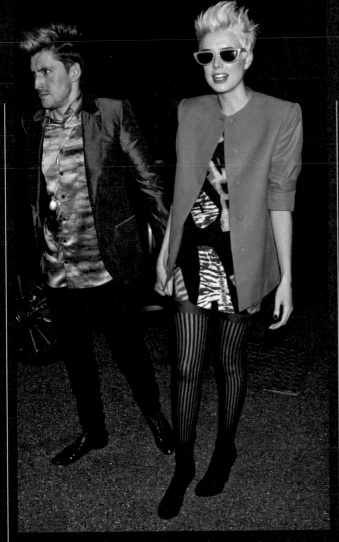

Even if you do evening on the cheap, you should really learn about GOOD HAIR AND MAKEUP. A one-time hair and makeup lesson is a worthwhile investment that will allow you to vamp it up a little bit for countless evenings. Before your lesson, grab a pile of your favorite magazines and rip out the pages you respond to. Although I'm happy to hear suggestions from a stylist, I have never been happy letting someone else's opinion shape my look completely.

A collection of ECCENTRIC ACCESSORIES—gloves, belts, scarves—that suit your style is worth having. They can be just that little something that your outfit is lacking or the perfect thing to throw off an otherwise predictable combination.

Since I don't collect real jewelry with serious intent, FRESH FLOWERS are my favorite way to add richness to my look (not to mention luscious color and personality). When I see a girl with fresh flowers in her hair, I almost always like her look, no matter what she is wearing. I also happen to *love* fresh flower corsages, attached to a ribbon around your wrist or pinned to your dress.

Looking for SOMETHING TO COVER YOUR SHOULDERS is a great excuse to add another layer to your evening look. I have a whole collection of bits and pieces I have gathered over the years that add a bit of drama and decoration. I am a big fan of the fur shrug, which can be found in affordable abundance at thrift stores and flea markets. If you don't wear fur, an elaborate shawl can be equally effective as long as it has some personality: embroidery, fringe, double-face satin, etc. A cape can also work to great effect in the right situation.

Accessorize with SOME GREAT COSTUME JEWELRY (see page 230).

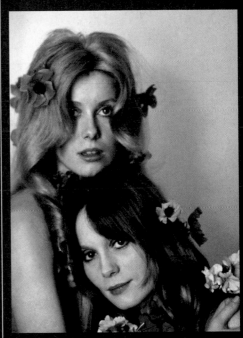

WHEN I SEE A GIRL WITH FRESH FLOWERS IN HER HAIR, I ALMOST ALWAYS LIKE HER LOOK, NO MATTER WHAT SHE IS WEARING.

CHEAP CHIC
Where to Find It

When it comes to cheap chic shopping, you have to be willing to look for things in the unlikeliest of places. Just because you don't like the overall aesthetic of a brand or store doesn't mean that there isn't something in there that will work for you.

CHEAP AND TRENDY CHAIN STORES

Cheap chic chain stores have changed the face of American fashion. It used to be that fashion trends were only for those who could afford to buy designer clothing. However, with the invention of inexpensive stores that carry high-end trends, fashion-forward clothes can be found at shockingly good prices. If you depend on these stores, you must go regularly and be prepared to make decisions on the spot. Their turnover is amazingly fast, and if they have something really good it's usually sold out within a few days. Also, don't expect the clothes themselves to last very long. They just are not durable. If you find something you think you'll wear over and over, buy multiples.

MY FAVORITE CHAIN STORES:

Zara
They carry the best fit and quality for tailored clothes—blazers, overcoats, trousers, and fitted dresses—perfect for the office. While they do offer trends, their clothes have the most grown-up, long-lasting appeal. Even people I know who renounce cheap chic chains stores love Zara.

H&M
On the whole, the best of what they offer is for a young and very trendy customer. The fit is all over the place—I range from a 2 to a 10—but the prices are really low. I tend to have most success with very casual and colorful printed summer dresses in cotton or crepe. I also did *very* well with the Viktor and Rolf capsule collection.

Topshop
While it is very trendy, Topshop offers trends that feel more sophisticated and grown-up—very close to what you see in designer stores, albeit lower price and quality. I have bought everything at Topshop from bikinis to shoes (I almost never buy inexpensive shoes!) to jeans to winter coats. The size of the store and the selection are also huge. They truly have something for everyone.

J.Crew
While the overall aesthetic of J.Crew does little to mask my predictably preppy roots, they do have phenomenally well-priced classics: sweaters, shorts, T-shirts, and trousers that last both in quality and in style.

ETHNIC STORES
Ethnic stores of all kinds sell authentic, unique, hard-to-find clothes and accessories at really reasonable prices. I *love* cotton Mary Jane slippers and Chinese pajamas from Chinese stores, embroidered tunics and metallic sandals from Tibetan stores, dangly sparkly earrings from Indian stores, printed dashikis from African stores, and bangle bracelets and slippers from Moroccan stores.

Another option for cheap ethnic finds is to scour local shops when you travel. I recently went to Mexico on vacation and came back with a few years' supply of beach dresses and embroidered caftans. The most elaborate hand-stitched one of the lot only cost $40 U.S. And the leather sandals I bought to wear with them were $4.50!

ATHLETIC STORES
You'll find a big selection of Nike, Adidas, Puma, etc. While these brands put out hundreds of new styles each year, I am invariably attracted to the old-school remakes from the late 70s and early 80s.

STREET-STYLE STORES
For hip-hop icon shirts, funky vintage Nikes, and Kangol hats. I love mixing these more out-there pieces with something formal and classic, like a beautifully tailored pantsuit.

CHEAP CHIC
Inspiration

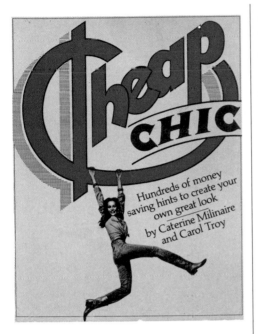

Hundreds of money saving hints to create your own great look by Caterine Milinaire and Carol Troy

BOOK

CHEAP CHIC

Cheap Chic is a book unlike any other. Published in the 70s, it is still the ultimate guide to achieving style on a budget. When I was in my early twenties I discovered it in a used book shop and fell in love with it immediately; it validated the way I'd been dressing all my life. The combination of high style and low prices makes this book a winner for anyone who buys it. In fact, rereading *Cheap Chic* a few years ago gave me the inspiration to write this book. If you are a cheap chic shopper, you *must* own this book. It is a cult favorite, and is therefore no longer a cheap chic purchase itself (if you Google it you'll find it on many collectible book Web sites for around $200) but it is absolutely worth buying. It is just a must must-have.

Two of the best points in *Cheap Chic* came from a woman named Ingeborg Day, a chic office worker who has a very practical attitude toward getting dressed. Both suggestions reduce shopping for clothes down to simple formulas and have simplified the decision-making process when you budget your purchases.

1. **Cost per wear.** It's not how much one item of clothing costs, but how much it costs to wear it each time. The formula goes like this:

$$\frac{Price}{Number\ of\ times\ worn} = Cost\ per\ wear$$

$$\frac{\$300}{100} = \$3\ per\ wear$$

So even if it seems like a lot to spend $300 on a pair of shoes, it's actually going to cost you much less per wear than if you buy $50 shoes and only wear them ten times.

2. Ingeborg also suggests making your own **pie chart** prioritizing the areas of your life you dress for. She narrows it down to six areas: work, play/casual, play/elegant, sports/exercise, social functions, and bedtime. It's really helpful to think about how much time you spend in each area, how important those areas are to you, and budget accordingly. For example, I used to spend most of my money on clothes for going out in the evening with my husband. But after taking this suggestion to heart, I realized that I spent way more time in my life dressed casually and that my casual clothes were suffering from neglect. So now I limit my tendency to buy only special things so I can afford also to buy some more casual things—like cashmere sweaters and great weekend pants—that are not only comfortable but also look good and make me feel attractive even if I'm just taking the kids to school.

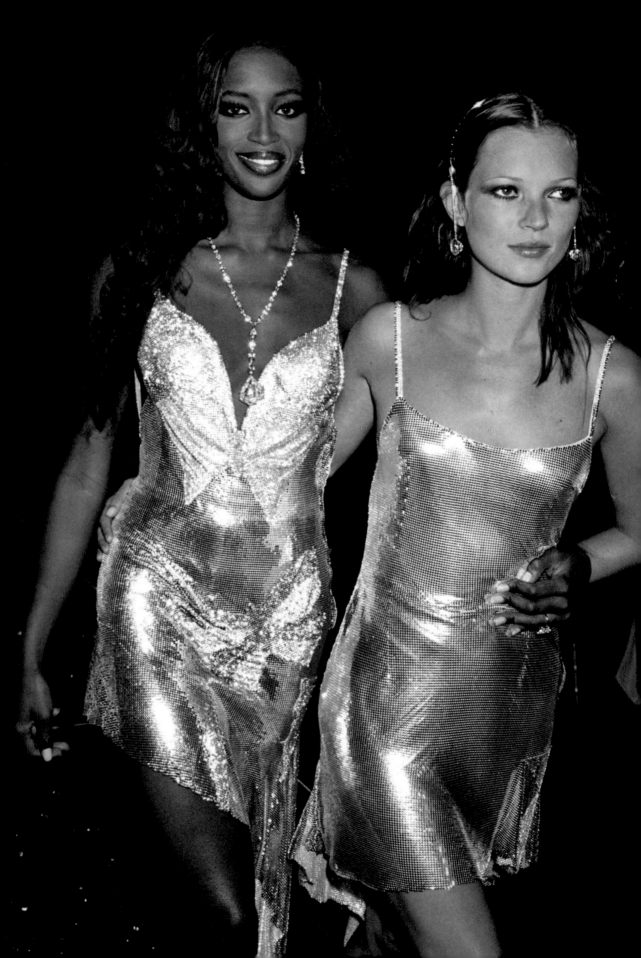

DESIGNER

//

I NEVER GO OUT IN SOMETHING THAT I AM UNCOMFORTABLE IN, WELL EXCEPT HIGH HEELS, AND THEY'RE TORTURE. AND THAT'S JUST SOMETHING I DEAL WITH."

—DIANE VON FURSTENBERG

There is an entire spectrum of women who buy designer labels. Some simply wear the perfume, or they save for months to get the handbag, while others have that same bag in every color. Some women buy just a single designer piece every once in a while, while others buy the whole look—or even the whole collection. When I worked at Tuleh we knew of a girl who had a standing order with Bergdorf Goodman to have every piece by Tuleh in her size charged to her account and sent directly to her house! Every piece! Another woman would buy two of everything she liked. She commuted between New York and Washington, D.C., and wanted to have everything she liked in both closets so she didn't have to think about packing! You gotta *love* these women. They are total fashion enthusiasts.

At the other end of the spectrum is the woman who splurges on one piece here and there and works it into an otherwise affordable wardrobe. My friend Venessa, a design assistant at Zac Posen, buys herself one pair of knockout designer shoes every season and wears them until they fall apart. Because she is young and

Naomi Campbell and Kate Moss wearing Versace, 1999.

trendy, she isn't choosing the tasteful black leather Manolo Blahnik pump; she wants the gold lamé Lanvin sandal on a wood platform or the highest Miu Miu Hawaiian-printed wedge heels. She goes for maximum impact with her shoes and wears them with everything from a Mexican sundress from the flea market to Prada short shorts found at a consignment shop.

The key to designer shopping is to make calculated decisions based on what you know about your style. Do you wear the same coat every winter for a decade? Then it's probably a good idea to invest in one. If you *love* trendy shoes but know you'll feel foolish wearing them when the trend has passed, limit yourself to one pair per season, and really work them with everything while they're hot. Buying designer clothes should always be a calculated decision.

DESIGNER
My Designer Shopping

I'VE NEVER BEEN A BIG DESIGNER CLOTHES SHOPPER, AT LEAST NOT AT FULL RETAIL PRICES.

1984

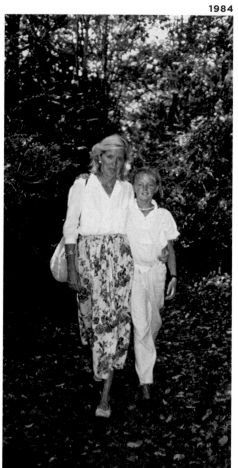

1977

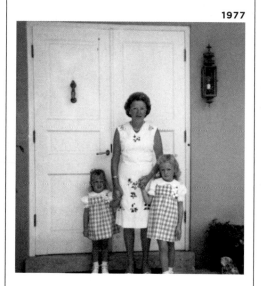

Though I covet designer things and sneak in a few splurges here and there—mostly shoes, tailored jackets, costume jewelry—the truth is that I've never been a big designer clothes shopper, at least not at full retail prices. Nevertheless, some form of "designer clothing" has always been present in my life. When I was a very little girl, to have anything by Florence Eiseman, the queen of preppy children's clothes, was an exciting treat. Every girl I knew wanted her clothes, which were all brightly colored and decorated with simple appliquéd flowers. Whenever I visited my grandmother, she would buy identical Florence Eiseman dresses for me, my sister, and my two cousins. You can imagine the family photo sessions that ensued.

In my early teens it was Esprit and Merona that captured my attention. Still preppy, still colorful, but less naive, these were the clothes that inspired oohs and aahs at school. The experience of going to a department store (Gimbels) to buy them added greatly to the excitement. One summer, my parents took us to France. The clothes I saw in Galeries Lafayette, the "Bloomingdales" of Paris, enthralled me. They were different, more sophisticated than the clothes I was used to back home. I chose two outfits—Ton Sur Ton yellow parachute pants with a matching sweatshirt and Et Vous overalls (pictured above)—but my sense of fashion possibility had been broadened and excited.

At thirteen I had another defining moment

This page: (Left) My sister Kim and me, with our grandmother Florence Whittemore, in our first designer dresses by Florence Eiseman, 1977.

(Right) Me, with my mother, in Et Vous overalls from Paris, 1984.

Opposite: Me, in a Zac Posen gown for a Vogue *photo shoot at my husband's family farm in England, 2005. My friend Duro sent me a vintage rhinestone pin, which I attached to the dress to make the look more personal. Photograph by Jonathan Becker.*

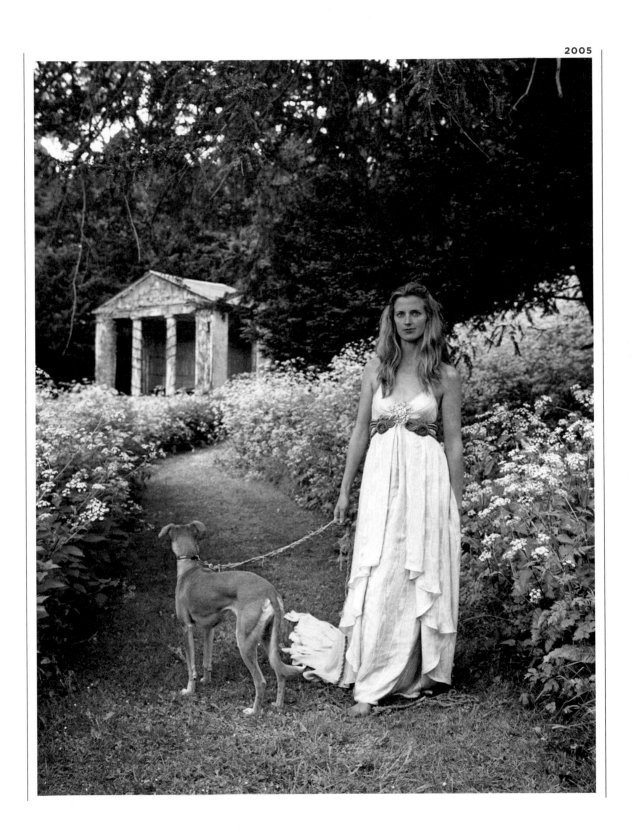

Amanda Brooks

DESIGNER
My Designer Shopping

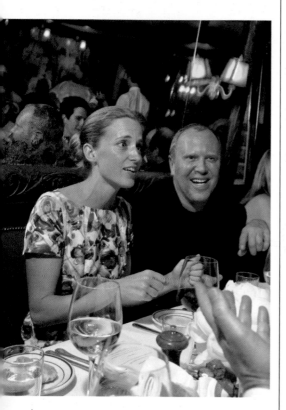

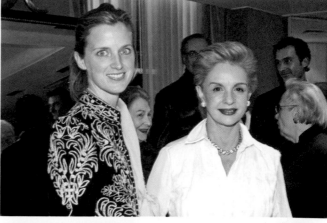

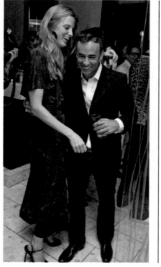

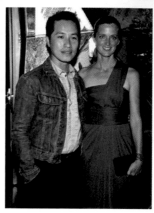

in my style and my relationship with fashion. It was brought about by an outfit by Norma Kamali, who I had never heard of at the time. It was three pieces: a long-sleeve T-shirt, a very short ruffled skirt, and leggings. They were all white and had washing instructions—yes, washing instructions—printed all over them in big red letters. I know it sounds weird, and believe me, it was weird, but I loved it. I begged and begged my mother, and she bought it for me on my birthday. This is the moment when I broke with what was cool at school and picked something that just felt right to me. My mom must have really had to bite her tongue when I wore that outfit, but I am really impressed—and grateful—that she let me find my own way around clothes.

I arrived at college wearing a Ralph Lauren dress from an outlet store, having learned to venerate the Polo look in boarding school. I was clearly not prepared for Brown's fashion parade. One friend I made in art class wore Chanel quilted combat boots with a matching backpack. Another girl who lived down the hall in my dorm, whose father was a real estate mogul, wore RalphLauren's bohemian collection to lunch only days after I'd seen it in *Vogue*. When I asked her how she had gotten hold of these clothes so quickly (and in Providence, Rhode Island), she said, "Oh, I flew down to the city last weekend to have my hair cut by Frederic [Fekkai], and I picked up

This page: (Clockwise from left) Me with Michael Kors, Carolina Herrera, Phillip Lim, Francisco Costa.

Opposite: (Clockwise from top left) Me with Tory Burch, Stefano Pilati, Diane von Furstenberg, Christian Louboutin, Thakoon and stylist Tina Chai, Zac Posen.

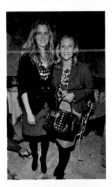

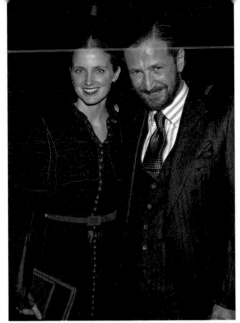

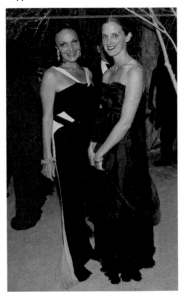

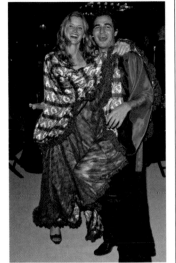

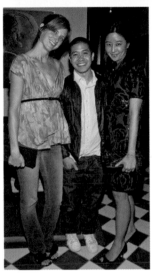

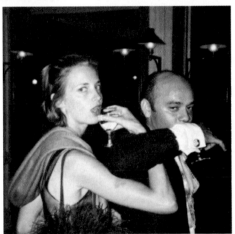

my spring order at Bergdorf's." There you go. I didn't know whether to be mortified or jealous.

My new college friends' enthusiasm for labels and accessories made me look at fashion in a way I never had before. Although I did my best to imitate their high style via thrift-store finds and cheap chic knockoffs, I couldn't afford any real designer clothes or accessories until a few years after I graduated and got a real job.

If I had piles of money, I imagine that I might be tempted to buy a lot more designer clothing than I do now (and I'll admit that I am very lucky to be friends with a lot of the designers whose clothes I adore, and they often give me things or let me order things from their studios at a discount). But part of me is secretly glad that I can't afford more; having a budget requires me to address trends in a more creative, less expected way. I know in my heart that a limited budget actually makes me a better, more personal dresser in the end.

DESIGNER
What to Look For

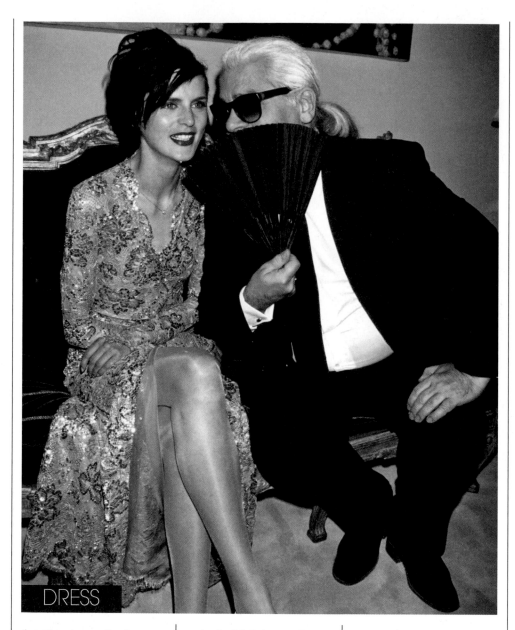

DRESS

Stella Tennant (channeling Coco Chanel) with Karl Lagerfeld, 1996.

A **DRESS** is usually the most signature piece a designer makes, but the level of wearability depends highly on the complexity of the design. If the design is simple—usually in a solid color with clean lines—a dress can be worn again and again and accessorized with belts, cardigans, and different jewelry each time to reinvent it. But if a dress is very specific—made in a noticeable print, has intricate details such as stitching, beading, and embroidery, or has a very noticeable construction such as large ruffles or complicated seaming—it might just be a one-hit wonder (until your daughter is a teenager and wants to steal it from you) in which case you have to ask yourself if the place or event you are going to is worth the money spent.

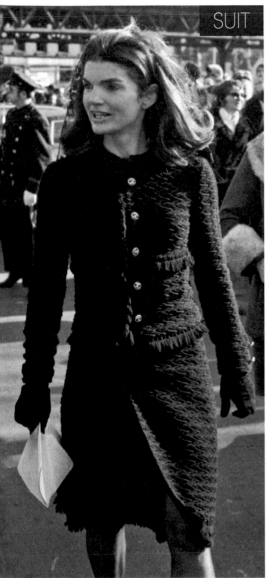

SUIT

Left:
I think about
this suit of
Jackie O's when
I wonder to
myself if I'll
ever buy a
Chanel suit.
If so, I'd like one
just like this,
1970.

There are a *lot* of what my mom calls **"FASHION COATS"** out there. Think patterned trench coats, cotton peacoats, capes, that kind of thing. They are neither warm nor water-proof, but the complexity of design makes it easy to wear as a statement piece with nothing of much interest underneath. I own countless fashion coats!

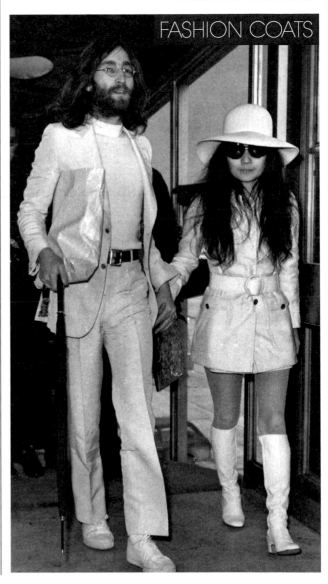

FASHION COATS

Designers seem to understand that **SUITS** are bought for prac-ticality—not on an impulse or for a one-time event—and so they are made for durability and flexibility. The suits tend to project both a classic sensi-bility and the designer's sig-nature. A black Chanel suit is the perfect example of this. I've probably worn a suit as a suit a sum total of about three times, but I have worn the pieces of a suit as separates over and over again.

Right:
Yoko Ono and
John Lennon
feeling the all-
white 60s vibe
at the London
airport, 1969.

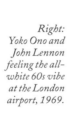

DESIGNER
What to Look For

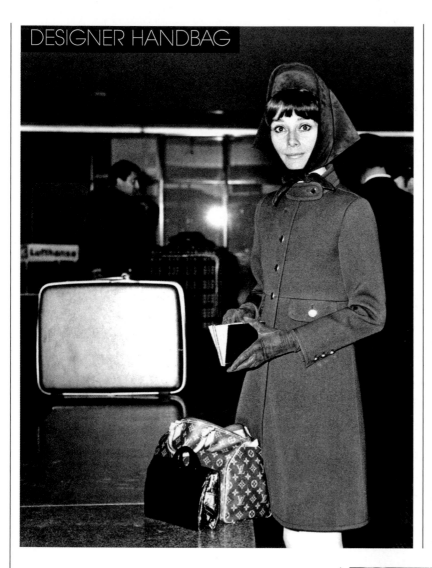

DESIGNER HANDBAG

If you are **THINKING ABOUT PURCHASING AN OVERTLY TRENDY BAG,** *ask yourself these questions before plunking down the cash:*

- *Do I have enough money that it won't matter if I wear this bag for only a few months and then get sick of it?*

- *Do I absolutely love this bag and intend to keep it for posterity, even if I won't actually carry it for very long?*

- *Do I feel an intense personal connection to this bag, such that I will keep carrying it for a long time, even if next season it is totally uncool?*

If you answer yes to any of these questions, just buy yourself the damn bag. But if you're just buying it to feel like the coolest girl in the room for ten minutes, maybe you should buy something that will contribute to more long-term happiness.

It really isn't my thing, but I understand that some people feel that they have to have an **OVERTLY TRENDY DESIGNER HANDBAG.**

"FASHION FADES, ONLY STYLE REMAINS THE SAME."
—COCO CHANEL

Above: It's amazing how Audrey Hepburn's Louis Vuitton bag, in 1968, looks every bit the same and as chic as it does today.

Right: A 2004 Louis Vuitton bag.

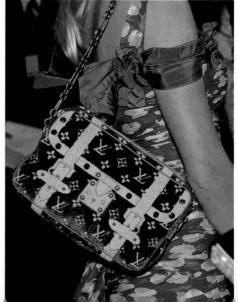

If you have the means and motivation to really splurge, buy a **CLASSIC CHANEL 2.55 BAG**. You will wear it the rest of your life. It looks good with everything, and it pulls together the rest of your outfit.

Clockwise from left: Elodie Bouchez, 2004.

Agyness Deyn in a Chanel "bicep" bag, 2008.

A minuscule Chanel evening bag.

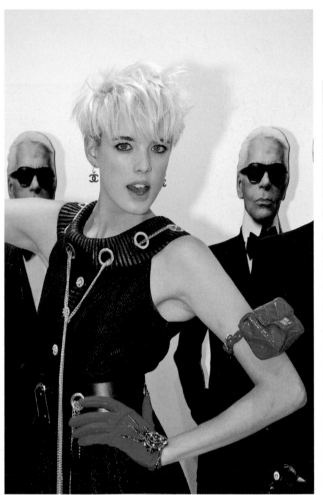

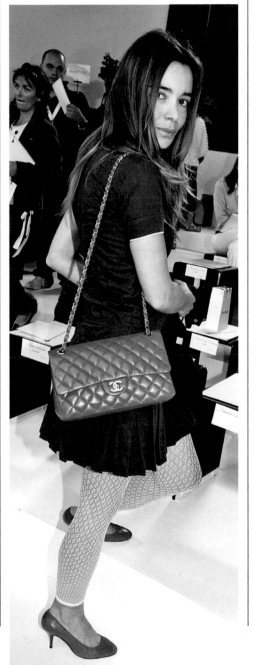

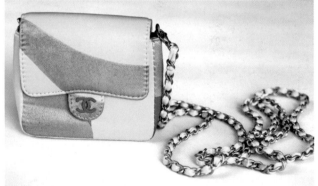

SMALL ACCESSORIES

Another alternative for girls pining for that ultra trendy purple ostrich bag is to buy the **WALLET**, the **EYEGLASS CASE**, the **KEY RING**, or the **CHANGE PURSE** instead. It will save you significant cash, and, being more discreet, it will be easier to keep using when the trend has passed.

DESIGNER
What to Look For

**"I LOVE TO TAKE
THINGS THAT ARE
EVERYDAY . . .
AND MAKE THEM
INTO THE MOST
LUXURIOUS
THINGS IN THE
WORLD."**
—MARC JACOBS

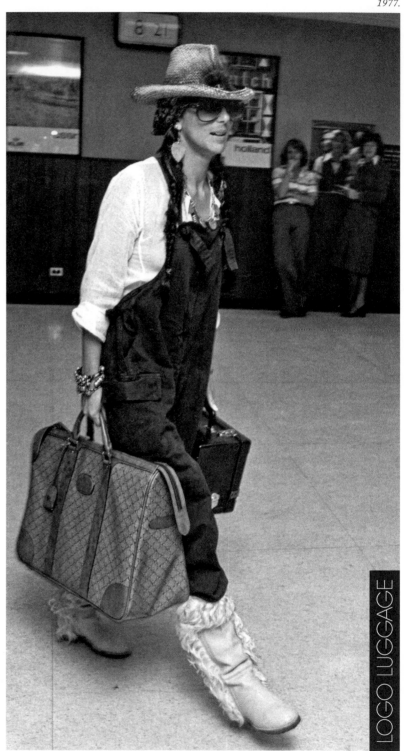

LOGO LUGGAGE

If you are a status lover, you could go for the full monty and buy **LOGO LUGGAGE**, which is actually quite classic. If I see someone in the airport with Louis Vuitton luggage, I don't think what a fashion victim they are. I think, "Oh, there's someone with fancy luggage." If I were to buy logo luggage I would buy vintage. Wouldn't it be cool to have a complete set of Gucci logo luggage from the 70s? I think that would be super chic.

ANALYZING A
DESIGNER'S COLLECTION

Shopping in the world of high fashion can be a full-time job (which presents a problem, since you probably need a full-time job in order to pay for it). Fashion today comes and goes more quickly than ever before, and it takes a trained and disciplined eye to follow and anticipate its changes: from fashion magazines, to runway shows, to finding what you want, to getting on the waiting list for what you want, to returning things you don't want, to figuring out what to wear it with, to calculate whether it's worth the price. Just writing about it exhausts me. But I do it. I do all of the above. Because I love fashion. I am a total addict. I am a slave. And I enjoy it. It's thrilling, it's rewarding, and it's creative. That's the key. You can only be devoted to fashion if you enjoy the entire process. If you don't, there are a million better ways to spend your time and money. In my mind I break down every fashion designer's collection I see (whether on the runway, in the showroom, or in the store) into three sections, listed below. When shopping for designer clothes, do the same for yourself. It helps to put things in perspective and prioritize where it's best to spend your money:

1. In the fashion world we call trendy things "editorial" because they are the pieces that grab the editors' attention and will most likely end up featured in big spreads in magazines. These are the pieces that give us fashion news—a new proportion, shape, color palette, or conceptual idea. These are also the pieces that will most likely end up in the designer's ad campaign and on red carpets.

2. Then there are the basics that work to bring the more attention-grabbing pieces back down to earth: the pants, the pencil skirts, the underpinnings for the suits, the basic dress that goes under the over-the-top coat.

3. In between the previous two categories are pieces that address the trends of the season but in a more subtle, toned-down way. For example there was a collection done by Proenza Schouler (one of my most favorite designers—they also did a line for Target) that was filled with the most stunning, intricately designed and decorated winter coats. I went to see the collection in the showroom and left with a few fabulous pieces but none of the coats from the runway. Even if I really splashed out to afford just one, I knew I would see it around a lot and likely be tired of it before long. What I did buy, though, was a wool toggle coat—completely classic in shape and fabric that had some of the detailing of the fancier coats on the sleeves. I was so satisfied buying the toned-down version of the inspiration piece, knowing that I could feel of-the-moment for this season but that I could also easily wear this more timeless version for seasons afterward.

DESIGNER
SHOPPING TIPS

BEWARE OF ANYTHING THAT APPEARS IN THE DESIGNER'S AD CAMPAIGN. *Because fashion is so global and we are all such magazine junkies these days, we will most likely grow tired of a designer's signature "look of the season" before it even hits the stores. Buy less highly visible pieces from a beloved collection or go with the full look with gusto and confidence.*

If I had a bigger clothing budget, I would buy a lot of **CLASSIC BASICS** *from high-end designers. The valuable thing about designer basics is that they're well made so they last a long time, and they make you look great without having to add a lot of accessories. Another advantage of designer classics is that their cut stays consistent so if you like a pair of pants from a certain designer one season you'll probably find that style again the following season. A good staple of high-end classic basics should include tailored shirts in silk and in cotton, cashmere sweaters, tailored pants in many neutral colors, a few different shapes of skirts in solid colors, a tailored jacket, and a winter coat in wool or cashmere.*

There are two approaches to **HANGING ON TO THINGS THAT ARE NO LONGER "IN FASHION."** *One option is to put them away for a while. I bought an Yves Saint Laurent leather "flower" bag three years ago. I loved it so much but never wore it once, because by the time I actually got it I was sick of seeing it in magazines and ads and on celebrities. But I bought it anyway, knowing that one day I would get over it and wear it when it was no longer the thing of the moment. Every six months or so I'd remember that I have that bag sitting in the back of the closet and I'd ask myself if I am ready to wear it yet. I haven't gotten there yet, but I can feel the day approaching. I do, though, have some things in storage that I haven't worn in ten years and whose appeal I can no longer imagine. Those go straight to Goodwill.*

A WORD ABOUT RETURNS: *Don't hesitate to return something if you are not happy with it. If the jeans you bought stretch too much, or the button falls off an overcoat the second time you wear it, or even if you just get that feeling that you'll never wear the four-inch heels that the pushy salesman talked you into, don't hesitate to correct the problem. Any store worth doing business with would want you to be happy with your purchase so that you will come back and shop again. Don't feel guilty about it! That said, serial returners, or people that buy things just to wear them and then return them, are a nightmare. Returns are fine, but return with integrity!*

"WHOEVER SAID MONEY CAN'T BUY HAPPINESS SIMPLY DIDN'T KNOW WHERE TO GO SHOPPING."
—BO DEREK

DESIGNER
What to Look For

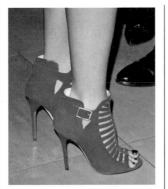

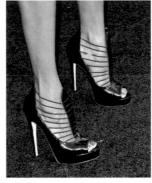

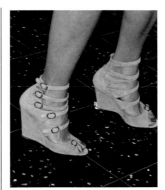

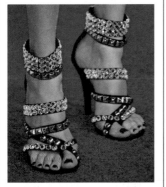

TRENDY SHOES

Unless you have an endless budget for **TRENDY SHOES**, it's best to buy trendy shoes that at least have a classic shape. I have a hard time getting behind asymmetrical toes and weird-shaped heels because it's inevitable that you'll grow tired of them very quickly. As for the boots that are laced up to the top of your thigh, the gigantic silk rose sitting on the end of your pump, the rhinestone-encrusted heel, or the Trojan sandal straps working their way up your calves—I say go for it. Fabulous shoes are a fantastically satisfying indulgence and speak volumes about your personality.

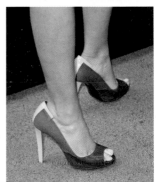

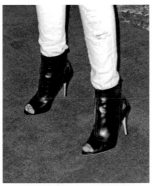

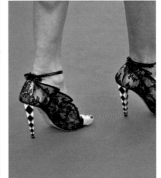

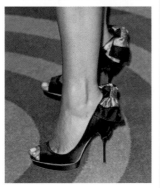

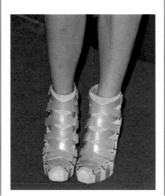

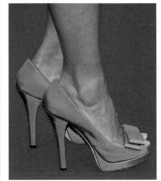

DESIGNER
Evening

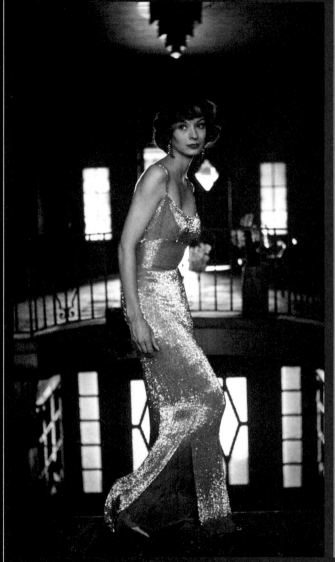

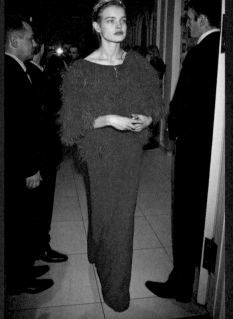

Natalia Vodianova in an iconic red Valentino gown, 2008.

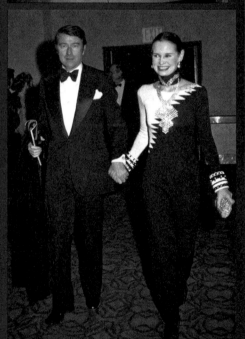

Fashion designers make some of the most enviable and drool-inducing evening clothes in the world. While I know how lucky I am to have access to borrowing designer gowns, I am not so lucky as to have the resources to buy them. In fact, I have never bought a designer evening gown. With my budget it's just not possible to justify that much money for something I will wear so few times. However I do have friends with lots of money who plan out their social schedules in advance and go to department store trunk shows to order their gowns for the season. I can just imagine how much fun that would be. But still, even if I had the money I don't think I would do it. I take so much pleasure from the challenges presented by getting dressed for evening on a budget—using my own personal mix of vintage pieces, something borrowed, something cheap chic, always with an element of classic mixed in. It's hard to imagine I would feel like myself if the process were just as easy as buying a fabulous dress off the rack.

Left:
A gold beaded sheath, 1959.

Above: Gloria Vanderbilt and her husband Wyatt Cooper at the premiere of Cabaret *at the Ziegfeld, New York City, 1972. I love the bangles and the choker with the zigzag gown.*

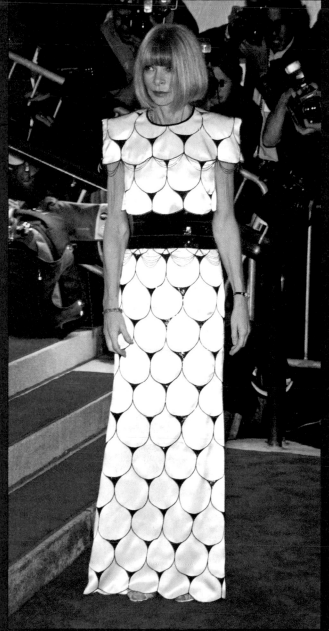

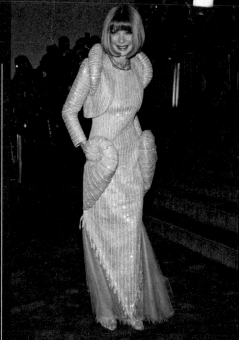

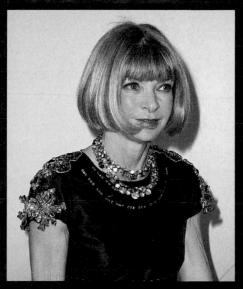

Clockwise from left: Anna Wintour, 2009, 2008, and 2008.

If I had to choose one person who inspires me most with designer evening clothes, it would be *Vogue* editor Anna Wintour. Even though she pretty much sticks to a uniform for day (skirt, cashmere sweater, Manolo Blahnik shoes), she absolutely pulls out all the stops for evening, boldly choosing elaborate over-the-top looks (sequined columns, feathered tea dresses, and jeweled and fur-trimmed riding jackets) with daring accessories. What enables her to pull this off is her resolute conviction of sticking to flattering shapes and keeping the hair and makeup at a minimum. Having watched Anna up close and from afar all my life I have never seen her change her haircut or hairstyle. Just because I admire her doesn't mean that we all have to afford couture to look as good as she does, but we can all learn from her self-knowledge, her daring sense of fashion adventure, and her discipline in sticking with what works.

DESIGNER
Where to Find It

DEPARTMENT STORES AND DESIGNER BOUTIQUES

In order to get the clothes you want each season, it is important to have a relationship with a **SALESPERSON** at the store where you intend to buy things. Many of the clothes that arrive at the store never make it to the shopping floor. Instead they are sent directly to clients who have reserved them in advance through their salespeople. When a client especially likes a specific designer, sometimes a sales person will send the client everything that arrives in the store by that designer in her size so she can try everything on at home and decide what she wants at her leisure. You don't have to be a *major* shopper to receive this kind of attention; you just have to develop a relationship with someone and hopefully buy a few things along the way.

If you see something in a magazine you want to buy but suspect it might be in high demand (as most items shown in ads and magazines are), go into the store a few weeks before its anticipated arrival and ask them to reserve it for you.

If you are a really ambitious shopper, **TRUNK SHOWS** can be the best way to shop. Here's how a trunk show works: Every season a given department store, let's say Bergdorf Goodman, hosts a trunk show for popular designers a month or two after the clothes have been shown on the runway, but long before the clothes will arrive in the store. A trunk show is an opportunity for a client to see an entire collection in person and reserve in advance the pieces she is interested in buying. If the clothes come in and don't fit or satisfy you, you can still return them. Shopping at a trunk show is a great way to ensure that you will get the pieces you want.

BARGAIN HUNTING

The key to all bargain shopping is to be a regular. One week a store may have nothing at all, and the next week they have three pairs of great Marc Jacobs shoes in your size. **EBAY** takes a lot of the pavement-pounding out of looking for designer discounts. You can check in as regularly as you like (maybe more regularly than you like!) and conduct very specific searches with immediate results.

DISCOUNT DESIGNER DEPARTMENT STORES

Like thrift shopping, hunting for clothes in discount designer department stores can be time-consuming. If, however, you have an hour or two to kill, you might wind up with some great pieces that you could otherwise not afford. The best approach is to keep your expectations low and go regularly. Whenever my niece is in town she gets so excited to go to Century 21, a New York City legend, and in the years I have taken her there she has sometimes left with one thing, other times with twenty. Don't buy just because you are there. But if you see something you instinctively like and the fit is good, don't be afraid to go for it, even if the price is a little more than you had in mind. Once at Century 21 I found an amazing pair of Viktor and Rolf sailor pants. The cut and fit were beautiful, but at $400 (60 percent off the original price) I passed. Now, when I am getting dressed for evening, I often think of the pants I left behind and how great they would have been. I still regret it! They were classic, the fit was perfect, and I would have worn them for years. My $400 would have been well spent.

HIGH-END DEPARTMENT STORE SALES

The majority of my designer clothes and accessories come from sales at my favorite department stores. Common wisdom says that the end-of-season sale is full of trends that didn't catch on, but I often find some really great and useful things that have more classic appeal. Again, time and patience and your editing eye are all necessary here. And beware the trap of buying something that you don't really love just because it's "designer" and it's affordable.

SAMPLE SALES

Designers in New York City hold their sample sales twice a year. These are one-day shopping opportunities with prices marked down significantly (at least 50 percent off). It is crucial to keep your expectations low, and it is, again, important not to fall into the trap of buying something crazy just because one of your favorite designers made it and (for once!) you can afford it. At sample sales I often end up feeling that I would rather pay full retail price for something I really love than get mediocre things for a bargain. That said, I have had some sample sale triumphs over the years— Christian Louboutin knee-high black lace boots, Manolo Blahnik for Lanvin brown leather pumps, and more recently a pair of *gorgeous* black leather gloves from Hermès—all for a fraction of their original price.

DESIGNER NAMES

André Courrèges
AHN-dray COO-rezh

Ann Demeulemeester
Ann De-MULE-uh-ME-ster

Anna Sui
Anna SWEE

Azzedine Alaia
Azz-UH-deen Ah-LIE-ah

Balenciaga
Buh-len-see-AH-guh

Balmain
BALL-meh

Bottega Veneta
Bo-TAY-guh VE-net-ah

Cacharel
CASH-ah-rell

Chanel
Sha-NELL

Chloe
CLO-ay

Christian Dior
CHRIS-tee-ahn Dee-OR

Christian Lacroix
CHRIS-tee-ahn La-KWAH

Christian Louboutin
CHRIS-tee-ahn Loo-boo-TAN

Commes des Garçons
COME day Gar-SAWN

Diane von Furstenberg
DIE-ann von FUR-sten-berg

Dolce and Gabbana
DOL-chay and Gah-BAH-nah

Dries van Noten
DREES van NO-ten

Giles Deacon
JYE-els DEE-cun

Hedi Slimane
Eddy Slim-MAN

Hermès
AIR-mezz

Hervé Leger
Air-VAY Le-ZHAY

Hubert de Givenchy
Hoo-BEAR de ZHEE-vawn-she

Hussein Chalayan
Hoos-AINE Sha-LIE-an

Issey Miyake
Is-ZEE Me-AH-kee

Junya Watanabe
JOON-ya Wa-TEN-a-bee

Lanvin
Lawn-VAN

Loewe
Lo-WAY-vay

Louis Vuitton
Loo-EE VUEE-tahn

Manolo Blahnik
Muh-NO-low BLAH-nick

Martin Margelia
Martin Mar-GHELL-uh

Miu Miu
Myoo Myoo

Moschino
Moss-SKI-no

Nicolas Ghesquière
Nicolas GUESS-kee-air

Nina Ricci
NEE-nah REE-chee

Paco Rabanne
PAH-co Ra-BAHN

Proenza Schouler
Pro-EN-za SKOO-ler

Pucci
POO-chee

Ralph Lauren
Ralf LOOR-en

Rodarte
Ro-DAR-tay

Stefano Pilati
Stef-UH-no Pil-AH-ti

Thakoon
Ta-KOON

Tse
Say

Veronique Branquinho
Vair-ron-EEK Bran-KEE-no

Versace
Ver-SAH-chee

Yohji Yamamoto
YO-jee Ya-ma-MO-to

Yves Saint Laurent
EEV Sahn Low-RAHN

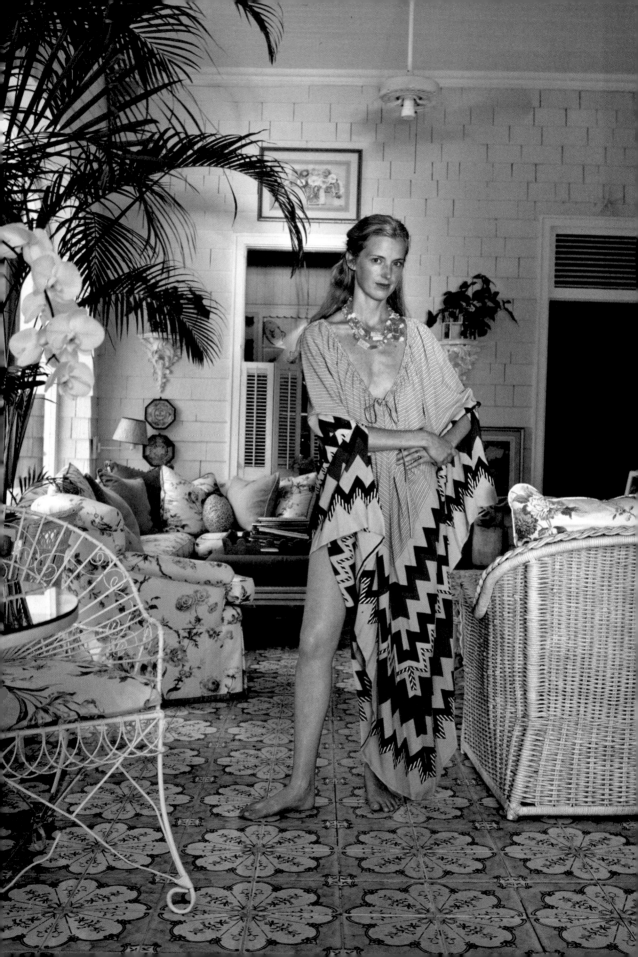

VINTAGE

"

AS EVERYONE IS DISCOVERING, IT FEELS GOOD TO WEAR EXPENSIVE CLOTHES, ESPECIALLY WHEN SOMEONE PAID FOR THEM THE FIRST TIME OUT."
—CAROL TROY

Vintage shopping has gone mainstream. In fact, it has practically become a competitive sport for women who love unique things. Twenty-first-century fashion, like it or not, borrows heavily from the iconic styles of the twentieth century, and the proliferation of vintage resources in our new millennium ensures that you can buy the original when a look comes back around. If the 70s are popular you can find a great vintage Gucci trench and a Giorgio Sant'Angelo caftan; when we're in a 60s moment you can buy a Courrèges shift dress or a Balenciaga coat. Instead of having the same trendy pieces as your friends, whether designer or knockoff, why not find the vintage original? You can also create a style that has nothing at all to do with the current fashion climate: 70s hippie clothes when 60s chic is all the rage, classic clothes when avant-garde is where it's at, or an over-the-top decorative cape when minimalism is the height of chic. Vintage clothes allow you to create the look you want, when you want, giving you greater freedom in your dress and more opportunities to express your personality. It requires you to think a little harder than girls who just buy this season's look right off the mannequin, but this experimentation is what eventually leads us to our truest stylish selves.

Vintage style is the ultimate test of how well you know yourself, because there is a lot less guidance out there for buying vintage than there is for buying new clothes or current trends. That said, creating a great look using vintage clothes is the ultimate coup. There is something about receiving compliments on vintage clothing that is way more satisfying than compliments on anything else. It's the fact that *you* found it, *you* chose it, *you* decided it was right for you, and most exciting is that it is highly unlikely that anyone else will ever have the same thing. Vintage clothes haven't been preapproved or promoted by designers and magazines, so even though you can often buy them from a store that has been curated according to current trends, there is still a lot potential for fashion disaster. And avoiding that disaster deserves commendation.

Me, in my great-aunt Molly's vintage Lanvin caftan, in Palm Beach, 2004. Photograph by Jonathan Becker.

VINTAGE
My Vintage Shopping

I'M FIRED UP BY THE MERE POSSIBILITY OF FINDING SOMETHING THAT REALLY SPEAKS TO ME.

2007

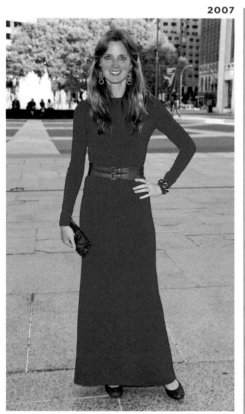

2001

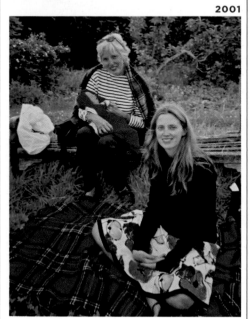

When I'm on my way to a vintage shop, a flea market, or even my computer to log on to eBay, I get this feeling in my stomach: excitement, promise, hope, and greed all at once. I don't even have to buy something to get that rush; it's really the anticipation of the hunt that I love. I'm fired up by the mere possibility of finding something that really speaks to me, inspires me, excites me, and is likely one of a kind.

The objects of my searching have been many. When I first got into thrift shopping as a skinny tomboy at age nine, finding a real Ralph Lauren polo shirt or a pair of worn Levi's that fit my curveless figure was the ultimate achievement. In junior high I was into 20s-style flapper dress and in high school my adrenaline peaked at the sight of cashmere cardigans.

By college my interest had shifted to the more fashionable designer items, and back in Palm Beach at the charity thrift shops I unearthed everything from a 70s Missoni maxiskirt to a Miss Dior canary-yellow feathered "chubby." Today thrift store shopping has become so popular that such treasures are rare, and when you do find them they are often outrageously priced. I knew Palm Beach thrift shopping had become a popular pastime in my late teens when I found a 60s Balenciaga leopard fur cropped coat at the Animal Rescue League shop and put it on hold to decide if I could come up with the $250 they were asking for it. I went back two days later, and it had been sold. Months later I was in New York and ran into Stephanie Seymour—wearing that coat! I asked where she had found it and sure enough it was the exact coat I had failed to snap up at the Palm Beach Goodwill. I'm still not over it.

When I moved to New York City I couldn't wait to discover the vintage scene, so you can imagine how disappointed I was by the steep prices. By 1996, vintage had become a

This page: (Left) Me, in a vintage skirt I bought in college, with my mom and daughter in England, 2001.

(Right) When I was in college there was an Alaïa "vintage" shop right around the corner from his Paris boutique. I got this dress and belt there, and I still wear it, like at the opening night of the New York City Ballet, 2007.

Opposite: Me, in 1930s Norman Hartnell, at my husband's family's farm in England, 2008. Photograph by Jonathan Becker.

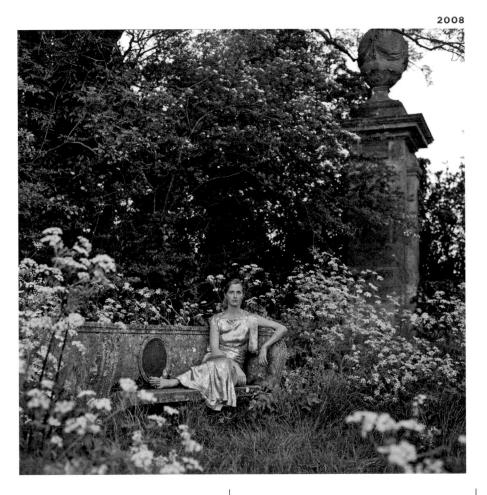

widespread trend and New York was, of course, leading the way with highly curated stores and prohibitive (at least for me) prices. It seemed like the end of an era for me, but in truth it was just time to discover a happier hunting ground: the still affordable and wildly diverse Chelsea flea market. The junky quality of the displays and stands was familiar and comforting and seemed to promise reasonable prices. A dark purple wool military coat, a floor-length crocheted skirt, suede fringed Indian boots, and handfuls of amazing costume jewelry are among my most valued flea market finds.

This same flea market also deepened my relationship with designer vintage. There was one woman with a stand of well-edited clothes whom I always sought out and occasionally bought things from. When she began to recognize me she would pull things out from the secret stash she kept for preferred customers. These pieces were more expensive than I was used to, but they were undeniably amazing and considered to be "collectible"—a term that had previously meant nothing to me. The exclusivity, the fact that she had chosen me to be a part of it, and, of course, the clothes themselves were all highly seductive, and I continued to haunt her stand. Over the years, a strapless floral Emanuel Ungaro dress, a Pierre Cardin fur-trimmed coat, and three perfectly cut Adolfo secretary blouses all found their way into my closet thanks to her.

Today I draw on all the phases I've been through with vintage shopping. I still love the challenge of burrowing into uncurated displays, the relative ease of flipping through well-edited racks, and the occasional splurge on a collectible designer piece. And today we have eBay offering everything from the most basic wool sweater to the most covetable Balenciaga vintage coat. The thrifting landscape may change, but the thrill of the hunt never does.

VINTAGE
What to Look For

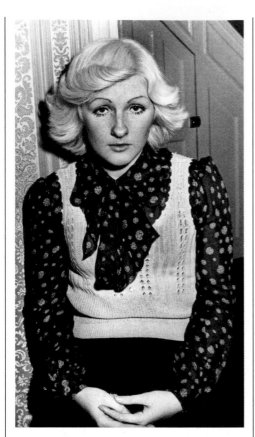

*Left:
Judy Cavanaugh
at home, 1975.
I love that 70s
look of putting a
sweater vest over
your blouse.*

*Below:
I got this vintage
Dior dress for
$30 at a vintage
store. It was long
to the floor,
but I cut it off.*

*Opposite:
Sabrina
Guinness in
a lovely summer
floral dress
while on a date
with Prince
Charles, 1979.*

DESIGNER
DRESS

A great **DESIGNER VINTAGE DRESS** is a worthy purchase. It's an exciting discovery to make, for one thing. Imagine that you're swimming through a sea of overpriced Pucci dresses and suddenly you behold a sequined Ungaro sheath from the late 70s that's just your size. My heart beats faster just thinking about it! It's also a lot of fun when someone asks you what you are wearing. I *love* saying, "It's old Dior," "It's vintage Balenciaga," "It's 60s Pierre Cardin." Best of all, designer clothes are usually made and designed so well that once they've gone out of style and come back in again, they tend to remain classic forever.

SILK
BLOUSES

The first things I look for in any vintage store are **SILK BLOUSES**. There is always a wide variety of old styles that look relevant to me today: peasant, sexy secretary, button-down, and tunics are all great styles. I also love to look for great prints such as floral, polka dots, and stripes.

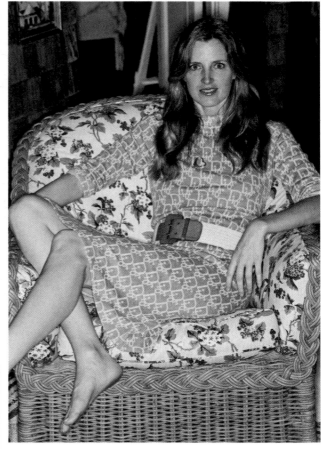

**I *LOVE* SAYING,
"IT'S OLD DIOR,"
"IT'S VINTAGE BALENCIAGA,"
"IT'S 60s PIERRE CARDIN."**

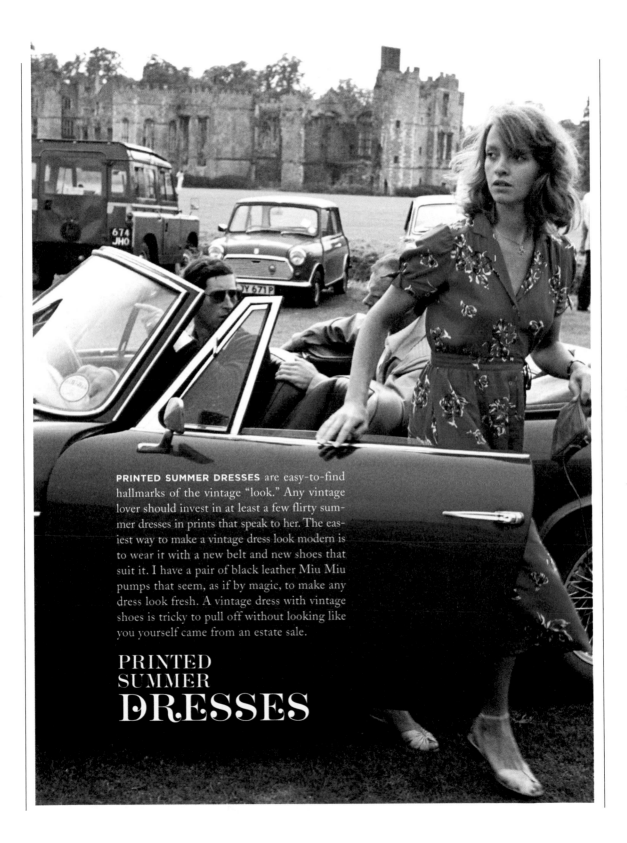

PRINTED SUMMER DRESSES are easy-to-find hallmarks of the vintage "look." Any vintage lover should invest in at least a few flirty summer dresses in prints that speak to her. The easiest way to make a vintage dress look modern is to wear it with a new belt and new shoes that suit it. I have a pair of black leather Miu Miu pumps that seem, as if by magic, to make any dress look fresh. A vintage dress with vintage shoes is tricky to pull off without looking like you yourself came from an estate sale.

PRINTED SUMMER DRESSES

VINTAGE
What to Look For

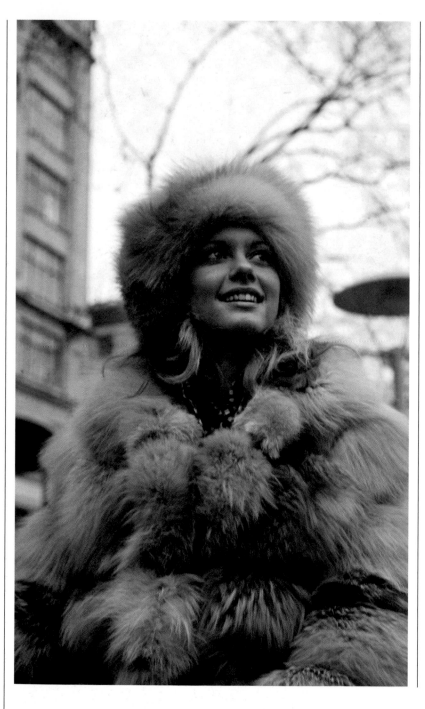

FUR COATS

Vintage stores are a great source of affordable **FUR COATS** and **ACCESSORIES**. People usually take good care of their fur, and the styles are for the most part fairly classic. Some vintage styles look really new on the right person (Peter Pan collars, three-quarter sleeves), but other styles simply look too dated (exaggerated shoulders, over-sized proportions). If you're not 100 percent pleased with the shape and styling, keep looking. There are more of them out there, and it's expensive and tricky to have a fur coat tailored.

Shopping Tip:
MAKE SURE IT FITS.
Some serious vintage collectors don't dare alter an original designer dress for fear of reducing its value. I can sympathize with the desire to preserve something great and old, but I also believe that if you can't wear it and look great in it, then there isn't much point in having it. Even the most collectible piece should be altered if it improves the way it looks on you.

EVEN THE MOST COLLECTIBLE PIECE SHOULD BE ALTERED IF IT IMPROVES THE WAY IT LOOKS ON YOU.

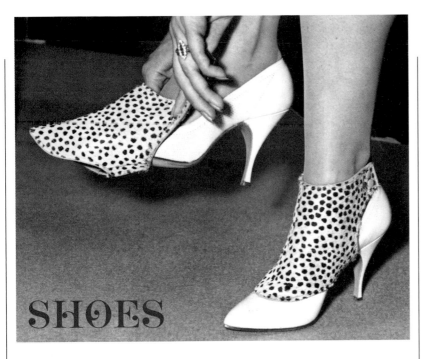

SHOES

Although I'm tempted to say that I never, ever buy **VINTAGE SHOES**, I know deep down that's not entirely true. I have some 80s wood-heeled platform sandals by Candie's that I've worn a surprising amount, and I covet my 70s Yves Saint Laurent black leather knee-high boots. But on the whole I tend to pass over vintage shoes unless a pair really jumps out and catches my eye. The trouble is that shoes somehow look more "of an era" than almost anything else and can really date your look if the heel or the last is the wrong shape. It's a subtle thing to notice but a very important one.

Opposite: Olivia Newton John really going for it with the fur, outside the Savoy hotel, London, 1980.

This page: (Above) Aren't these leopard spats amazing? 1959.

(Right) A stunning Madame Grès coat, 1951.

Coats stay in fashion longer than most other clothes, so **VINTAGE COATS** are a great investment. Look for wool military coats, Burberry trench coats, Gucci suede "car coats," cashmere wrap coats, or anything that suits your style.

COATS

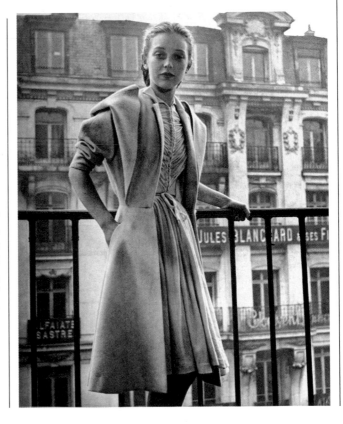

VINTAGE
What to Look For

HANDBAGS

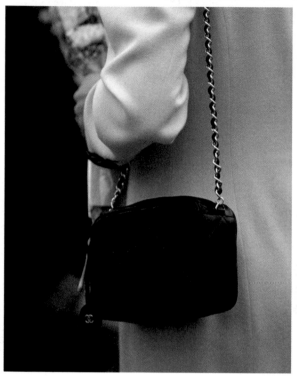

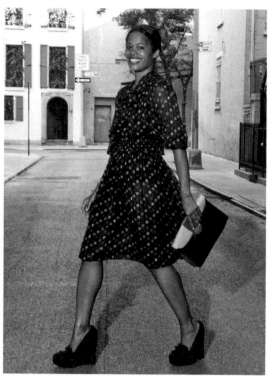

I've had slightly better experiences with vintage handbags than with shoes, but I still think you should proceed with caution.

I always like **VINTAGE DESIGNER BAGS**. I guess it's a testament to the success and talent of fashion designers that their designs stand up to the test of time. I also like the authenticity of an original that is not so easily attainable today. For example, I wouldn't carry a new Gucci logo-printed handbag, but I would carry a vintage one. There is something about finding an original one that makes me feel more unique, more individual.

If you can't afford a new one, eBay has a big selection of reasonably priced vintage Chanel bags. I also haven't completely lost my teenage fondness for the old **"CHANEL-INSPIRED" BAGS** at the thrift store: quilted leather, gold chains, but with an entirely different logo. Somehow these bags seem more honest, self-confident, and witty than straight-up Chanel knockoffs.

Left: Princess Diana's Chanel bag, 1992.

Right: Bonnie Morrison, 2008.

I also really love **ANONYMOUS VINTAGE HANDBAGS**. I can't actually say I love all of them, but there are some really good ones out there. Look for good quality leather in a rich color, well-made hardware, and a shape that suits you and your style. I prefer the 70s styles for vintage bags.

Shopping Tip:
DON'T TRY TO BUY AN ENTIRE OUTFIT FROM THE VINTAGE STORE.
The key to wearing vintage clothes is to buy great pieces and wear them one at a time. Wearing a vintage dress with vintage accessories looks old-fashioned, or just old, period.

JEWELRY

BELTS

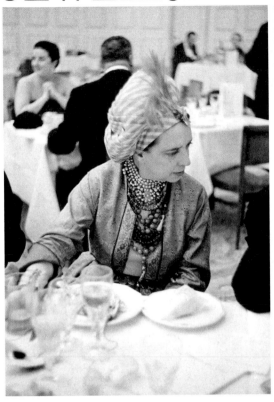

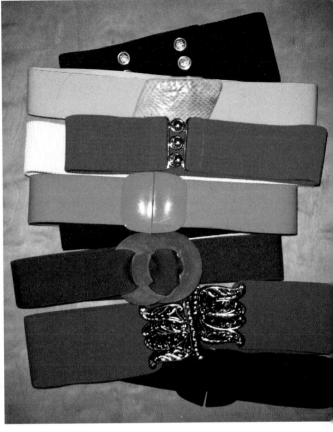

Nearly all my favorite **VINTAGE COSTUME JEWELRY** comes from flea markets, thrift stores, and eBay. The great thing about costume jewelry is that it usually isn't a big investment and therefore doesn't have to be so classic. I have a friend who collects vintage owl jewelry, another who raves about 60s cocktail rings, and I collect jewelry made of wood. When it comes to vintage jewelry, bold is best, so look for big strong pieces that make a real impact or multiples that reinforce an idea and make it stand out.

Left: Alber Elbaz must be inspired by this photo of Jeanne Lanvin from 1940 when he designs all that amazing jewelry for Lanvin today.

Right: Zandy Forbes's collection of vintage belts, 2006.

Shopping Tip:
GO EASY ON THE ACCESSORIES.
Most vintage clothes are quite decorative and don't require much accessorizing. Kate Moss wears vintage simply and therefore looks modern, not retro or tired. A simple clutch and classic pumps are always a great way to go with vintage clothes.

I've shared my reservations about vintage bags and shoes, but I think **VINTAGE BELTS** are fantastic. They are easy to come by at great prices, and there are loads of good ones out there. My friend Zandy Forbes, a very fashionable scientist (yes, she is a scientist!), has a thing for brightly colored wide elastic belts. They're a product of the 80s, but she thinks they're perfect over a summery dress to add a bit of bright solid color and to define the waist. She also loves that they usually have a metal clasp in a charming shape such as a flower or a butterfly, or even just a graphic row of circles. They look amazing on her. Because there are limited ways to design a belt, trends in belt design are usually reinterpretations of the past. So when wide waist belts come into style, you can find something similar from the 80s or the 50s. Or when low-slung hippie belts seem cool, look to the 70s to find a more authentic version.

VINTAGE
Evening

A GREAT
DRESS

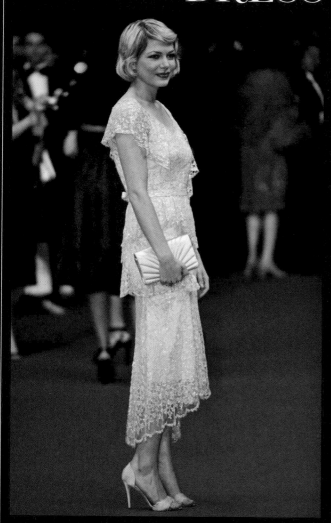

Left: Michelle Williams in vintage Chanel at the Cannes Film Festival, 2008.

Below: Kate Moss, 2007.

I have two **DESIGNER VINTAGE EVENING JACKETS** that I have worn over and over with everything from jeans to men's tailored trousers to a ball-gown skirt. One is my mom's old Oscar de la Renta from the 80s: black velvet with outrageous, baroque gold ribbon embroidery. The other is a 70s Yves Saint Laurent black sequined bolero with black ostrich feather sleeves. These may sound unwearably eccentric, but a little jacket with a lot of punch is incredibly useful. Just make sure you wear it with something simple and classic and with restrained makeup and hair. This can go kitsch in the blink of an eye if you are not careful about refining the rest of your look.

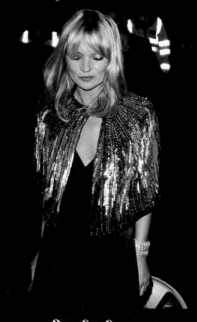

EVENING
JACKET

To make vintage work in the evening, all you need is a **GREAT DRESS**. If it fits and flatters and is a pretty color, put on mascara and lip gloss and go: a marvelous look. I once saw a *stunning* vintage YSL dress on eBay; I wanted it badly but it soon skyrocketed out of my price range, eventually selling for something like $1,500. It was a navy silk jersey evening gown with one shoulder and a scarf that tied around the neck. It was just the thing to wear over and over again throughout your life. Something like that (but hopefully less expensive) is the goal.

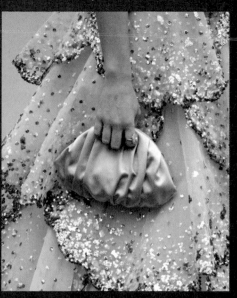

I like a vintage silk **EVENING COAT** from the 50s or 60s that has a simple but beautifully structured shape. Black is always chic and useful, but they also come in really amazing colors like pink, yellow, and red. If you could find one that was cream colored and stainless that would be a major score. Evening coats look good on any figure and can be worn with all kinds of things underneath: trousers, a short dress, a long dress. For a super easy signature evening look, build up a collection of vintage evening coats and rotate them over black trousers and a black blouse.

EVENING
COAT

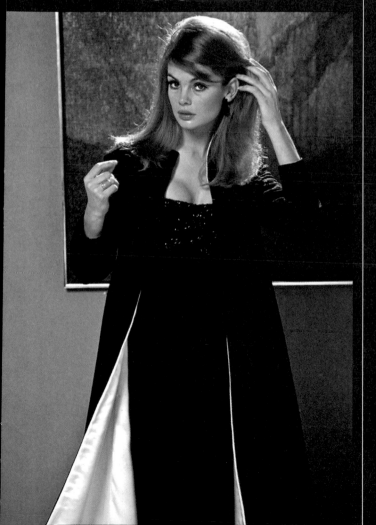

Left: Jean Shrimpton, 1965.

Above: A vintage-inspired handbag, 2009.

There is a glut of **VINTAGE EVENING BAGS** in the marketplace, making them generally well priced (unless they are rare in design or made of an expensive material like crocodile). Why don't you start a little collection of vintage evening bags? A great evening bag can personalize and pull together the simplest outfit. Look for good quality, strong colors that you are attracted to, and simple design, unless you specifically want something over-the-top. My favorite evening bags are a silver mesh clutch, a burgundy suede clutch (for more casual evening looks), and a very simple brown lizard clutch. (I only like clutches. Those little handles or straps on vintage bags just don't do it for me.)

EVENING
BAG

VINTAGE
Where to Find It

Vintage shopping must be a passion. You must feel that tingle of hope and promise when you walk into a vintage store you've never been to, that irresistible pull toward eBay or that exhilaration when you finally find something you've always hoped to find, whether it's a Christian Dior opera cape or the anonymous 70s sundress that somehow says everything about you. Otherwise it isn't worth the effort. And it can be quite an effort.

FLEA MARKETS are hands-down the best place to find something unexpected. If you go with the hope of finding something specific you will probably be disappointed, so keep an open mind. Flea market shopping is a fun social activity and a great opportunity to haggle. Do not hesitate to haggle! It is expected. Chat up the people who run your favorite stands, establish relationships, and they might give you a peek at the secret stash of gems they have hidden away for good customers.

THRIFT STORES offer rock-bottom prices but usually require strenuous digging and editing. The typical sea of holiday sweatshirts may reveal an unexpected pearl from time to time (I've found new Manolos at a Salvation Army and a cashmere Sonia Rykiel sweater in a suburban "bargain box"), but you're more likely to come home with an anonymous brand 70s ruffled blouse, a worn-in Mickey Mouse T-shirt, and a groovy braided rope belt. The best thing about thrifting is that the prices allow you to play. Most items are under $20 and you'll rarely see anything over $100. When you a buy a blouse for $7, it's not a tragedy if you wear it only once before deciding that it isn't right for you. For me, thrifting trial and error was the single most important part of establishing a style and fashion identity.

CURATED VINTAGE is similar to thrift, but someone with an eye for style and trends has done all the hardest weeding for you, ridding the racks of sacklike dresses, blouses with shoulder pads, and unflattering jeans. These stores exist mainly in larger cities and college communities where people take an interest in style, and in the last decade curated vintage stores have sprung up like mushrooms all over the younger, trendier neighborhoods of New York. They tend to have a better selection of 40s, 50s, 60s, and 70s outfits than thrift stores and the clothes tend to be in better condition. For the most part these stores carry no-name clothes with great style, which is just fine with me. I don't want to pay more for that designer label unless it's attached to something truly, truly special.

The **"DESIGNER" VINTAGE STORES** cropping up in major cities are full of well-kept clothes with significant labels and price tags to match, offering a much more high fashion vintage experience. Cherry and Resurrection in New York, Decades and Lily et Cie in Los Angeles, and Didier Ludot in Paris put this kind of shopping on the map, but most major cities have good copycat stores today, organized by people who have a great knowledge of fashion history, good taste, and a sense of current (and soon-to-be-current) trends.

While I *love* designer vintage with all my heart, I try to avoid buying it from designer vintage stores. I find the high prices hard to swallow after all the success I've had on eBay (a 60s Lanvin pendant necklace for $40, 70s Gucci ostrich knee-high boots for $400) or in more obscure vintage stores in smaller cities (a stunning brown wool Courrèges suit for $300 from a resale store in Palm Beach). It's hard to fork over significantly more cash for something just because it's in a well-designed boutique with good lighting and a chic salesperson. But designer vintage is perfect for people who love the labels but can't afford to buy them new. It's also great for people who love (and buy) designer clothes but want to add some more personal, unexpected pieces to their closets.

VINTAGE
THRIFTING TIPS

The best thrift stores are typically found in wealthy neighborhoods
inhabited by senior citizens or in rural towns devoid of hipsters.

- *Scout out all the thrift stores in your area. Pick a few favorites and visit them often. Most thrift stores put out new merchandise every day, so stopping by regularly increases your odds of finding something amazing.*

- *Thrifting can be a fun social activity, but choose your partner carefully to avoid competition and fierce envy—preferably someone with a different body type and shoe size. This prevents any disputes over hot items. Usually.*

- *Belts, scarves, sunglasses, and other treasures are often stored in drawers, which tend to be overlooked by most shoppers. Poke around and don't be scared to open drawers.*

- *Check out the luggage section; there is a wealth of candy-colored leather luggage from the 60s out there, including flight bags and travel makeup cases that can double as purses.*

- *Don't be afraid to haggle. If an item you want has any kind of damage, try to negotiate a lower price.*

- *Look for messy shops, the kind with pants hanging out in the blouse bin. The very best bargains are found in stores where you have to roll up your sleeves. If everything is well organized, you are definitely paying extra for that little "luxury"!*

- *If you have the whole day and don't mind traveling, hit the outlying areas of the city, especially the old guard suburbs like Locust Valley, Long Island, Lake Forest, Illinois, and so on.*

- *Stake out five thrift stores instead of spreading yourself too thin over fifteen.*

- *Clean your purchases and take them to the tailor right away, or you'll never get around to it. (That goes for new purchases, too, come to think of it.)*

THE VERY BEST BARGAINS
ARE FOUND IN STORES WHERE YOU HAVE
TO ROLL UP YOUR SLEEVES.

VINTAGE
Where to Find It

CONSIGNMENT STORES allow you to exchange your old clothes for store credit, which can be a great incentive to clean out your closet. While you can find the odd great vintage piece at these stores, they are usually filled with gently used contemporary designer pieces. Slightly more expensive than thrift stores and vintage stores, consignment shops have high standards for quality and a pretty good eye for editing out the things no one in their right mind would want.

ANTIQUE STORES rarely sell clothing, but most of them have a good selection of jewelry. Many of them also sell evening bags and the occasional fur stole.

The idea of riffling through a recently deceased person's things in search of a bargain may seem a bit morbid, but **ESTATE SALES** are the best place to find good deals on vintage classics like fur coats, cashmere sweaters, jewelry, and even furniture. Again, keep an open mind. Like flea markets, estate sales are typically held on Saturdays and Sundays and they are always listed in the newspaper. They are almost always held in the house of the owner (or former owner) and you are free to wander from room to room. Most estate sales start early in the morning; get there five minutes early to beat or join the diehard estate sale fanatics who scoop up the good stuff before anyone else has gotten out of bed. Frankly I don't know whether haggling is appropriate in this particular setting—maybe polite haggling? Either way, estate sales are a great place to find bargains. Sometimes waking up early on a Sunday morning really pays off.

At a **VINTAGE FAIR** many, many different dealers set up stalls in a large venue such as a conference center or event space. It's like a more organized, curated flea market, with higher quality (and correspondingly more expensive) merchandise. When I go to a vintage fair I make a whole day of it. I love wandering through all the stands with ample time to take everything in, try things on, and then decide what I am going to buy. It's exhausting, but really more time efficient than visiting a bunch of stores that won't have half as much to offer. You can search for a vintage fair near you on the Internet.

While the clothing at most **VINTAGE FASHION AUCTIONS** is generally at the highest end of price range, the quality is unparalleled. Many things sold at auction are either haute couture or highly collectible and in great shape—in a word, mouthwatering. You might find an original 50s Chanel suit, an impeccable Madame Grès gown, or a beautifully tailored Balenciaga wool coat with fur trim. The price is high but, again, still a bargain compared with designer clothes today, and you're buying something very rare that you almost certainly won't see on anyone else.

The best thing ever to happen to vintage shoppers is **EBAY**. You can find things in any price range and the selection is second to none. Vintage designer clothes are, on the whole, much cheaper here than at any vintage store, and you don't even have to leave your house. I must warn you, however, that it is *addictive*. Seriously. I go through eBay phases, spending a couple of hours trolling through all my favorite searches, bidding on four or five things, maybe winning one or two. Then I force myself not to do it again for a few weeks. I have a life to lead!

EBAY
SHOPPING TIPS

POPULARITY
- *Look for things that are not insanely popular. Everyone is bidding on Marc Jacobs handbags, but far fewer people are after vintage Biba (which is more unique anyway).*

MEASUREMENTS
- *If you're shopping for clothes on the Internet, you must know your exact measurements. You should also determine the ideal skirt and sleeve length for your body.*

NOTIFICATIONS
- *Find a few of your favorite searches and sign up to be e-mailed when new merchandise appears that matches them.*

AUTHENTICITY
- *If you care about a bag's authenticity, ask for a photo of the serial number or the proof of authenticity card that comes with the bag when purchased. You can also look at the seller's "feedback score" to see whether previous buyers have been happy and reported the seller to be reliable. I once bought what was advertised as a vintage Chanel bag on eBay, and it turned out not to be real (I could tell by the quality of the interior that it was not up to Chanel standards). But I loved the bag's design. It's a classic brown suede ladylike bag from the 70s but has big interlocking C's in brown lizard and a long gold chain strap. I felt a bit cheated, having paid $250 for something that wasn't real, but the truth is that I have worn it so much now that the authenticity and price no longer matter to me.*

"OLD CLOTHES GIVE YOU A FEELING THAT IN THIS THROWAWAY WORLD THERE ARE STILL SOME THINGS AROUND THAT CAN LAST TEN, TWENTY, THIRTY, FORTY YEARS, OR MORE, AND REMAIN BEAUTIFUL. AND IF YOU HAVE THE INSTINCTS OF A BLOODHOUND THEY CAN BE IN YOUR VERY OWN CLOSET."
—CAROL TROY

VINTAGE
Finding Your Decade

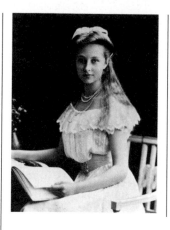

10s

Designers: Paul Poiret, Jeanne Lanvin, Mariano Fortuny
It Girls: Pola Negri, Mary Pickford, Theda Bara
Body Type: S-shaped
The Look: short hair, corsets, hobble skirts, feathered hats, long sleeves, long skirts, turbans, embroidery, and beading
The Movies: *Cleopatra* (with Theda Bara), *Broken Blossoms*, *Poor Little Rich Girl*
The Music: ragtime, opera

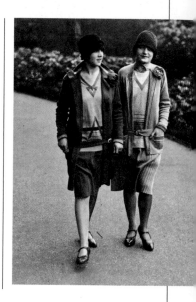

20s

Designers: Madeleine Vionnet, Jean Patou, Coco Chanel
It Girls: Louise Brooks, Clara Bow, Josephine Baker
Body Type: boyish and athletic
The Look: loose garments, drop waists, cloche hats, neutral colors, elaborate evening wear (feathers, fur, beading, lace), short hair, flapper dresses
The Movies: *Metropolis*, *It*, *Flesh and the Devil*
The Music: Bessie Smith, George Gershwin, jazz

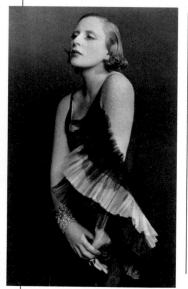

30s

Designers: Elsa Schiaparelli, Madame Grès, Mainbocher
It Girls: Wallis Simpson, Greta Garbo, Lee Miller, Marlene Dietrich
Body Type: statuesque
The Look: wide-legged pants, calf-length skirts, fur, bias-cut dresses, wavy hair, puffed sleeves
The Movies: *The Women*, *The Blue Angel*, *The Wizard of Oz*
The Music: Edith Piaf, Billie Holiday, Louis Armstrong

40s

Designers: Christian Dior, Charles James, Claire McCardell
It Girls: Veronica Lake, Joan Crawford, Katharine Hepburn
Body Type: statuesque
The Look: Dior's "new look," suits, trousers, structured clothes, shoulder pads, curled hair, jackets with a peplum, hats, platform shoes, alligator skin accessories
The Movies: *Philadelphia Story*, *Casablanca*, *Cover Girl*
The Music: Andrews Sisters, Bing Crosby, Doris Day

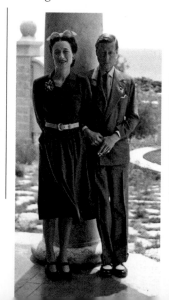

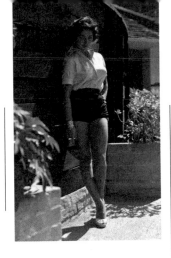

50s

Designers: Hubert de Givenchy, Cristobal Balenciaga, Marcel Rochas
It Girls: Grace Kelly, Elizabeth Taylor, Marilyn Monroe, Audrey Hepburn
Body Type: hourglass, voluptuous
The Look: full skirts, sweater sets, pedal pushers, pastels, pillbox hats, pinched waists, strapless "prom gowns," Peter Pan collars, scarf-tied ponytails
The Movies: *And God Created Woman*, *How to Marry a Millionaire*, *Vertigo*
The Music: Peggy Lee, Elvis, Nina Simone

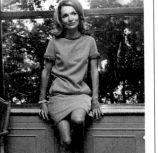

60s

Designers: André Courrèges, Emilio Pucci, Mary Quant, Pierre Cardin
It Girls: Jackie O, Mia Farrow, Julie Christie, Twiggy
Body Type: childlike and leggy
The Look: short skirts, chain belts, go-go boots, beehive hairstyles, boxy suits, brightly colored prints, hot pants, space-age fabrics (metallics), contrasting colors
The Movies: *Blow-Up*, *Darling*, *Breakfast at Tiffany's*
The Music: Nancy Sinatra, Serge Gainsbourg, the Beatles

70s

Designers: Halston, Yves Saint Laurent, Biba
It Girls: Catherine Deneuve, Anita Pallenberg, Bianca Jagger
Body Type: tall and thin
The Look: platform shoes, bell-bottoms, loud colors, peasant blouses, ethnic fabrics, wide lapels, polyester, long free-flowing hair, pantsuits, maxiskirts
The Movies: *Performance*, *Klute*, *3 Women*
The Music: Joni Mitchell, Blondie, David Bowie

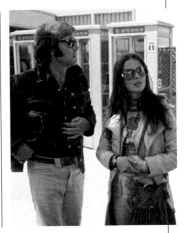

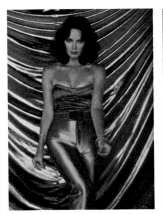

80s

Designers: Azzedine Alaia, Gianni Versace, Norma Kamali
It Girls: Madonna, the cast of *Dynasty*, Grace Jones
Body Type: amazon, athletic
The Look: tight jeans, spandex, leggings, fingerless gloves, shoulder pads
The Movies: *The Hunger*, *Desperately Seeking Susan*, *Heathers*
The Music: Siouxsie Sioux, the Smiths, the Go-Go's

90s

Designers: Tom Ford, Miuccia Prada, Helmut Lang, Calvin Klein
It Girls: Kate Moss, Winona Ryder, Chloe Sevigny
Body Type: waif
The Look: vintage clothing, grunge fashions, mini-backpacks, baby-doll dresses
The Movies: *Clueless*, *Unzipped*, *Buffalo 66*
The Music: Nirvana, Sonic Youth, Pavement

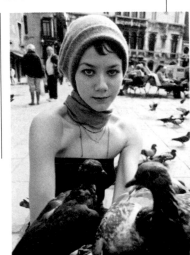

Amanda Brooks

EBAY
FAVORITE SEARCHES

"Vintage Lanvin," especially for jewelry.

"Vintage Saint Laurent" for sunglasses, blouses, and over-the-top evening dresses.

"Louboutin Wedge" for wedge-heel espadrilles and sandals.

"Miu Miu platform" and "Prada platform" for platform shoes.

"Kenneth Jay Lane" for the greatest, gaudiest costume jewelry. Ever. And it's super-cheap on eBay.

"Marc by Marc Jacobs," "See by Chloe," "Sonia by Sonia Rykiel." Diffusion lines are even more affordable on eBay.

"Vintage (Gucci, Chanel, Prada) purse." There is no need for a bag-of-the-moment or an inexpensive knockoff if you can find a classic designer bag for a fraction of its original price.

"Gold (lion, owl, snake, etc.)." Use this search in the jewelry category. EBay is great for jewelry because the market is oversaturated and you can find unique pieces that are extremely inexpensive. Animal-themed jewelry can be really chic or fantastically tacky. Either way works in my book. Also check out deco jewelry, rhinestone bib necklaces, and Bakelite bangles.

"Vintage (Marc, Sex and the City or SATC, Nicole, Sienna)" are keywords are often used to attract eBay shoppers to vintage clothes that mirror the aesthetic of designer or celebrity fashions.

"Snakeskin, tortoiseshell, alligator" can glean vintage accessories or jewelry on eBay made out of luxurious materials that are traditionally expensive or flat-out illegal (like ivory) for a fraction of the cost.

OTHER DESIGNERS TO SEARCH FOR

Chanel	Adolfo	Oscar de la Renta
Vionnet	Bonnie Cashin	Givenchy
Balenciaga	Sonia Rykiel	Holly Harp
Christian Dior	Courrèges	Biba
Loris Azzaro	Cardin	Mary Quant
Fiorucci	Rudi Gernreich	Norma Kamali
Thea Porter	Geoffrey Beene	Stephen Burrows
Madame Grès	Bill Blass	Giorgio Sant'Angelo
	Diane von Furstenberg	

VINTAGE
Inspiration

BOOKS

Harriet Love's Guide to Vintage Chic
by Harriet Love

This book was written by the owner of one of the first trendy vintage stores in New York City. She gives very specific advice and information about buying vintage clothes, such as how to alter and launder them, where to find them, and how to put vintage looks together. The photos have the charm of casual snap shots. I was so amused to discover pictures of Geena Davis and Madonna (pre-fame) casually mixed in. They must have been friends or clients of the author.

Cheap Chic
by Caterine Milinaire and Carol Troy

I'm going to write about this book again because I love it so very much. It overflows with great inspiration for thrift shopping and wonderful stories and photos of women who wear vintage clothing. So funny and genuine. Find yourself an old copy of it. Go! Now!

Cheap Date
('zine) by Kira Jolliffe and Bay Garnett

Cheap Date was a wonderful 'zine, published in New York City from 2001 to 2004, primarily devoted to the joys of thrift shopping. It also included features on stylish women (such as Anita Pallenberg and Karen Elson) and quirky fashion spreads.

Thrift Score
by Al Hoff

This is a very humorous book about thrifting. It's a great read with *loads* of tips, some just funny, others quite useful, such as answers to the questions: "What to do with clothes that no longer fit you?" "Who to go thrift shopping with?" "How to decorate your house from the thrift store?"

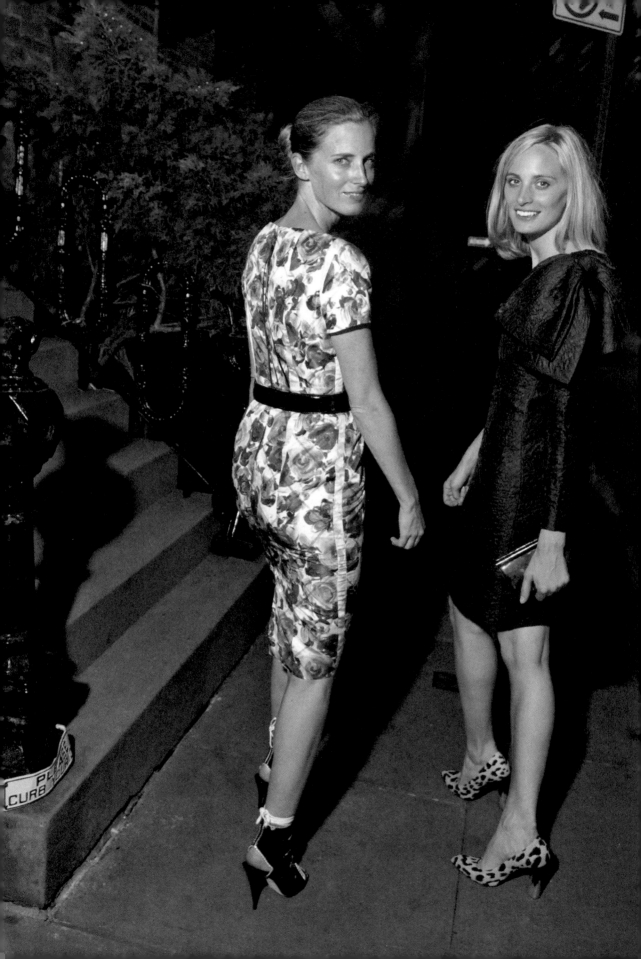

Final Thoughts

By now you know that, for me, real style is not about rules or thoughtless emulation. Style is a public display of your most intimate idea of self and your truly unique personal history. Your personal look can be inspired by countless combinations of concrete things—images (magazine tear sheets, favorite books, and movies), characters (the sexy secretary, hippie goddess, Park Avenue prepster), favorite places, memories, and aspirations. But also know, personal fashion can incorporate pure imagination and fantasy as well.

Take Cinderella, as weird as it may sound. This story plays a part in practically *every* little girl's childhood, and remarkably, I've found it offers both aesthetic inspiration and useful guiding principles. While some may see the moral as: dutiful goodness will be rewarded, let's be honest—a huge part of the story's appeal is its *glamour*: the romance, the dresses, the magic of transformation. That delicate glass slipper has surely inspired more than a few love affairs with shoes! Although Cinderella rises above the people who are keeping her down and wins true love without betraying her innate decency, she still needs the right clothes to do it. You can't go to the ball in rags, however sweet and beautiful you are, and you won't fool anyone by trying to cram your foot into a shoe that doesn't fit, however much you want to. You have to be yourself, so why not be your best-dressed self?

Fairy godmothers are hard to come by these days, but if this book has done its job then you should have some ideas about how to make your own magic. Whether you're trying to land the prince or the job, struggling to write a novel or to get the kids to school on time, finding the wardrobe that works for you will make your life simpler (and even more creative and fun). Be confident. If you aren't confident, fake it!

If you've come this far, but still don't know where to start, go clean out your closet. Play with what you have. Try things on in ways you haven't before. Don't worry if it looks silly—no one's watching. Get rid of anything that doesn't fit. Get rid of anything that fills you with regret. Take note of the things that make you look and feel best. Develop a relationship with a tailor. Grab a friend and go shopping. Explore a neighborhood or store you've never visited. Read, look, copy, tweak. If something works, don't be afraid to wear it over and over. If something doesn't work, don't be afraid to throw it overboard, even if it's something you've always thought you "had" to have. Don't let yourself get bored. Open yourself up to inspiration and experimentation. Soon you might find yourself inspired by your own past triumphs and amused by your own mistakes. Soon you'll be able to look in the mirror and say, "I love your style!"

Lauren Santo Domingo, in vintage YSL, and me, in Thakoon, leaving dinner at the Waverly Inn, 2008.

ACKNOWLEDGMENTS

To Honky, Beast, and Bucky, for giving me my own world outside of fashion,
and for always having an honest opinion about my outfits.

To Papa, Grandy, Carrie, and Little Carrie, for your encouragement and belief in me.

To Richard Pandiscio, for being the first person to get behind this book. For all the years
I've hung out at Pandiscio, I've always wanted to see my name on that project board behind your desk.
Thank you for giving me the honor.

To Bill Loccisano, for putting up with me sitting next to you all that time,
and for your long, long hours of incredibly hard work. It was "fun."

To Ira Silverberg, for giving me excellent advice and support throughout.

To Cal Morgan, Brittany Hamblin, Carrie Kania, Andrea Rosen, Joseph Papa
and everyone at HarperCollins who worked on this project, for making sure this book saw the light of day.
I know it was *your* faith in this project that made it happen.

To Chelsea Fairless, the best researcher in the world—you really are a walking, talking encyclopedia
of fashion! So much of what is cool in this book I owe to you.

To Caroline Mullen, for keeping all the balls up in the air at once and getting me to the finish line.

To Anna Wintour and all the editors at *Vogue*, for your tireless and invaluable support of me.

To Diane von Furstenberg, for taking an interest in me when I was still an awkward teenager,
and for teaching me and inspiring me ever since. I love you, DVF.

To all my friends who allowed me to interview and/or photograph them for this book.

To Hannah Thompson, Chris Floyd, Charles Thompson, Debra Sherer, Todd Eberle, Inez and Vinoodh,
Adam Woodward, and Sarah Wilmer, for being so generous with your photos.

To Robin Bellinger, for making everything I wrote sound better and more efficient.

To Josh Patner, for advising me along the way.

To Betsy Pearce, for telling me to write a book.

To Tim Blanks, for showing me that I could write this book myself.

To Sasha, Nellie, and Celerie, for making "dress up" so much fun.

And finally, to Judith Regan, for originally taking this book on. Without you it wouldn't exist.

THANK YOU

PHOTOGRAPHIC CREDITS

Note: For pages with several photographs, credits are provided in clockwise order, from top left.

5 Courtesy of Amanda Brooks
8 Debra Sherer
10 Courtesy of Amanda Brooks
12 Courtesy of Amanda Brooks
13 Courtesy of Bert and Richard Morgan Studio
14 Courtesy of Amanda Brooks
15 Illustration by Beatrice Bowry, courtesy of Amanda Brooks; courtesy of Bert and Richard Morgan Studio
16, 17, 19 Courtesy of Amanda Brooks
20 Eric Ryan/Getty Images
23 Iain Macmillan; courtesy of Yoko Ono
24 Rabbani and Solimene Photography/WireImage (top left); courtesy of Amanda Brooks (top center, center, far right); all others courtesy of Patrick McMullan
27 Ray Tamarra/Getty Images
29 Jeremy Kost/WireImage; Brian Hamill/Getty Images; Andrew Maclear/Hulton Archive/Getty Images; Bernard Gotfryd/Getty Images
30 Terry O'Neill/Hulton Archive/Getty Images
32 Courtesy of Amanda Brooks
33 Courtesy of Amanda Brooks; Debra Sherer
34 Pascal Le Segretain/Getty Images
35 Evening Standard/Getty Images
36 AP Images/Disneyland
37 M. McKeown/Daily Express/Hulton Archive/Getty Images; Stefan Tyszko/Hulton Archive/Getty Images
38 James Devaney/WireImage
39 Larry Ellis/Express/Getty Images
40 Alfred Eisenstaedt/Time & Life Pictures/Getty Images
41 Courtesy of Everett Collection/Rex Features; Fotos International/Getty Images
42 Baron/Getty Images
43 Eric Ryan/Getty Images
44 Hannah Thomson
45 Alan Band/Keystone/Getty Images; Marcel Thomas/FilmMagic
46 Sharland/Time & Life Pictures/Getty Images
47 Media Press/Rex Features; Paul Ashby/Getty Images
48 © Alain DeJean/Sygma/Corbis
49 Alfred Eisenstaedt/Pix Inc./Time & Life Pictures/Getty Images; Mike Franklin/FilmMagic; Hannah Thomson
50 Express/Express/Getty Images
51 Chaloner Woods/Getty Images; Hannah Thomson
52 Chris Moore/Catwalking/Getty Images; James Devaney/WireImage

53 David Cairns/Express/Getty Images
54 Frank Driggs/Getty Images; Amanda Brooks
55 Time & Life Pictures/Pictures Inc./Time & Life Pictures/Getty Images
56 Courtesy of Haynsworth Photography
57 Slim Aarons/Getty Images; Eric Ryan/Getty Images
58 Terry O'Neill/Hulton Archive/Getty Images; Everett Collection/Rex USA
59 Anwar Hussein/Getty Images
60 Alfred Eisenstaedt/Time & Life Pictures/Getty Images
61 Reginald Davis/Rex Features; Evan Agostini/Liaison; Keystone/Hulton Archive/Getty Images
62 Victor Blackman/Getty Images; Evening Standard/Getty Images
63 Courtesy of Patrick McMullan
64 Tom Wargacki/WireImage
65 Keystone/Getty Images; Rex Features/Blackbrow/Rex Features
66 Hulton Archive/Getty Images; Michael Webb/Keystone/Getty Images; John Kobal Foundation/Getty Images
67 Keystone/Getty Images
68 Slim Aarons/Getty Images
69 Evening Standard/Getty Images; Hulton Archive/Getty Images; Allan Grant/Time & Life Pictures/Getty Images
70 New York Times Co./Getty Images; Topical Press Agency/Getty Images
71 Richard Harrison/Fotos International/Getty Images; Julian Wasser/Time & Life Pictures/Getty Images; Julian Wasser/Time & Life Pictures/Getty Images
72 Jonathan Becker
73 Hannah Thomson; Charles Thompson
74 Keystone/Hulton Archive/Getty Images; Keystone/Hulton Archive/Getty Images; Weegee (Arthur Fellig)/International Centre of Photography/Getty Images
75 Alistair Guy; Syndication International/Getty Images
76 Mike Stephens/Central Press/Getty Images; courtesy of Amanda Brooks
77 Arthur Schatz/Time & Life Pictures/Getty Images; Slim Aarons/Hulton Archive/Getty Images; Bob Thomas/Popperfoto/Getty Images
80 Gisela Torres/Tank magazine
82 Courtesy of Amanda Brooks; Courtesy of Bert and Richard Morgan Studio
83 Courtesy of Amanda Brooks; Jonathan Becker
84 Everett Collection/Rex Features
85 Evan Agostini/Getty Images

86 Susan Wood/Getty Images; Lipnitzki/Roger Viollet/Getty Images
87 Jason Kempin/FilmMagic
88 Keystone Features/Getty Images
89 Harry Benson/Getty Images; Crollalanza/Rex Features
90 Courtesy of Amanda Brooks; Michael Ochs Archives/Getty Images
91 Ron Galella, Ltd./WireImage
92 Courtesy of Amanda Brooks; Hulton Archive/Getty Images
93 Universal Pictures/Getty Images
94 Cynthia Macadams/Time & Life Pictures/Getty Images
95 Terry Richardson
96 Fotos International/Getty Images
97 Astrid Stawiarz/Getty Images
98 Jack Robinson/Hulton Archive/Getty Images; Nils Jorgensen/Rex Features
99 Will Ragozzino/Getty Images
100 Image of the Marchesa Casati © Ryersson & Yaccarino/Casati Archives; Hulton Archive/Getty Images
101 Burt Glinn/Magnum Photos; Todd Eberle
102 Michael Ochs Archives/Getty Images
103 Hulton Archive/Getty Images; Nickolas Muray © Nickolas Muray Archives
104 Adam Woodward
105 Chris Floyd; Gisela Torres/Tank magazine
106 Jemal Countess/WireImage; Hulton Archive/Getty Images
107 Ron Galella/WireImage; Janis Joplin by Michael Ochs Archives/Getty Images; Ralph Crane/Time & Life Pictures/Getty Images
108, 109 Covers courtesy of Amazon.com
112 © Bettmann/Corbis
115 Debra Sherer
116 © Robert Mapplethorpe Foundation/Art + Commerce
117 Eric Ryan/Getty Images; Francois Durand/Getty Images
118 Leon Morris/Hulton Archive/Getty Images; Julien Hekimian/WireImage
119 Collexxx-Lex van Rossen/Redferns
120 Chaloner Woods/Getty Images
121 Luca Ghidoni/Getty Images; illustration by Chelsea Fairless
122 Alan Band/Keystone/Getty Images
123 Reg Lancaster/Getty Images
124 Chris Kleponis/AFP/Getty Images; Clarence Sinclair Bull/John Kobal Foundation/Getty Images
125 Keystone/Getty Images
126 Inez van Lamsweerde & Vinoodh Matadin; John Kobal Foundation/Getty Images; Archive Photos/Getty Images
127 CBS Archive/Getty Images
128 Henry Clarke/Musee

PHOTOGRAPHIC CREDITS

Galliera/ADAGP/Collection *Vogue* Paris/Getty Images
129 RDA/Getty Images; Michael Tighe/Hulton Archive/Getty Images
130 MPI/Getty Images; John Loengard/Time & Life Pictures/Getty Images
131 George Hurrell/Hulton Archive/Getty Images
132 Rex Features; courtesy of Patrick McMullan
133 Courtesy of Patrick McMullan
134 Sarah Wilmer
135 Ray Tamarra/Getty Images; James Devaney/WireImage
136 Eric Ryan/Getty Images; Jim Smeal/WireImage; Eric Ryan/Getty Images
137 Hulton Archive/Getty Images
140 Hannah Thomson
142 Courtesy of Amanda Brooks; Hannah Thomson
143 Miles Aldridge/Condé Nast
144 Central Press/Getty Images; Mat Szwajkos/Getty Images
145 Keystone/Getty Images
146 Keystone/Getty Images
147 Roger Kisby/Getty Images; Dave Hogan/Getty Images (right)
148 Christopher Simon Sykes/Hulton Archive/Getty Images; Gareth Cattermole/Getty Images (right)
149 Murray Garrett/Getty Images; Slim Aarons/Hulton Archive/Getty Images; Eric Ryan/Getty Images
150 Slim Aarons/Hulton Archive/Getty Images; Dave M. Benett/Getty Images
151 Mike Lawn/Getty Images
152 Mike Marsland/WireImage
153 Keystone/Getty Images
154 Ron Galella/WireImage; Rabbani and Solimene Photography/WireImage
155 Ray Tamarra/Getty Images; J. A. Hampton/Topical Press Agency/Getty Images; Michael Ochs Archives/Getty Images
156 *Evening Standard*/Hulton Archive/Getty Images; Popperfoto/Getty Images; Keystone/Getty Images
157 Robin Platzer/Time & Life Pictures/Getty Images
158 RB/Redferns
159 Ron Galella/WireImage; artwork courtesy of Motown Records
160 General Photographic Agency/Getty Images; Everett Collection/Rex Features
161 Dave Benett/Getty Images; courtesy of Amanda Brooks
162 Courtesy of Patrick McMullan
163 Hannah Thomsom
164 Gustavo Caballero/WireImage for Dan Klores Communications; Gustavo

Caballero/Getty Images; Dominique Charriau/WireImage
165 Julien M. Hekimian/Getty Images
166 Tony Vaccaro/Hulton Archive/Getty Images; *Evening Standard*/Getty Images
167 *Evening Standard*/Getty Images; Ron Galella/WireImage; Max B. Miller/Fotos International/Getty Images
168 John Rawlings/*Vogue* © Condé Nast Publications Inc.; Eduardo Garcia Benito/*Vogue* © Condé Nast Publications Inc.; Eric Boman/*Vogue* © Condé Nast Publications Inc.; Javier Vallhonrat/*Vogue* © Condé Nast Publications Inc.
169 Clifford Coffin/*Vogue* © Condé Nast Publications Inc.; Herbert Matter/*Vogue* © Condé Nast Publications Inc.; Patrick Demarchelier/*Vogue* © Condé Nast Publications Inc.; Richard Avedon/*Vogue* © Condé Nast Publications Inc.
172 © Tony Frank/Sygma/Corbis
174 Courtesy of Amanda Brooks
175 Courtesy of Amanda Brooks (left); Lawrence Lucier/Getty Images (right)
176 David Mcgough/DMI/Time & Life Pictures/Getty Images
177 Robin Platzer/Time & Life Pictures/Getty Images; Hulton Archive/Getty Images
178 Sherman/Getty Images; Graham Wiltshire/Getty Images
179 Hulton Archive/Getty Images
180 Rob Loud/Getty Images
181 James Devaney/WireImage: Fred Duval/FilmMagic; Danny Martindale/WireImage; Fred Duval/FilmMagic
182 Courtesy of Patrick McMullan
183 Courtesy of Patrick McMullan
184 Ray Stevenson/Rex Features
185 Christopher Furlong/Getty Images; Brian Rasic/Rex Features; Eric Ryan/Getty Images
186 Paul Popper/Popperfoto/Getty Images; Gai Terrell/Redferns
187 Frank Micelotta/Getty Images
190 Dave Benett/Getty Images
192 Courtesy of Amanda Brooks
193 Courtesy of Patrick McMullan
194 © Horst Horst / Art + Commerce
195 Morgan Collection/Getty Images; *Evening Standard*/Getty Images; Bernard Gotfryd/Getty Images
196 Harry Dempster/Express/Getty Images; Ron Galella/WireImage; Tom Wargacki/WireImage
197 Express Newspapers/Getty Images
198 Amanda Brooks; courtesy of Laura Bailey
199 Dana Lixenberg/*Sunday Telegraph*
200 Richard Young/Rex Features (bottom left); all others courtesy of Patrick McMullan

201 Courtesy of Patrick McMullan (top left, top middle); Stephen Butler/Rex Features (top right, bottom middle); Rex Features (bottom left, bottom right)
202 Amy Graves/WireImage; Chris Weeks/WireImage
203 Venturelli/WireImage
206 Susan Wood/Getty Images
208 A Di Crollalanza/Rex Features
210 Photos courtesy of Amanda Brooks
211 Photo courtesy of Amanda Brooks
212 Ralph Crane/Time & Life Pictures/Getty Images
213 Terry O'Neill/Getty Images; Tim Boxer/Hulton Archive/Getty Images
214 Julian Wasser/Time & Life Pictures/Getty Images
215 Rex Features; Ron Galella, Ltd./WireImage
216 Everett Collection/Rex Features; courtesy of Amanda Brooks; Lipnitzki/Roger Viollet/Getty Images
217 Dave Benett/Getty Images
218 Melvin Simon/The Kobal Collection
220 Jo Hale/Getty Images
222 Courtesy of Amanda Brooks
223 Hannah Thomson; courtesy of Patrick McMullan
224 Bouzad/Atkins/Rex Features
225 Courtesy of Amelie Hegardt; Everett Collection/Rex Features
226 Robin Platzer/Twin Images/Time & Life Pictures/Getty Images
227 Terry O'Neill/Hulton Archive/Getty Images; Hulton Archive/Getty Images
228 Andrea Blanch/Getty Images
229 © Jeffrey Thurnher/Corbis Outline
230 Al Freni/Time & Life Pictures/Getty Images; Rabbani and Solimene Photography/WireImage
231 Terry Smith/Time & Life Pictures/Getty Images
232 Bill Ray/Time & Life Pictures/Getty Images
233 David Mcgough/DMI/Time & Life Pictures/Getty Images; Alan Davidson/WireImage
234 Michael Tran/FilmMagic; Time & Life Pictures/DMI/Time & Life Pictures/Getty Images
235 Slim Aarons/Hulton Archive/Getty Images
236 Fred Duval/FilmMagic; Terry Disney/Express/Getty Images
237 Roger Viollet Collection/Getty Images
238 Terry O'Neill/Hulton Archive/Getty Images
239 JAB Promotions/WireImage Rex Features; Rex USA
241 Cover courtesy of Amazon.com
242 Dave Benett/Getty Images
244 Courtesy of Amanda Brooks

PHOTOGRAPHIC CREDITS

245 Jonathan Becker
246 Hannah Thomson (left); Dafydd Jones/WireImage (bottom center); courtesy of Patrick McMullan
247 Rabbani and Solimene Photography/WireImage for LaForce and Stevens (top right); courtesy of Amanda Brooks (bottom right); courtesy of Patrick McMullan
248 Dave Allocca/DMI/Time & Life Pictures/Getty Images
249 Ron Galella/WireImage; *Evening Standard*/Getty Images
250 Everett Collection/Rex Features; Lester Cohen/WireImage
251 Jorge Herrera/WireImage; Hannah Thompson; Eric Ryan/Getty Images
252 Ron Galella/WireImage
255 Jason Merritt/Getty Images; Kevin Winter/Getty Images; Jason LaVeris/FilmMagic; Jason Merritt/Getty

Images; Anne-Christine Poujoulat/AFP/Getty Images; Francois Durand/Getty Images; Steve Granitz/WireImage; Gareth Cattermole/Getty Images; Jason LaVeris/FilmMagic; Frederick M. Brown/Getty Images
256 Chris Jackson/Getty Images; Tim Boxer/Getty Images; Gordon Parks/*Life* Magazine/Time & Life Pictures/Getty Images
257 Kevin Mazur/WireImage; Dimitrios Kambouris/WireImage; Andrew H. Walker/Getty Images
260 Jonathan Becker
262 Courtesy of Amanda Brooks; courtesy of Patrick McMullan
263 Jonathan Becker
264 *Evening Standard*/Getty Images; Debra Sherer
265 Tim Graham/Getty Images
266 Hulton Archive/Getty Images

267 Fox Photos/Getty Images; Nina Leen/Time & Life Pictures/Getty Images
268 Tim Graham/Getty Images; Hannah Thomson
269 Roger Viollet Collection/Getty Images; courtesy of Amanda Brooks
270 Anne-Christine Poujoulat/AFP/Getty Images; Harold Cunningham/WireImage
271 Robyn Beck/AFP/Getty Images; Popperfoto/Getty Images
276 Keystone/Getty Images; Brooke/Getty Images; Thomas D. McAvoy/Time & Life Pictures/Getty Images; Imagno/Getty Images
277 Hulton Archive/Getty Images; Max B. Miller/Fotos International/Getty Images; Evan Roberts/Aurora/Getty Images; Hulton Archive/Getty Images; Dennis Oulds/Getty Images
280 Hannah Thomson

INDEX